Spinal Arthroplasty
A New Era in Spine Care

SPINAL ARTHROPLASTY
A NEW ERA IN SPINE CARE

EDITED BY

RICHARD D. GUYER, MD, FAAOS

Co-Founder, Texas Back Institute, and Co-Director, Spine Fellowship Program, Texas Back Institute, Plano, Texas; Associate Clinical Professor, Department of Orthopedic Surgery, University of Texas Southwestern School of Medicine, Dallas, Texas

JACK E. ZIGLER, MD, FACS, FAAOS

Co-Director, Spine Fellowship Program, Texas Back Institute, Plano, Texas; Associate Clinical Professor, Department of Orthpaedic Surgery, University of Texas Southwestern School of Medicine, Dallas, Texas

QMP

Quality Medical Publishing, Inc.

ST. LOUIS, MISSOURI • 2005

Printed in Canada

This book presents current scientific information and opinion pertinent to medical professionals. It does not provide advice concerning specific diagnosis and treatment of individual cases and is not intended for use by the layperson. Medical knowledge is constantly changing. As new information becomes available, changes in treatment, procedures, equipment, and the use of drugs becomes necessary. The editors/authors/contributors and the publisher have, as far as it is possible, taken care to ensure that the information given in this text is accurate and up to date. However, readers are strongly advised to confirm that the information, especially with regard to drug usage, complies with the latest legislation and standards of practice. The authors and publisher will not be responsible for any errors or liable for actions taken as a result of information or opinions expressed in this book.

The publishers have made every effort to trace the copyright holders for borrowed material. If they have inadvertently overlooked any, they will be pleased to make the necessary arrangements at the first opportunity.

PUBLISHER Karen Berger
DIRECTOR OF EDITING Suzanne Seeley Wakefield
EDITOR Michelle Berger
DIRECTOR OF PRODUCTION Carolyn Garrison Reich
PRODUCTION Barbara Northcott, Cindy Thurman, Brett Stone
COVER DESIGN Amanda Behr

Quality Medical Publishing, Inc.
2248 Welsch Industrial Court
St. Louis, Missouri 63146
Telephone: 1-800-348-7808
Web site: *http://www.qmp.com*

LIBRARY OF CONGRESS CATALOGING-IN-PUBLICATION DATA

Spinal arthroplasty : a new era in spine care / edited by Richard D. Guyer, Jack E. Zigler.
p. ; cm.
Includes bibliographical references and index.
ISBN 1-57626-190-5 (hardcover)
1. Intervertebral disk prostheses.
[DNLM: 1. Arthroplasty, Replacement—methods. 2. Intervertebral Disk—surgery. 3. Arthroplasty, Replacement—instrumentation. 4. Joint Prosthesis. 5. Spinal Diseases—surgery.
WE 740 S7565 2005] I. Guyer, Richard D. II. Zigler, Jack E.
RD755.7.S665 2005
617.5'6059—dc22

2005009271

QM/F/F
5 4 3 2 1

We dedicate this book

To the people who got us to this point in our careers:
our parents, parents-in-law, wives, siblings, and children

To the people who challenge us every day to excel:
our fellows, our partners, and our international colleagues

To the people for whom we strive to be better and better,
and for whom we believe arthroplasty will be a significant
life-improving technology: our patients

And to each other, who are not just partners
but also share a lifetime of friendship

CONTRIBUTORS

Howard S. An, MD
The Morton International Professor, Director of Spine Surgery, Department of Orthopaedic Surgery, Rush University Medical Center, Chicago, Illinois

Qi-Bin Bao, PhD
Vice President, Spine Development, Pioneer Surgical Technologies, Marquette, Michigan

Andrew R. Block, PhD
Clinical Assistant Professor, Department of Psychiatry, University of Texas Southwestern Medical Center, Dallas, Texas; Director, The Wellbeing Group, Plano, Texas

Scott L. Blumenthal, MD
President, Texas Back Institute, Plano, Texas

Salvador A. Brau, MD, FACS
Visiting Clinical Assistant Professor of Surgery, Department of Surgery, Keck School of Medicine, University of Southern California; Clinical Instructor of Surgery, Department of Surgery, Geffen School of Medicine, University of California Los Angeles, Los Angeles, California

Vincent Bryan, MD
Department of Neurosurgery, Swedish Medical Center, Seattle, Washington

Karin Büttner-Janz, MD, PhD
Director of Orthpaedic Clinic, Hospital im Friedrichshain, Vivantes Healthcare Network, Berlin, Germany

Timothy A. Burd, MD
Associate Faculty, Orthopaedic Spine Surgeon, Department of Orthopaedic Surgery, Creighton University School of Medicine; Volunteer Faculty Instructor, Department of Orthopaedic Surgery and Rehabilitation, Omaha, Nebraska

Andrew Cappuccino, MD, FACS, FAAOS
Attending Spine Surgeon, Department of Orthopedics, Catholic Medical System; Attending Spine Surgeon, Department of Orthopedics, Kaleida Health System, Buffalo; Lockport Memorial Hospital, Department of Spine Surgery, Lockport, New York

Joseph C. Cauthen, MD, FACS, FACSS
President, Neurosurgical and Spine Associates, Gainesville, Florida

Junius Clawson, MD
Orthopaedic Surgeon, Department of Orthopaedics, Cottonwood Hospital, Marray, Utah

Bryan W. Cunningham, MSc
Director of Spinal Research, Department of Orthopedic Surgery, Union Memorial Hospital, Baltimore, Maryland

Lukas Eisermann, BS
Principle Engineer, Product Development, Medronic Sofamor Danek, Memphis, Tennessee

Lisa A. Ferrara, PhDc
Director, Spine Research Laboratory, Department of Neurosurgery, The Cleveland Clinic Foundation, Cleveland, Ohio

Tai Friesem, MD
Department of Orthopaedic Service, University Hospital of North Tees, Stockton-on-Tees, United Kingdom

Rolando Garcia, Jr., MD, MPH
Chairman, Department of Orthopedic Surgery, Aventura Hospital and Medical Center, Aventura, Florida

Richard D. Guyer, MD, FAAOS
Co-Founder, Texas Back Institute, and Co-Director, Spine Fellowship Program, Texas Back Institute, Plano, Texas; Associate Clinical Professor, Department of Orthopedic Surgery, University of Texas Southwestern School of Medicine, Dallas, Texas

Stephen H. Hochschuler, MD
Chairman, Texas Back Institute, Plano Texas

Jean-Charles LeHuec, MD, PhD
Professor of Orthopedic Surgery; Spine Unit Chief, Bordeaux University Hospital, Bordeaux, France

Koichi Masuda, MD
Associate Professor, Departments of Orthopedic Surgery and Biochemistry, Rush Medical College at Rush University Medical Center, Chicago, Illinois

Hallett H. Mathews, MD
Associate Clinical Professor, Department of Orthopaedic Surgery, Medical College of Virginia, Richmond, Virginia

Paul C. McAfee, MD
Chief of Spinal Surgery, Department of Orthopedic Surgery, St. Joseph's Hospital, Baltimore, Maryland

Robert C. Mulholland, MB, BS, FRCS
Professor of Trauma and Orthopaedics, University of Nottingham; Emeritus Consultant Spinal Surgeon, Queen's Medical Center, University Hospital, Nottingham, United Kingdom

Donna D. Ohnmeiss, Dr Med
Director of Research Education, Texas Back Institute Research Foundation, Plano, Texas

Luiz Pimenta, MD, PhD
Assistant Professor, Orthopedics Institute, University of São Paulo; Vice-Chairman, World Spine Society, São Paulo, Brazil

Mark Reiley, MD
Private Practice, Berkeley Orthopedic Medical Group, Berkeley, California

Barton L. Sachs, MD, MBA, FACS
President, Texas Back Institute Research Foundation, Plano, Texas; Adjunct Professor of Orthopaedic Surgery, Albany Medical College, Albany, New York

Dilip K. Sengupta, MD, Dr Med
Assistant Professor, Department of Orthopaedics, Spine Center, Dartmouth-Hitchcock Medical Center, Lebanon, New Hampshire

James Q. Spitler, BS
Development Engineer, Research and Development, Innovative Spinal Technologies, Plano, Texas

Hansen A. Yuan, MD, FACS
Professor, Department of Orthopaedic and Neurological Surgery, SUNY, Upstate Medical University, Syracuse, New York

Jack E. Zigler, MD, FAAOS
Co-Director, Spine Fellowship Program, Texas Back Institute, Plano, Texas; Associate Clinical Professor, Department of Orthpaedic Surgery, University of Texas Southwestern School of Medicine, Dallas, Texas

FOREWORD

Every 5 to 10 years, a notable change in philosophy and actions occurs in the management of degenerative spinal disorders. Twenty years ago the spinal community witnessed the explosion of pedicular fixation, which allowed rigid segmental control of the "force nucleus" of the spine and three-column manipulation of the spinal elements. Following this, surgeons realized the importance of the anterior intervertebral disc as a potential pain generator in symptomatic degenerative disc disease. This led to the introduction of stand-alone intervertebral fusion cage devices of all shapes and sizes (cylindrical, rectangular, and trapezoidal). A subset of patients responded very well to this intervention, but it was clear many patients continued to be symptomatic, and further stability (posterior stabilization) was necessary. Subsequently, spinal care providers became aware of the adverse consequences of fusion, such as stiffness, loss of mobility, and junctional degeneration and disease.

A logical evolution of intervention to these morbidities has been the concept of providing controlled or stable motion to a symptomatic degenerative interspace. This can be accomplished in many novel ways, such as through nucleus replacement, total disc replacement, facet replacement, segmental posterior dynamic implants, or nonsegmental interspinous process spacers.

The editors of *Spinal Arthroplasty: A New Era In Spinal Care* have organized a comprehensive overview of the philosophy of motion-sparing technology as well as its origin and evolution over the last decade. Drs. Guyer and Zigler are internationally renowned thought leaders who have been at the forefront of the study of disc arthroplasty in North America. The experience and wisdom they share here give the reader a balanced understanding of the importance of motion preservation and stability in the management of degenerative disease, especially in the younger patient population.

The editors and authors should be congratulated for filling the void in our understanding of this relatively new concept of care for symptomatic spinal degenerative disorders. This textbook will serve as an introduction to the less experienced in this philosophy of care as well as a reference tool for more experienced spinal care providers endeavoring to gain a greater understanding of the science which supports the preservation of motion in spinal reconstruction.

ALEXANDER R. VACCARO, MD, FACS
Professor, Department of Orthopaedics, Rothman Institute,Philadelphia, Pennsylvania;
Co-Director, Delaware Valley Regional Spinal Cord Injury Center;
Co-Chief, Spinal Surgery; and Co-Director, Spinal Fellowship Program

FOREWORD

This is a most exciting time for those involved in the care of patients with back pain—a major paradigm shift is underway in the basic precepts of surgical management of the spine. This book attempts to provide a comprehensive overview of the current aspects of the evolving arena of spinal arthroplasty.

Generally, the goal in treating back pain patients is to reduce pain and increase function. Traditionally in treatment of the spine, as was the case many years ago for other joints, this goal has been pursued by eliminating motion of the symptomatic joint. Great progress was made years ago for hips and knees with the development of dependable total joint replacements that allowed painless motion of what had been a painful and disabling degenerative joint. Only since the mid-1980s has similar progress been made for the spine. At that time, Drs. Kurt Schellnack and Karin Büttner-Janz in Berlin, Germany designed the first clinically viable total disc replacement. The third generation of that design is in use today.

Texas Back Institute's interest in artificial discs began in the early 1990s and led to our hosting a visit by Dr. Büttner-Janz to our institute. We immediately embraced the technology and sent researchers to Europe to review the results at several centers which had been using the device. This experience confirmed our enthusiasm for spinal arthroplasty, and we worked with the Link company to bring the technology to the United States. This relationship led to our having the honor of implanting the first Charité device in the United States in March 2000, and the first ProDisc in the United States in October 2001. Since that time, the surgeons at the Texas Back Institute have been actively involved with the evaluation of three of the four lumbar disc replacement devices undergoing FDA study as well as with the evaluation of cervical total disc replacements.

In the more than 25 years that I have been practicing spine care, there has been no greater excitement than that which is presently occurring. The topics in this textbook address many of the stimulating aspects of spine care, including disc replacements, posterior dynamic stabilization devices, and the future potential of tissue engineering and microelectronic applications in spine. Motion will not totally replace fusion but will have a significant impact in providing better care for the spine patient. This compendium is the first attempt by our institute to document what is occurring in this new world of spine. We welcome you on this journey.

STEPHEN H. HOCHSCHULER, MD
Chairman, Texas Back Institute
Plano, Texas

Preface

For years, spinal fusion has been the standard for treating discogenic pain. While fusion is an appropriate treatment for some patients, scientists, and clinicians have been searching for an alternatives that retain, rather than restrict, the natural motion of the spine and allows for the sharing of loads among the spinal segments as is demonstrated in a normal intact spine. The development of artificial discs and other motion-preserving implants are a result of this quest. The possibility of an artificial disc became a clinical reality in the 1980s, and in 2000, the first total disc replacement was performed in the United States as part of an FDA clinical trial. In addition to total disc replacements, other motion-retaining spinal implants such as disc nucleus replacements, posterior stabilization devices, facet joint replacements, anular repair procedures, and cervical disc replacements are under development and in various stages of laboratory and clinical evaluation. These advancements offer exciting alternatives for treating discogenic pain.

As we enter this new era of motion retention and total disc replacement, there is no comprehensive publication incorporating current information on various arthroplasty devices. With the rapid evolution of motion-preservation technology in spine surgery, we recognized the need for book that incorporated the design goals, technology, and clinical results of current spinal arthroplasty devices. This book represents a collaborative effort bringing together experts with unique experience and wisdom in a number of different technologies.

This book is organized is organized into four parts that, when taken together, form a foundation for learning about this exciting technology. Part I describes essential background information and begins with a discussion on the evolution of the treatment of lumbar disc related pain and the history of the artificial disc. Careful patient selection is one of the most important keys to ensure successful device implantation and good outcomes; in arthroplasty procedures, it is of even greater importance because this is pioneering surgery in which many of the standard approaches require modification and new thinking. Therefore the two remaining chapters in this first part describe the physical and psychological evaluation of patients and define indications and contraindications for spinal arthroplasty.

With the engineering and development of motion-preservation devices an understanding of spine biomechanics becomes critically important not only to the engineers and developers but also to the surgeons who implant the devices. For example, from a clinical standpoint the device must possess methods of attachment to the vertebral body endplate; from a biomechanical perspective, issues such as biocompatibility and load bearing are important. Part II discusses these design goals and subsequent chapters describe how these goals have been addressed by various arthroplasty devices.

Part III is devoted to the techniques and technologies of spinal arthroplasty. The discussion begins with an in-depth description of the anterior approach to the spine. The remaining chapters offer detailed discussions of arthroplasty technologies for both the cervical and lumbar regions. In each chapter the authors have included updated information on clinical trials and results. An understanding of this information will aid surgeons in evaluating the benefits of this new technology.

The book concludes with a consideration of future technologies that are likely to bring even more exciting treatments for back pain, including biologic disc repair as well as the merging of medicine and electronic technology in the form of microelectromechanical systems (MEMS), nanoelectromechanical systems (NEMS), and robotics.

Spinal arthroplasty represents a long-awaited advancement in the care of patients with back pain. The development and use of motion-retaining spinal implants represent one of the greatest innovations in spine care surgical treatment. It is our hope that this book will provide young and experienced surgeons alike with a basis for learning as they explore this exciting, new technology.

RICHARD D. GUYER
JACK E. ZIGLER

Contents

PART IV Future Considerations

PART

I

FUNDAMENTALS

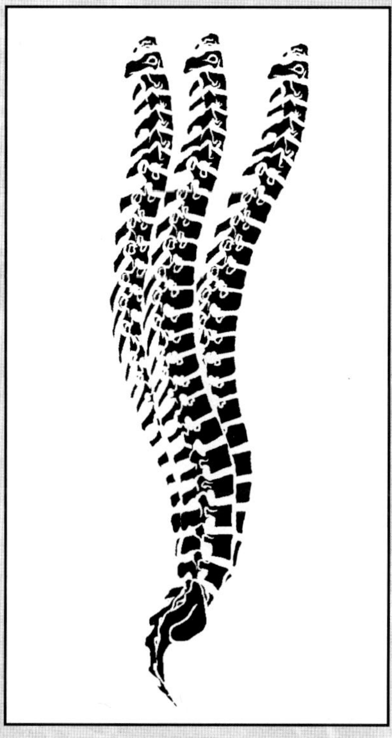

CHAPTER

1

EVOLUTION OF THE TREATMENT OF LUMBAR DISC–RELATED PAIN

Donna D. Ohnmeiss ▪ Scott L. Blumenthal

The intervertebral disc is an intellectual, diagnostic, and treatment challenge. The body of knowledge associated with the disc and its role in back pain has been slow to evolve. Also slow to develop is a firm understanding of the most appropriate approaches to diagnosing and treating pain related to this disc. It is difficult to differentiate normal aging-related disc changes from changes related to clinical symptoms in patients with back pain. Throughout the study of the intervertebral disc, there have been controversies concerning the innervation of the disc, the diagnosis of discogenic pain, and the treatment of such pain. Only if the surgeon understands disc-related pain mechanisms can patients with this condition be optimally treated. Optimal treatment is safe, adequately addresses and is limited to the source of symptoms, produces a predictable result, maximally reduces the chance of iatrogenic problems, and is affordable. These goals can only be achieved if the surgeon has a sound knowledge of the mechanisms of disc-related pain and the physiologic effects of treatments, and is familiar with clinical studies evaluating the results of various therapeutic interventions. This chapter presents the possible mechanisms of the disc as a pain generator; we will also briefly review the diagnostic tools for disc-related pain and the evolution of treatments for this condition. The discussion of treatments will focus on treatment for discogenic pain rather than on pain that is related to stenosis, spondylolisthesis, or the simple model of nerve root compression.

Pain Mechanisms in Lumbar Disc–Related Pain

Treatment of patients who have pain should be based on an understanding of the pain mechanism of their condition. As described by Ohnmeiss, there are at least three distinct mechanisms of lumbar disc–related pain.[74] Disc-related pain may arise from (1) disc tissue compressing the nerve root, (2) leakage of neurotoxic agents from the disc irritating the nerve root, and (3) true discogenic pain arising from the disc itself, independent of nerve root involvement. Part of the difficulty in accurately diagnosing disc-related pain is that these three problems may be present at the same disc level, or in the same patient at different disc levels. Also, disc-related pain may occur in conjunction with other painful pathology such as stenosis or spondylolisthesis, or facet joint pain at the same or different motion segment. Only through a thorough evaluation of physical examination findings, imaging studies, and injections can the pain generators be identified and other possibilities be ruled out. However, there is no perfect evaluation, and the definitive identification of the source of symptoms remains elusive in many patients.

Nerve Root Compression

In 1934 Mixter and Barr published an article on the role of disc prolapse resulting in nerve root compression.[68] Although this was not the first description of this phenomenon (Middleton and Teacher had described disc rupture as early as 1911),[66] this article established the role of the disc in generating radicular pain by compressing a nerve root; the article thereby sparked an interest in the role of the disc in patients with back pain. The primary point of the article was that nerve root compression in many patients with radicular pain was caused by disc tissue, not tumors, as had previously been diagnosed. Mixter and Barr reported that the prolapsed disc tissue could easily be removed surgically, thus relieving the patient's pain.

Our knowledge of the effects of compression on nerve roots has expanded greatly in recent years. We now know that nerve root compression results in severe nutritional compromise[77,86] as well as vascular changes.[52] These physiologic alterations are likely to play a role in the production of radicular pain; the compression may be produced by displaced disc tissue or by bony compression.

Chemical Irritation

The model of the disc causing radicular pain by compression of the nerve roots was readily accepted; however, it was clear that it was not adequate to explain all low back and radicular pain originating from spinal structures. As early as 1958, Smyth and Wright investigated the influence of nerve root compression via manipulation of a suture placed around nerve roots.[95] They found that compressing the nerve root by constricting the suture around it did not cause pain in a normal nerve root; however, the same maneuver did produce pain in an irritated nerve root. Years later, Kuslich confirmed this finding in a study using local progressive anesthesia during discectomy.[54] Manipulation of a normal nerve root was not painful; however, manipulation of an inflamed nerve root did provoke pain, which led researchers to wonder about the source of the inflammation that sensitized the nerve roots to compression.

The inflammation of nerve roots and the dorsal root ganglion has been the topic of much investigation. In 1987 on a study in canines McCarron et al found that autogenous nucleus pulposus placed in the epidural space induced an inflammatory response,[64] but no such response was noted in a control group. The importance of inflammation caused by disc tissue was further verified by

Olmarker et al,[78] who found that placing autologous nucleus pulposus tissue on a nerve root caused a significant reduction in nerve conduction velocity. No similar change occurred in the control group in which a fat graft was placed on the nerve root. This study confirmed that chemical irritation induced by the nucleus disc tissue could create changes in nerve root function independent of nerve root compression. These findings were later tested by Kayama et al,[48] who created a disc disruption model in which incision of the anulus allowed nucleus tissue to leak out into the epidural space, resulting in significantly reduced nerve root conduction velocities. The findings from these studies are important in the clinical situation because in humans it was found that 98% of extruded disc material samples contained nucleus tissue, and nucleus was the predominant tissue in 89% of the samples.[70] Such findings support the notion that tissue herniating or leaking from the disc nucleus comes in contact with the nerve roots and becomes a source of pain because of chemical irritation of the neural tissue.

Several specific agents have been identified in the process of nucleus-induced chemical irritation of the nerve roots. In 1990 Saal et al[88] reported on the high levels of phospholipase A_2 found in herniated disc tissue that was removed at the time of surgery. This study established biochemical inflammation related to disc herniation. Since that time several studies have sought to identify specific inflammatory mediators that have a role in disc-related pain. Tumor necrosis factor-alpha (TNF-α) has been found to be an important mediator in nerve root inflammation related to disc tissue.[41] Some of the other proinflammatory mediators that have been identified as likely to have a role in disc-related pain include interleukin-6, interleukin-8, and interleukin-1 beta.[13,79]

Disc-Related Pain (Without Nerve Root Compression or Irritation)

The role of the disc, independent of compressing nerve roots, as a potential pain generator has been questioned for many years, primarily because of the debate over whether or not the disc was innervated. If the disc was not innervated it would be impossible for it to be a primary source of the patient's symptoms. The possibility of pain being referred from the disc was not well accepted because the early literature regarding the innervation of the disc was inconsistent.[37,42,62,85,104] However, as investigative methods improved, studies providing identification of nerve endings in the outermost one third of the layers of the anulus,[9] and possibly up to one half of the anulus,[106] supported the possibility that pain could arise from within the disc itself, independent of nerve roots. Kuslich reported that among a group of patients with radicular pain undergoing discectomy with the use of a local progressive anesthesia, in about two thirds of the patients stimulation of the disc anulus provoked symptoms.[54] These symptoms were similar in intensity to the patient's preoperative back pain. The earliest studies identified nerve endings in the outer layers of the disc anulus. More recent studies reported that an injured disc may have vascular structures and nerve endings deep into the annular tissues and possibly into the nucleus.[23,31] It has also been reported that neovascularization along the edge of the nucleus pulposus occurs in prolapsed discs but not in control discs.[80] Freemont et al compared discs in which pain was provoked during discography with those that were not painful during discography.[32] Microvascular blood vessels accompanied nerve fibers growing into the painful discs, and these expressed nerve growth factor. Some of the nonpainful disc had vessels, but these entered from the anulus fibrosus; the nonpainful discs did not express nerve growth factor and did not have nerves passing into the disc. This study provides much insight into a possible mechanism of discogenic pain.

The finding of nerve endings in the anulus, particularly in injured discs, combined with the previous findings of the neurotoxic effect of inflammatory agents in the disc nucleus supports the model for pain arising from within the disc itself. It may be that once an injury has occurred, the number of nerve endings within the injured disc increases. The inflammatory agents from the nucleus may irritate these new nerve endings, producing pain. Another possibility is that the inflammatory agent sensitizes the nerve endings in the disc and makes them more sensitive to mechanical stimulation at a level that would not be painful in normal discs.

There is a general belief that leg pain is related to nerve root compression, and back pain is indicative of disc pathology not involving the nerve root but this may be an overly simplistic view of the situation. The concept of pain originating in spinal structures, such as facet joints and ligaments, and being referred to other areas of the body has been established for decades.[27,49,69] Saal described chemically mediated discogenic pain in patients with low back and possibly referred lower extremity pain that was often burning in sensation in patients with no evidence of mechanical nerve root compression.[87] He speculated that such pain is related to inflammation causing sensitization of anulus or peridiscal nociceptive afferents. There have been several studies suggesting that pain may be referred from the disc into the lower extremity.[67,73,76] These studies support the notion that lower extremity pain, including that passing below the knee, may be caused by the disc in the absence of nerve root compression. Milette et al reported on a population of patients with lower extremity pain but with no evidence of nerve root compression.[67] The patients' clinical symptoms could be provoked by injection of contrast medium into the disc during discography and relieved by injection of an analgesic agent into the disc. Ohnmeiss et al[76] compared the pain drawings from patients with pain arising from discs with no outer annular wall deformation and no leakage of contrast material from the disc space (discs not affecting the nerve root) to the drawings from patients with outer annular wall deformation and/or leakage of contrast material from the disc space (possibility of nerve root involvement). They found no difference in the distal extent of pain, thus confirming that the disc may refer pain into the lower extremity. In a study using intradiscal electrothermal therapy (IDET),

O'Neill et al[73] increased the distal extent of leg pain, sometimes passing below the knee, by increasing the temperature of the probe in the disc. There was no increase in temperature around the nerve roots. Although these three studies employ very different methods, all three support the concept that pain may arise from the disc and be referred into the lower extremities, independent of nerve root involvement.

Diagnosis of Symptomatic Disc Disruption

New insights concerning the structure of the disc and possible pain mechanisms and diagnostic methods were evolving in Sweden during the 1940s. Lindblom injected the nuclei of cadaveric discs with red lead,[59] after which he observed the pattern of spread of the injected material. He noted that in some discs the lead remained in the center of the disc. In other discs, the lead passed from the nucleus into fissures in the anulus. To determine whether these fissures could be related to producing pain in patients, clinical investigations were performed using radiographic contrast material. The development of discography was slowed because of concerns about injecting material into the disc, that is, concerns about injuring the disc and complications arising from the technique of disc injection. However, so far there has been no evidence of discography harming the disc. In an animal study, histologic analysis failed to identify any changes in disc tissue following disc injection.[45] Several clinical studies have not found any injury to the discs of animals undergoing discography.[3,16,29,44] In the study by Flanagan and Chung, the length of follow-up ranged from 10 to 20 years, and the researchers did not find any more changes among the discs that had previously undergone discography than in those that did not have discography.

The controversy over discography continues today and is often refuted based on studies by Carragee et al.[17,18] However, careful review of the studies identifies problems in trying to apply the findings to the clinical situation. The primary problem with several of the studies is that clinically, discographic pain provocation is interpreted in terms of the similarity of the pain provoked to that of the patient's clinical symptoms. In any study that uses asymptomatic subjects, no such comparison can be made. In the Carragee studies, the subjects in whom the reports of significant pain occurred were those with psychological problems.[17] These findings confirmed those reported earlier in studies investigating the influence of psychological factors on discographic pain provocation. Block et al[6] reported that elevated scores on the hysteria and hypochondriasis scales of the Minnesota Multiphasic Personality Inventory (MMPI) were significantly associated with reports of pain during the injection of a nondisrupted disc. Ohnmeiss et al[75] reported that abnormal pain drawings were associated with a greater percentage of patients reporting pain during the injection of a nondisrupted disc.

Initially it was hoped that MRI could replace discography. However, the high rate of abnormal images in subjects without back pain has limited its use in differentiating the source of pain in patients with back pain.[8,11,19,43] The rate of abnormalities in subjects without back pain has been reported to be as high as 76%.[11] The lack of image findings with back pain emphasizes the need for pain provocation tests such as discography to help differentiate which visualized abnormalities are related to the patient's pain.

Treatment of Symptomatic Disc Disruption

The treatment of symptomatic disc disruption has changed and continues to change over time. The reported results are inconsistent and difficult to analyze. This is not surprising considering the many variables that can influence outcome. Also, there have been inconsistencies in the understanding of the physiology of pain as well as in the diagnosis of lumbar disc–related pain. Over the years, many surgical methods have been introduced to treat pain that arises from the intervertebral disc.

Fusion

Although many articles have been published on various fusion techniques, relatively few studies deal specifically with symptomatic disc disruption or symptomatic disc degeneration confirmed by discography.

Originally, the primary strategy for treating disc-related pain was to remove part of the pain generator—that is, the disc. Although this could possibly relieve symptoms, it also had the potential to destabilize the spinal segment. Removal of disc tissue also allowed collapse of the disc space, which could create problems with the facet joints as well as cause collapse of the neuroforaminal space, resulting in nerve root compression. To address these potential difficulties, distracting the disc space following the removal of disc tissue and stabilizing the operated segment seemed like good ideas and were the goal of interbody fusion. The other primary strategy was to fuse the spine posteriorly, which was based on the belief that stabilizing the painful motion segment would eliminate the load on the disc and thus the patient's pain.

Interbody Fusion

Perhaps the most widely used treatment for symptomatic disc disruption is interbody fusion via either an anterior or posterior approach to the spine. This procedure was introduced for the treatment of disc prolapse by Cloward in 1945.[21] Interbody fusion allows direct access to the disc space for removal of the pain-causing tissue. Fusing the vertebral bodies of a painful motion segment imparts a great deal of stability to the segment. Whether there is any preference for anterior or posterior interbody fusion is not clear. The anterior approach has the potential benefit of allowing easier and wider access to the disc space, and the removal of a greater amount of disc tissue. It also avoids the potential problem of overretracting the nerve roots while accessing the disc from the posterior approach. However, the anterior approach has an increased risk of injury to the major vascular structures located just in front of the spinal column. Also, the risk of sympathetic injury, such as that resulting in retrograde ejaculation, is greater. Posterior interbody fusion has the benefit of reducing potential injury to the vascular structures and sympathetic chain. It also allows easy access to the posterior elements to address stenosis or free disc fragments in the spinal canal. The primary disadvantages of this approach are the risk of injury to the nerve roots related to possible overdistraction of these structures and that the access to the disc space is not as wide and thus interbody implant options may be limited. Also, damage is inflicted on the muscles that are dissected to gain access to the spine.

Several studies find that the total evacuation of the disc space may have benefits in the treatment of symptomatic disc disruption. Total evacuation provides removal of the tissue that is causing the pain.[58,63] McAfee et al[63] reported a higher fusion rate among patients in whom a total versus a partial discectomy was performed. They compared the fusion rates in procedures in which the disc space was evacuated to those in which only enough disc tissue was removed to insert threaded fusion cages. Support for this finding was identified in an animal study by Li et al.[58] Using a swine model, they found that disc tissue mixed with autograft results in reduced bone formation compared to a group in which the entire disc was removed before the graft was placed.

Although there are many studies reporting on the results of interbody fusion, there are few that deal specifically with discogenic pain. However, in these studies the percentage of patients with favorable results generally ranged from 64% to 86%.[7,60,72] Worse results were reported in a small series of 23 patients; none of the two-level cases had a good result and only 35% of single-level cases were successful.[51] However, the poor fusion rate in the study (0% for two-level procedures and 36% fusion in single-level cases) may account, at least in part, for the poor results.

There have been very few reports specifically on posterior interbody fusion for discogenic pain. However, in two studies from the same center, a favorable result was achieved in more than 90% of cases.[56,92] Although they are promising, these results are from relatively small case series.

Derby et al[26] investigated the outcome of various treatments delivered to patients with chemically sensitized discs identified by discography (concordant pain provoked with low injection pressure). They found that 89% of patients receiving an interbody procedure, with or without intertransverse fusion, had a successful result. This was significantly better than the 20% success rate among patients undergoing posterior intertransverse fusion and the 12% success rate noted among patients who did not undergo surgery.

For many years, autogenous iliac crest was used as the graft for interbody fusion. In the middle to late 1980s, the use of a femoral ring allograft was introduced.[39] This allograft had the potential to provide stability to the segment while eliminating the pain and potential complications related to harvesting the iliac crest. However, there was some concern about the bony incorporation of the dense cortical femur ring. At our institution this was addressed by filling the hollow center of the femur with a cancellous bone plug; this construct provided the stability of the femur and a scaffold for bone growth into the less dense plug.

The 1990s saw the development of threaded fusion cages packed with autogenous iliac crest graft for anterior or posterior interbody fusion. The primary theorized benefit of the cages was that they would provide stability of the spine while the bone graft was incorporating. Also, the cages should provide better distraction of the disc space than autogenous bone graft alone. The devices could be implanted using an endoscopic approach anteriorly. The published results for the fusion cages were very favorable.[55,84] However, there has been concern as to whether these devices can be used as stand-alone devices—that is, without posterior stabilization. There has been no clinical study published comparing the results of cages with and without posterior stabilization, nor any studies with an appreciable number of patients describing a high rate of reoperation or poor results when using cages alone. There is a suggestion that cages are not reliable as stand-alone implants; however, this is not supported by studies reported in the literature.

There are potential difficulties with the cages in that the cylinders may not ideally fit into the disc space. At L5-S1, the high lordotic angle forces the cages to penetrate the cancellous bone in the posterior aspect of the vertebral body. Ideally, the cages would be implanted into the vertebral body endplates, not penetrating very deeply into the cancellous bone, reducing support. Another metal cage design emerged during the late 1990s: a modular system that has struts to allow adjustment of the obliquity of the device endplates.[35]

Also during the 1990s, the use of threaded cylindrical allograft was introduced.[38] This graft had the potential benefit of more closely matching the physiologic properties of the vertebral bodies and would not create artifact on imaging studies, which has been encountered with metal implants. Years later, similar implants have been marketed. Another cage design consists of a carbon fiber rectangular cage designed to be used with pedicle screws.[12]

One of the newest cage systems approved for marketing includes a tapered threaded fusion cage combined with a bone morphogenetic protein (BMP); no posterior stabilization was used. In a prospective randomized study, Burkus et al reported that this treatment resulted in significant improvement in pain and self-reported disability scores.[14] This was noted in both the treatment and control groups. However, the use of the BMP avoided the pain and complications noted in the control group in whom the cages were packed with autogenous iliac crest graft.

Posterior Fusion

There have been few reports on the results of posterior fusion specifically for the treatment of symptomatic disc degeneration. The rationale for performing the procedure is not clear because the disc is only indirectly addressed. The assumption is that stabilizing the posterior spinal column will stabilize the anterior column sufficiently to unload the painful tissue and to prevent mechanical stimulation of the sensitized disc tissue and prevent pumping or leaking of the neurotoxic agents from the disc nucleus to nociceptors in the anulus or onto the nerve roots. The results of posterior lumbar fusion (PLF) for discogenic pain have been reported in two studies with relatively small numbers of patients. The results in both studies were poor,[81,103] which may be attributable, at least in part, to the failure to address the pain generator directly.

With respect to the stability of the anterior column achieved with posterior fusion alone, despite a solid posterior fusion, there may well be a "sugar-tong" effect, which allows small degrees of motion anteriorly. In studies with small numbers of patients, Weatherley and Barrick have both described patients with persistent symptomatic disc degeneration, identified by discography, in the disc included in a posteriorly fused segment.[2,102] In such patients, pain relief was achieved after the patient underwent an anterior interbody fusion procedure. Such cases further support the theory that posterior fusion alone may not be adequate to address symptomatic disc degeneration.

The "sugar tong" effect, that is, allowing significant mechanical stimulation of the disc under a posterior fusion, is supported in biomechanical studies. Abe et al[1] reported that posterolateral fusion and pedicle screws decreased intradiscal pressure during axial compression and extension. However, during flexion, the intradiscal pressure reached values as high as those measured in the intact spine. Thus posterior fusion alone may not adequately reduce the intradiscal pressure that is either directly stimulating nerve endings in the disc and/or pushing neurotoxic agents from the nucleus to the neural tissue in or beyond the disc.

Developments in posterior fixation devices have led to many designs of hooks, rods, plates, and screws. Most of these developments have evolved for the canal

treatment of spinal conditions other than lumbar disc–related pain. However, there is some crossover in light of combined anteroposterior fusion for the treatment of disc-related pain, which is discussed next.

Combined Anteroposterior Fusion

The role of combining anterior lumbar interbody fusion (ALIF) with posterior fusion, with or without internal fixation, in the treatment of disc-related pain has not been well defined. In the 1980s this was sometimes criticized as simply being too much surgery. The disadvantage of combining PLF with ALIF is the injury to the musculature associated with the posterior procedure. Also, there is additional cost and risk associated with performing two procedures. There may also be concern that making the operated segment too stable could result in accelerated degeneration of the adjacent vertebral disc or the sacroiliac joints. In response to this concern, there have been some reports on the use of translaminar facet screw fusion to supplement the ALIF. Recently, percutaneous pedicle fixation systems have come into clinical use; these methods offer benefits over traditional open pedicle screw placement such as reduced tissue trauma, less blood loss, shorter operating time, and shorter hospital stay.[90] However, there has been no investigation to determine whether these devices offer any benefit over ALIF alone.

Minimally Invasive Procedures

To avoid the potential complications of open spine surgery and to reduce operating time, blood loss, and length of hospital stay, surgeons became interested in percutaneous spine surgery. Over the years, several minimally invasive methods have been introduced for treating disc-related pain. The rationale for the use of the first percutaneous devices was that removing a small amount of disc tissue reduces disc pressure, thus reducing the pain. As a result, treatments could only be offered to patients with contained disc herniations.

The first percutaneous chemical therapy for radicular pain arising from an intervertebral disc was introduced in 1964 when Smith described the use of chymopapain, an enzyme, to degrade disc tissue.[94] The results of this intervention were promising. However, the treatment carries with it a risk of anaphylactic shock. In the United States the use of chymopapain was abandoned because of the risk involved and the medical-legal implications associated with its use.

The earliest percutaneous discectomy system used on a widespread basis was developed by Hijikata et al.[36] This system used a 5 mm cannula placed against the lateral aspect of the intervertebral disc. Instruments were passed through the cannula to remove disc tissue. A later instrument was designed with a cutting device to speed the disc tissue removal process; other percutaneous disc devices have included lasers to ablate disc tissue.

One of the most recent treatments for symptomatic disc disruption is intradiscal electrothermal therapy (IDET), a procedure that involves placing a thermal catheter into the disc and heating the tissue. The hypothesized mechanism of action that this treatment results in pain relief is that heat destroys nociceptors in the outer layers of the disc anulus and shrinks collagen tissue in the disc. It is thought that as the tissue remodels, the rupture in the disc heals or closes. Favorable results of IDET have been reported in a study with 2-year follow-up.[89] Karasek et al[61] supported the use of IDET, although they acknowledge that depending on how success is defined, the success rate following the procedure is in the range of 20% to 60%.[46] Lutz et al[61] also reported a favorable outcome from IDET, but other authors have had less favorable results with it.[22,98] Recently two prospective, randomized, blind, controlled trials were presented.[30,83] Pauza et al found that in a highly select group of patients, IDET patients had a significantly greater improvement in pain and disability scores than did the control group. However, several patients were lost to follow-up and the relative gain from IDET compared with the control group was only 1.3 points on the visual analog scale (VAS) and 6.3% on the Oswestry scale. The clinical relevance of such a small difference is questionable. Freemen et al[30] found no difference in outcome between IDET and a placebo control group.

These treatments have not proved to be a replacement for interbody fusion. Although these procedures were embraced with great enthusiasm, the results have not held up in the long term or with widespread use. In general, it appears that the percutaneous procedures are beneficial to a small subgroup of patients with early-stage symptomatic disc disruption. These devices have not generally undergone rigorous evaluation in randomized studies to determine whether they produce results comparable to those achieved with the more invasive procedures.

The mechanisms of action of these various percutaneous disc therapies differ greatly. It appears that if such therapeutic interventions are effective, they are applicable to only a very select subgroup of patients with early stages of disc disruption. For such patients, it is greatly preferable to undergo a minimally invasive procedure rather than a fusion procedure, or possibly having to delay a fusion for several years.

Artificial Discs

The primary rationale for artificial discs compared to fusion is to allow motion of the operated segment and to provide pain relief. There is an intuitive desire to have the operated segment function more normally, and one of the advantages is that the patient can avoid or delay adjacent segment breakdown related to the increased stresses placed on the discs adjacent to a fused segment.

In the 1950s the desire for devices that could maintain disc space height and maintain movement of a spinal motion segment was realized. The first patent for an artificial disc was issued to van Steenbrugghe in France in 1956.[99] The first reported use of an intervertebral arthroplasty device was published by Fernström of Sweden in 1966.[28] He implanted metal spheres into the disc space following discectomy. In the 1980s the Link SB Charité artificial disc was developed,[15] which was a biconvex polyethylene sliding core sandwiched between two metal endplates that interfaced with the vertebral bodies. The device allowed motion by articulation between the concave inner surfaces of the endplates and the biconvex core. The first two designs of the Charité device had problems with subsidence into the vertebral endplates. A third design of the device incorporated larger, oval endplates and this design remains in use today. The clinician results reported for it are that a good outcome is achieved in 62% to 79% of patients.[20,25,57,107] A prospective study[40] reports significant improvement in preoperative to postoperative scores on visual analog scales assessing pain and on the Oswestry disability questionnaire.

About 1990, Marnay of France patented a device with two metal endplates and a core that was convex on the superior surface and flat on the inferior surface. The inferior surface fit into the lower endplate, and the motion occurred through articulation between the concave and convex surfaces. Although the device has been used for quite a few years, there have been few European reports on its outcome. Bertagnoli and Kumar reported a very high rate, 91%, of excellent/good results following arthroplasty with the ProDisc.[4] However, the authors did not describe how outcome was defined. In a prospective study, significant improvement was noted in the pain and disability scores in patients who received this device.[108]

In addition to total disc replacements, several disc nucleus replacements have also been invented. These devices may have application in the treatment of early-stage symptomatic disc disruption. Another application may be as a discectomy adjunctive procedure to help prevent disc space collapse or instability after the removal of disc tissue. Nucleus replacement devices are designed to fill the nuclear cavity after disc nucleus tissue has been removed. Ray described the use of a hydrogel as a disc nucleus replacement; this material expands as water is absorbed. The hydrogel is contained in a restrictive jacket to control the maximal size of the implant. The Prosthetic Disc Nucleus (PDN) is designed for two devices to be implanted at each operated level. Since 1996, a total of 423 patients have received the device.[50] Although the authors report a 90% success rate, this is only the percentage of patients not requiring explanation of the device; no clinical success rate was reported. However, the authors did report significant improvements in pain and Oswestry scores. Other nucleus replacements have been described, but have not yet been used clinically on a widespread basis.

Soft Stabilization

During the past several decades, much of the focus in spine care has been on improving fusion rates. This goal has brought about the development of metal screw and rod systems, bone graft supplements, BMPs, gene therapy, fusion cages of various shapes and materials, posterior screws for facet fusion, and other various materials and devices. However, during this time there also developed a recognition of the potential iatrogenic problems related to stabilizing a spinal segment. Such problems include accelerated degeneration at the adjacent spinal segment or the sacroiliac joints, and stenosis at the adjacent segment. The rationale is that if a segment is solidly fused, the forces that had previously passed through that segment are now transferred to adjacent segments, stressing them beyond the loads they had previously borne. This additional stress results in these adjacent segments degenerating earlier than they otherwise would have. The incidence of adjacent segment breakdown is not known because there are only a few studies with truly long-term follow-up (i.e., more than 10 years) that investigate the condition of the adjacent segment. Attempts to provide the degree of stability needed to reduce the patient's pain while avoiding potential iatrogenic problems led to the development of what is now termed "soft stabilization."

Soft stabilization treatment is based on the concept of using implants that provide stability to the spine but allow controlled motion. One of the first such devices was the Graf ligament system, which consists of a polyester band connecting pedicle screws placed in adjacent segments. A report on early results of the system indicated that 72% of patients had a good or excellent outcome, but 34% required revision.[34] The results of a 7-year follow-up of patients with Graf ligaments was recently published in which 52% of the 40 patients, either had a second procedure or considered themselves to have either a poor or fair result from the surgery.[33] Mulholland and Sengupta have noted that a problem with this system is that too much load is placed on the posterior anulus of the disc.[71] They propose the use of a fulcrum-assisted soft stabilization (FASS) system that consists of an elastic band connecting pedicle screws as adjacent segments, and includes a flexible fulcrum placed in front of the band. The purpose of the fulcrum is to decrease the load on the posterior anulus. The FASS system was found to reduce disc pressure, and the reduction was maintained throughout the flexion-extension range of motion.[93]

Disc Repair and Healing

Perhaps one of the most exciting developments in spine care will be the ability to help the disc heal and restore its normal hydrostatic properties. Gene therapy may have applications in the treatment of pain related to the intervertebral disc, which primarily applies to pain related to disc degeneration. Although disc degeneration is a part of the normal aging process and is not always painful, it may also represent the late stage of symptomatic disc disruption with potentially painful nerve endings developing in the disc. One characteristic of disc degeneration is dehydration related to the reduction of water-imbibing proteoglycans in the disc nucleus. Genetic therapy may eventually provide a treatment method to increase or maintain the proteoglycan content within the nucleus.

In addition to dehydration, another characteristic of disc degeneration is changes in the collagen in the disc, and gene therapy may offer a therapeutic intervention in this area. Paul et al[82] recently reported that gene therapy increased type II collagen synthesis in human in vitro samples. Using the same therapy in a rabbit model, the architecture of the nucleus was maintained over time, unlike in the control discs. This work, as well as many other studies on gene therapy, may some day produce a viable nonoperative treatment for symptomatic disc degeneration. However, as described by Wallach et al,[101] the transfer of gene therapy from the laboratory into the clinical setting must be carefully guided by rigorous safety and efficacy studies for each gene of interest. These researchers found deleterious effects, including paralysis, associated with doses greater than those they had previously determined to be therapeutic, whereas the same dose of another agent did not demonstrate any deleterious effects.

Disc Tissue Transplants

In addition to gene therapy to restore tissue in the degenerated disc, another treatment approach is the direct transplantation of tissue into the disc. In a recent study using a canine model, autologous disc chondrocyte cells were transplanted back into the harvest sites 6 weeks later.[65] The authors reported that the implanted cells were viable and produced extracellular matrix similar to normal disc tissue. Proteoglycans, as well as types I and II collagen were present. These early findings suggest that more work investigating disc tissue transplantation is merited.

Pharmacologic Treatment

With the role of inflammation being identified in disc-related back pain, a natural step in seeking effective treatment was to look to antiinflammatory agents.

Cornefjord et al[24] investigated the effects of injections of diclofenac or ketoprofen into pigs in which nerve root inflammation was induced by placing autologous nucleus pulposus tissue around the first sacral nerve root. The researchers found that nerve root conduction velocity was significantly greater in the group receiving diclofenac than among the control animals receiving saline injections. The ketoprofen group did not demonstrate nerve conduction velocities that were better than the control group. This study demonstrated that nucleus pulposus–induced nerve root dysfunction could be reduced by antiinflammatory medication; however, the type of antiinflammatory drug used for treatment had a dramatic influence on the results. Such studies lay the framework for introducing nonoperative therapies for the treatment of radicular pain caused by inflammatory agents from the disc nucleus leaking or herniating onto the nerve roots.

The expanding knowledge concerning the mechanisms of inflammatory disc-related pain is leading to the development of mediator-specific treatments. Recently Karppinen and colleagues[47,53] reported on the intravenous infusion of a TNF-α monoclonal antibody in the management of severe sciatica in a group of 10 patients. They found that the treatment resulted in 50% pain relief in 1 hour. Favorable results were maintained during a 3 month follow-up period.[47] An update on this study found that the initial dramatic improvements of leg pain and disability were maintained during the 12 month follow-up.[53] One of the 10 patients had undergone surgery. These results are encouraging; however, caution must be exercised in further evaluation of the safety and efficacy of this therapy.

Psychological Evaluations

Although the development of new treatments is promising, devices and cellular-based therapy alone cannot guarantee improved clinical outcomes. There is strong evidence supporting the role of psychological factors in surgical treatment outcome.[5,96,97,105] Block[5] et al reported that structured psychological evaluation was strongly predictive of surgical outcome. Although factors such as previous spine surgery may be obviously related to treatment outcome, other less obvious factors such as abuse during childhood[91] and spousal support have also been identified as having a significant impact on treatment outcome.[100] Understanding of the disc as a pain generator has increased; likewise, further investigation into psychological factors and treatment outcome will expand and lead to more effective patient screening and improved outcomes.

Conclusion

The origins, diagnosis, and treatment of disc-related pain have been controversial and, in some instances, continue to be so. The details of the mechanisms of origin for disc-related pain are being better understood, and ongoing advancements in basic science will continue to increase the understanding of disc-related pain mechanisms. The treatment of disc-related pain will continue to evolve, with new designs and materials developed for total disc replacements, disc nucleus replacements, "soft" posterior stabilization systems, and treatments designed to promote the healing of injured or torn disc tissue. Progress in all areas of study in back pain brings us closer to the ideal treatment model for understanding the details of the pain generator in individual patients, having reliable diagnostic tests to correctly identify the pain generator, and then matching the best possible treatment from a large armamentarium of options to address the patient's symptoms. The ongoing advances in diagnosis and treatment should ultimately generate better results than those in the range of approximately 75% to 79% that have been reported in a review of the results of lumbar fusion.[10]

Beginning in the 1970s, much of the focus in spine surgery was on improving the chances of achieving a solid spinal fusion; this endeavor continues today. This era saw the development of a variety of screw and rod constructs, proliferation of bone graft supplements, a variety of fusion cage designs, and finally BMPs. In the first decade of the twenty-first century, the focus is shifting toward dynamic stabilization of the spine including total disc replacements, disc nucleus replacements, facet joint prostheses, and dynamic posterior stabilization systems. This era of mechanical treatments is likely to be followed by a generation of tissue-engineering applications that will promote healing of injured or degenerated disc tissue. However, the ability of these potential treatments to heal an injured, painful disc and address the potential problems created by the neurovascularization noted in injured discs remains to be investigated. Currently there are potential pharmacologic treatments for radicular pain related to inflammation. In addition to biologic and pharmaceutical therapies, microelectromechanical systems (MEMS) and nanotechnology are likely to play important roles in the treatment of patients with back pain. The future of back pain care is promising; however, enthusiasm must be tempered with careful and thorough assessment of these new technologies rather than giving in to the temptation to embrace the newest available treatment simply because it is innovative. Such therapies must be carefully evaluated in the basic research arena and then in the clinical setting.

The role of careful patient selection, including psychological screening, appropriately matching treatment with the patient's pain generator(s), technically correct execution of treatments, and appropriate posttreatment rehabilitation will remain critical to achieving good outcomes for patients with back pain. Not only is the future likely to bring exciting developments in mechanical therapies, we are already on the verge of therapies targeting specific inflammatory agents, tissue transplantation, and gene therapy.

REFERENCES

1. Abe E, Nickel T, Buttermann GR, Lewis JL, et al. Lumbar intradiscal pressure after posterolateral fusion and pedicle screw fixation. Tohoku J Exp Med 86:243-253, 1998.
2. Barrick WT, Schofferman JA, Reynolds JB, et al. Anterior lumbar fusion improves discogenic pain at levels of prior posterolateral fusion. Spine 25:853-857, 2000.
3. Bernard TN Jr. Lumbar discography and post-discography computerized tomography: Refining the diagnosis of low-back pain. Spine 15:690-707, 1990.
4. Bertagnoli R, Kumar S. Indications for full prosthetic disc arthroplasty: A correlation of clinical outcome against a variety of indications. Eur Spine J 11(Suppl 2):S131-S136, 2002.
5. Block AR, Ohnmeiss DD, Guyer RD, et al. The use of presurgical psychological screening to predict the outcome of spine surgery. Spine J 1:274-282, 2001.
6. Block AR, Vanharanta H, Ohnmeiss DD, et al. Discographic pain report. Influence of psychological factors. Spine 21:334-338, 1996.
7. Blumenthal SL, Baker J, Dossett A, et al. The role of anterior lumbar fusion for internal disc disruption. Spine 13:566-569, 1988.
8. Boden SD, Davis DO, Dina TS, et al. Abnormal magnetic-resonance scans of the lumbar spine in asymptomatic subjects: A prospective investigation. J Bone Joint Surg Am 72:403-408, 1990.
9. Bogduk N, Tynan W, Wilson AS. The nerve supply to the human lumbar intervertebral discs. J Anat 132:39-56, 1981.
10. Bono CM, Lee CK. Critical analysis of trends in fusion for degenerative disc disease over the last twenty years: Influence of technique on fusion rate and clinical outcome. Presented at the Annual Meeting of the International Society for the Study of the Lumbar Spine, Vancouver, Canada, May 2003.
11. Boos N, Rieder R, Schade V, et al. The diagnostic accuracy of magnetic resonance imaging, work perception, and psychological factors in identifying symptomatic disc herniations. Spine 20:2613-2625, 1995.
12. Brantigan JW, Steffee AD, Lewis ML, et al. Lumbar interbody fusion using the Brantigan I/F cage for posterior lumbar interbody fusion and the variable pedicle screw placement system. Spine 25:1437-1446, 2000.
13. Burke JG, Watson RW, McCormack D, et al. Intervertebral discs which cause low back pain secrete high levels of proinflammatory mediators. J Bone Joint Surg Br 84:196-201, 2002.
14. Burkus JK, Gornet MF, Dickman CA, et al. Anterior lumbar interbody fusion using rhBMP-2 with tapered interbody cages. J Spinal Disord & Tech 15:337-349, 2002.
15. Büttner-Janz K. The Development of the Artificial Disc: SB Charité. Dallas: Hundley & Associates, 1992.
16. Carragee E. Prospective controlled study of the development of LBP in previously asymptomatic subjects undergoing experimental discography. Presented at the Annual Meeting of the International Society for the Study of the Lumbar Spine, Vancouver, Canada, May 2003.
17. Carragee EJ, Tanner CM, Khurana S, et al. The rates of false-positive lumbar discography in select patients without low back pain. Spine 25:1373-1381, 2000.
18. Carragee EJ, Tanner CM, Yang B, et al. False-positive findings on lumbar discography: Reliability of subjective concordance assessment during provocative disc injection. Spine 24:2542-2547, 1999.
19. Cheung KMC, Karppinen J, Yang E, et al. Prevalence of intervertebral disc degeneration: A MRI study of 769 volunteers. Presented at the Annual Meeting of the International Society for the Study of the Lumbar Spine, Vancouver, Canada, May 2003.
20. Cinotti G, David T, Postacchini F. Results of disc prosthesis after a minimum follow-up period of 2 years. Spine 21:995-1000, 1996.

21. Cloward RB. New treatment of ruptured intervertebral discs. Presented at the Annual Meeting of the Hawaii Territorial Medical Association, May 1945.
22. Cohen SP, Larkin T, Abdi S, et al. Risk factors for failure and complications of intradiscal electrothermal therapy: A pilot study. Spine 28:1142-1147, 2003.
23. Coppes MH, Marani E, Thomeer RTWM, et al. Innervation of "painful" lumbar discs. Spine 22:2342-2350, 1997.
24. Cornefjord M, Olmarker K, Otani K, et al. Nucleus pulposus-induced nerve root injury: Effects of diclofen and ketoprofen. Eur Spine J 11:57-61, 2002.
25. David TJ. Lumbar disc prosthesis: Five years follow-up study on 96 patients. Presented at the Annual Meeting of the North American Spine Society, New Orleans, Oct 2000.
26. Derby R, Howard MW, Grant JM, et al. The ability of pressure-controlled discography to predict surgical and nonsurgical outcomes. Spine 24:364-371, 1999.
27. Feinstein B, Langton JNK, Jameson RM, et al. Experiments on pain referred from deep somatic tissues. J Bone Joint Surg Am 36:981-997, 1954.
28. Fernström U. Arthroplasty with intercorporal endoprosthesis in herniated disc and in painful disc. Acta Chir Scand 357(Suppl):154-159, 1966.
29. Flanagan MN, Chung BU. Roentgenographic changes in 188 patients 10 to 20 years after discography and chemonucleolysis. Spine 11:444-448, 1986.
30. Freeman BJC, Fraser RD, Cain CMJ, et al. A randomized double-blind controlled efficacy study: Intradiscal electrothermal therapy (IDET) versus placebo. Presented at the Annual Meeting of the International Society for the Study of the Lumbar Spine, Vancouver, Canada, May 2003.
31. Freemont AJ, Peacock TE, Goupille P, et al. Nerve ingrowth into diseased intervertebral disc in chronic back pain. Lancet 350:178-181, 1997.
32. Freemont AJ, Watkins A, Le Maitre C, et al. Nerve growth factor expression and innervation of the painful intervertebral disc. J Pathol 197:286-292, 2002.
33. Gardner A, Pande KC. Graf ligamentoplasty: A seven-year follow-up. Eur Spine J 11(Suppl 2):S157-S163, 2002.
34. Grevitt MP, Gardner AD, Spilsbury J, et al. The Graf stabilisation system: Early results in 50 patients. Eur Spine J 4:169-175, 1995.
35. Guyer RD, Davis R, Songer M. et al. The efficacy of a new modular cage for anterior lumbar interbody fusion. Presented at the World Spine Meeting, Chicago, Aug 2003.
36. Hijikata S, Yamagishi M, Nakayama T. Percutaneous discectomy: A new treatment method for lumbar disc herniation. J Toden Hospital 5, 1975.
37. Hirsch D, Ingelmark B, Miller M. The anatomical basis for low back pain. Acta Orthop Scand 33:1-17, 1963.
38. Hochschuler SH, Griffith SL, Weinhoffer SL, et al. Compressive strength of hollow, allograft bone cylinders proposed for lumbar interbody fusion. Presented at the Annual Meeting of the North American Spine Society, San Diego, Oct 1993.
39. Hochschuler SH, Guyer RD, Ohnmeiss DD, et al. Anterior lumbar interbody fusion using donor femur bone grafts. Presented at the Annual Meeting of the North American Spine Society, Monterey, Calif, Aug 1990.
40. Hochschuler SH, Ohnmeiss DD, Guyer RD, et al. Artificial disc: Preliminary results of a prospective study in the United States. Eur Spine J 11(Suppl 2):S106-S110, 2002.
41. Igarashi T, Kikuchi S, Shubayev V, et al. 2000 Volvo award winner in basic science studies: Exogenous tumor necrosis factor-alpha mimics nucleus pulposus-induced neuropathology: Molecular, histologic, and behavioral comparisons in rats. Spine 25:2975-2980, 2000.
42. Jackson HC, Winkelmann RK, Bickel WH. Nerve endings in the human lumbar spinal column and related structures. J Bone Joint Surg Am 48:1272-1281, 1966.
43. Jensen MC, Brant-Zawadzki MN, Obuchowski N, et al. Magnetic resonance imaging of the lumbar spine in people without back pain. N Engl J Med 331:69-73, 1994.

44. Johnson RG. Does discography injure normal discs? An analysis of repeat discograms. Spine 14:424-426, 1989.
45. Kahanovitz N, Arnoczky SP, Sissons HA, et al. The effect of discography on the canine intervertebral disc. Spine 11:26-27, 1986.
46. Karasek M, Bogduk N. Twelve-month follow-up of a controlled trial of intradiscal thermal annuloplasty for back pain due to internal disc disruption. Spine 25:2601-2607, 2000.
47. Karppinen J, Korhonen T, Malmivaara A, et al. Tumor necrosis factor-α monoclonal antibody, infliximab, used to manage severe sciatica. Spine 28:750-754, 2003.
48. Kayama S, Konno S, Olmarker K, et al. Incision of the anulus fibrosus induces nerve root morphologic, vascular, and functional changes: An experimental study. Spine 21:2539-2543, 1996.
49. Kellgren JH. On the distribution of pain arising from deep somatic structures with charts of segmental pain areas. Clin Sci 4:35-46, 1939.
50. Klara PM, Ray CD. Artificial nucleus replacement: Clinical experience. Spine 27:1374-1377, 2002.
51. Knox BD, Chapman TM. Anterior lumbar interbody fusion for discogram concordant pain. J Spin Disord 6:242-244, 1993.
52. Konno S, Arai I, Aoki Y, Olmarker K, et al. Compensatory neovascularisation in cauda equina nerve roots subjected to chronic compression. Presented at the Annual Meeting of the International Society for the Study of the Lumbar Spine, Brussels, Belgium, June 1998.
53. Korhonen T, Karppinen J, Malmivaara A, et al. Efficacy of infliximab for disc herniation-induced sciatica. One-year follow-up. Presented at the Annual Meeting of the International Society for the Study of the Lumbar Spine, Vancouver, Canada, May 2003.
54. Kuslich SD. The tissue origin of mechanical low back pain and sciatica as identified by spinal microsurgery. In SH Hochschuler et al, eds. Rehabilitation of the Spine: Science and Practice. St Louis: Mosby–Year Book, 1993, pp 595-600.
55. Kuslich SD, Ulstrom CL, Griffith SL, et al. The Bagby and Kuslich method of lumbar interbody fusion. History, techniques, and 2-year follow-up results of a United States prospective, multicenter trial. Spine 23:1267-1278, 1998.
56. Lee CK, Vessa P, Lee JK. Chronic disabling low back pain syndrome caused by internal disc derangements: The results of disc excision and posterior lumbar interbody fusion. Spine 20:356-361, 1995.
57. Lemaire JP, Skalli W, Lavaste F, et al. Intervertebral disc prosthesis. Results and prospects for the year 2000. Clin Orthop 337:64-76, 1997.
58. Li H, Zou X, Laursen M, Egund N, et al. The influence of intervertebral disc tissue on anterior spinal interbody fusion: an experimental study on pigs. Eur Spine J 11:476-481, 2002.
59. Lindblom K. Diagnostic puncture of intervertebral disks in sciatica. Acta Orthop Scand 17:213-239, 1948.
60. Linson MA, Williams H. Anterior and combined anteroposterior fusion for lumbar disc pain. A preliminary study. Spine 16:143-145, 1991.
61. Lutz C, Lutz GE, Cooke PM. Treatment of chronic lumbar diskogenic pain with intradiskal electrothermal therapy: A prospective outcome study. Arch Phys Med Rehabil 84:23-28, 2003.
62. Malinsky J. The nontogenetic development of nerve terminations in the intervertebral disc of man. Acta Anat 38:96-113, 1959.
63. McAfee PC, Lee GA, Fedder IL, et al. Anterior BAK instrumentation and fusion: Complete versus partial discectomy. Clin Orthop 394:55-63, 2002.
64. McCarron RF, Wimpee MW, Hudkins PG, et al. The inflammatory effect of nucleus puplosus. A possible element in the pathogenesis of low back pain. Spine 12:760-764, 1987.

65. Meisel HJ, Libera J, Moos V, et al. Disc chondrocyte transplantation in a canine model: A treatment for damaged or degenerated intervertebral disc? Presented at the Annual Meeting of the International Society for the Study of the Lumbar Spine, Vancouver, Canada, May 2003.
66. Middleton GS, Teacher JH. Injury of the spinal cord due to rupture of an intervertebral disc during muscular effort. Glasgow Med J 76:1, 1911.
67. Milette PC, Fontaine S, Lepanto L, et al. Radiating pain to lower extremities caused by lumbar disk rupture without spinal nerve root involvement. Am J Neuroradiol 16:1605-1613, 1995.
68. Mixter WJ, Barr JS. Rupture of the intervertebral disc with involvement of the spinal canal. N Engl J Med 211:210-215, 1934.
69. Mooney V, Robertson JA. The facet syndrome. Clin Orthop 115:149-155, 1976.
70. Moore RJ, Vernon-Roberts B, Fraser RD, et al. The origin and fate of herniated lumbar intervertebral disc tissue. Spine 21:2149-2155, 1996.
71. Mulholland RC, Sengupta DK. Rationale, principles and experimental evaluation of the concept of soft stabilization. Euro Spine J 11(Suppl 2):S198-S205, 2002.
72. Newman MH, Grinstead GL. Anterior lumbar interbody fusion for internal disc disruption. Spine 17:831-833, 1992.
73. O'Neill CW, Kurgansky ME, Derby R, et al. Disc stimulation and patterns of referred pain. Spine 27:2776-2781, 2002.
74. Ohnmeiss DD. Pain drawings in the evaluation of lumbar disc-related pain. Dissertation. Stockholm: Karolinska Institute, 2000.
75. Ohnmeiss DD, Vanharanta H, Guyer RD. The association between pain drawings and computed tomographic/discographic pain responses. Spine 20:729-733, 1995.
76. Ohnmeiss DD, Vanharanta H, Ekholm J. The relationship between pain location and disc pathology: A study of pain drawings and CT/discography. Clin J Pain 15:210-217, 1999.
77. Olmarker K, Rydevik B, Hansson T, et al. Compression-induced changes of the nutritional supply to the porcine cauda equina. J Spin Disord 3:25-29, 1990.
78. Olmarker K, Rydevik B, Nordborg C. Autologous nucleus pulposus induces neurophysiologic and histologic changes in porcine cauda equina nerve roots. Spine 18:1425-1432, 1993.
79. Özaktay AC, Cavanaugh JM, Asik I, et al. Dorsal root sensitivity to interleukin-1 beta, interleukin-6 and tumor necrosis factor in rats. Euro Spine J 11:467-475, 2002.
80. Pai RR, D'sa B, Raghuveer CV, et al. Neovascularization of nucleus pulposus. A diagnostic feature of intervertebral disc prolapse. Spine 24:739-741, 1999.
81. Parker LM, Murrell SE, Boden SD, et al. The outcome of posterolateral fusion in highly selected patients with discogenic low back pain. Spine 21:1909-1916, 1996.
82. Paul R, Haydon RC, Cheng H, et al. Potential use of Sox9 gene therapy for intervertebral degenerative disc disease. Spine 28:755-763, 2003.
83. Pauza K, Howell S, Dreyfuss P, et al. A randomized, double-blind, placebo-controlled trial evaluating intradiscal electrothermal anuloplasty (IDETTM). Presented at the Annual Meeting of the International Society for the Study of the Lumbar Spine, Vancouver, Canada, May 2003.
84. Ray CD. Threaded titanium cages for lumbar interbody fusions. Spine 22:667-680, 1997.
85. Roofe PG. Innervation of anulus fibrosus and posterior longitudinal ligament. Arch Neurol Psychiatry 44:100-103, 1940.
86. Rydevik B, Brown MA, Lundborg G. Pathoanatomy and pathophysiology of nerve root compression. Spine 9:7-15, 1984.
87. Saal JS. The role of inflammation in lumbar pain. Spine 20:1821-1827, 1995.
88. Saal JS, Franson RC, Dobrow R, et al. High levels of inflammatory phospholipase A_2 activity in lumbar disc herniations. Spine 15:674-678, 1990.

89. Saal JA, Saal JS. Intradiscal electrothermal treatment for chronic discogenic low back pain. Spine 27:966-974, 2002.
90. Sachs BL, Hisey MS, Zigler JE, et al. Clinical comparison of percutaneous (minimally invasive) placement of pedicle screws versus standard open pedicle screw placement. IMAST, Rome, July 2003.
91. Schofferman J, Anderson D, Hines R, et al. Childhood psychological trauma correlates with unsuccessful lumbar spine surgery. Spine 17(6 Suppl):S138-S144, 1992.
92. Schechter NA, France MP, Lee CK. Painful internal disc derangements of the lumbosacral spine: Discographic diagnosis and treatment by posterior lumbar interbody fusion. Orthopedics 14:447-451, 1991.
93. Sengupta DK, Ohnmeiss D, Webb J, et al. Can soft stabilization in the lumbar spine unload the disc and retain mobility? A biomechanical study with fulcrum-assisted soft stabilization on a cadaver spine. Presented at the International Society for the Study of the Lumbar Spine, Edinburgh, Scotland, 2001.
94. Smith L. Enzyme dissolution of the nucleus pulposus in humans. JAMA 197:137-140, 1964.
95. Smyth MJ, Wright V. Sciatica and the intervertebral disc: An experimental study. J Bone Joint Surg Am 40:1401-1418, 1958.
96. Sørensen LV, Mors O. Presentation of a new MMPI scale to predict outcome after first lumbar discectomy. Pain 34:191-194, 1988.
97. Spengler DM, Ouellette EA, Battié M, et al. Elective discectomy for herniation of a lumbar disc. J Bone Joint Surg Am 72:230-237, 1990.
98. Spruit M, Jacobs WC. Pain and function after intradiscal electrothermal treatment (IDET) for symptomatic lumbar disc degeneration. Eur Spine J 11:589-593, 2002.
99. van Steenbrugghe. French Patent FR1122634, 1956.
100. Wacholtz E, Block AR, Ohnmeiss DD. Responsiveness to spine surgery: Effects of spousal solicitousness on short-term recovery. Presented at the Annual Meeting of the North American Spine Society, New Orleans, Oct 2000.
101. Wallach CJ, Kim JS, Lattermann C, et al. Investigation into therapeutic window and safety issues of intradiscal gene transfer. Presented at the Annual Meeting of the International Society for the Study of the Lumbar Spine. Vancouver, Canada, May 2003.
102. Weatherley CR, Prickett CF, O'Brien JP. Discogenic pain persisting despite solid posterior fusion. J Bone Joint Surg Br 68:142-143, 1986.
103. Wetzel FT, LaRocca SH, Lowery GL, et al. The treatment of lumbar spinal pain syndromes diagnosed by discography. Lumbar arthrodesis. Spine 19:792-800, 1994.
104. Wiberg G. Back pain in relation to the nerve supply of the intervertebral disc. Acta Orthop Scand 19:211-221, 1949.
105. Wiltse LL, Rocchio PH. Pre-operative psychological tests as predictors of success of chemonucleolysis and treatment of low back syndrome. J Bone Joint Surg Am 57:478-483, 1975.
106. Yoshizawa H, O'Brien JP, Thomas-Smith W, Trumper M. The neuropathology of intervertebral discs removed for low-back pain. J Pathol 132:95-104, 1980.
107. Zeegers WS, Bohnen LM, Laaper M, et al. Artificial disc replacement with the modular type SB Charité III: 2-year results in 50 prospectively studied patients. Eur Spine J 8:210-217, 1999.
108. Zigler JE, Vialle EN, Burd TA, et al. Lumbar spine arthroplasty: Early results using the ProDisc II—a prospective randomized trial of arthroplasty versus fusion. J Spinal Disord Tech 16:352-361, 2003.

CHAPTER

2

HISTORY OF THE ARTIFICIAL DISC

Rolando Garcia, Jr.

If I have seen farther than others, it is because I was standing on the shoulders of giants.
SIR ISAAC NEWTON

The idea of an artificial disc is not new, and the field of disc replacement is not in its infancy; rather, it has just hit puberty, and this is a time of rapid and rebellious growth. This chapter will review the key figures in and early attempts to make an artificial intervertebral disc and provide readers with a solid background to help them understand the current state of the art. The early history of some of the currently used prostheses such as the Link and ProDisc prosthesis will be discussed, but the more contemporaneous experience will be covered in later chapters on specific prostheses.

The history of the artificial disc begins in 1934 in Boston, Massachusetts with Mixter and Barr's "discovery" of the herniated disc.[26] This discovery served as a catalyst for the development of our understanding of the disc as a common cause of radiculopathy and mechanical back pain.

Shortly after its introduction, the technique of discectomy or nucleotomy was widely accepted by many surgeons around the world. Initially surgeons were satisfied with the ability of a nucleotomy to resolve nerve compression and radiculopathy. It was not long, however, before surgeons like Barr himself began to realize that "a disc which has been surgically removed is no longer anatomically or mechanically normal."[2] It was the less than ideal results of nucleotomy or discectomy that led surgeons to attempt to treat disc dysfunction with a fusion. In 1947, Barr published a paper on the treatment of ruptured intervertebral disc and sciatic pain, in which he concluded "that the thesis that every patient should have a spine fusion done at the time of laminectomy is tenable."[1]

Indeed, the initial attempts at "replacing" an intervertebral disc were made with the use of bone with the goal of obtaining a fusion. Although other investigators had earlier reported on the anterior lumbar interbody technique for spondylolisthesis, in 1948 Lane and Moore first described the operation of anterior lumbar discectomy and fusion for the specific indication of disc degeneration.[20] Whereas Lane and Moore used a transperitoneal approach, in 1950 Paul Harmon was the first to describe the technique through a retroperitoneal approach.[15]

In 1955 David Cleveland of Milwaukee published the first paper on replacing a surgically excised disc with a material other than bone.[5] Cleveland applied methylacrylic into the disc space of 14 patients at the time of lumbar discectomy in an attempt to stabilize the operated segment through a bilateral keyhole laminotomy approach. After retracting the dura, a nucleotomy was made by removing the entire disc except for its anterior and lateral rims. He then injected sterile methylacrylic into the disc space in a liquid phase and allowed for polymerization. Of the 14 patients operated on by Cleveland, 10 had had no previous lumbar surgery and four had had a previous discectomy. Five months postoperatively all 10 patients with no previous surgery reported complete resolution of back pain and sciatica, whereas in the four patients who had had previous surgery, three had residual sciatica but all four patients had resolution of back pain.

Although Cleveland was the first to publish on disc replacement, he wrote that he developed his concept of disc replacement after visiting James Gardner, who had replaced hundreds of damaged lumbar discs with Lucite pegs 8 mm wide and 22 mm long. Although Cleveland did not provide any specific statistics, he wrote that Gardner's operation achieved "excellent results." Cleveland also referred to a surgeon who had used metallic implants made of tantalum. However, Cleveland did not mention the surgeon's name, nor did he reference an article.

In 1957 Wallace Hamby (Fig. 2-1) and Harry Glaser of Buffalo, New York presented a paper at the annual meeting of the American Academy of Neuro-

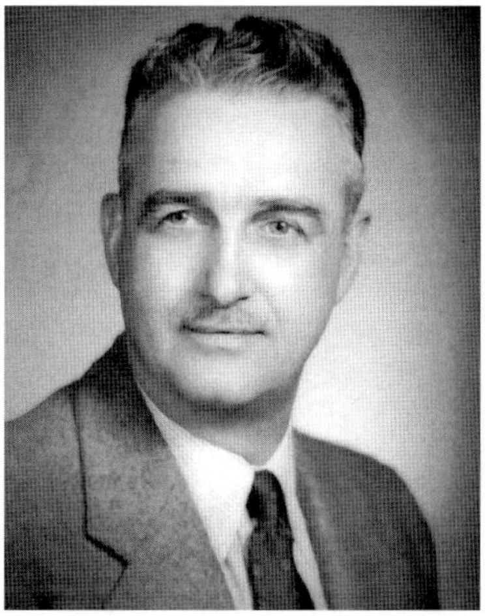

Fig. 2-1 Wallace Hamby, MD.

logical Surgery on their results of disc replacement with methylacrylic in the method previously described by Cleveland.[14] They compared the results of discectomy and replacement with methylacrylic to the results of discectomy alone. The authors followed the patients for 1 year postoperatively and found no difference between the two groups in length of hospital stay, return to work, or back pain. In addition, they found no difference in restoration or maintenance of disc height between the two groups.

Between 1959 and 1961, Paul B. Harmon, an orthopedic surgeon from northern California, implanted vitalium spheres in 13 patients at the time of anterior lumbar discectomy to replace the disc. Harmon (Fig. 2-2) pioneered the use of the retroperitoneal approach, which he first described in 1950.[15] Although he never published the results of replacement with his prosthesis, in a 1969 letter he indicated that the reason he abandoned the procedure was not because of poor clinical results but rather "largely that of the medical-legal climate in sunny Southern California."[16]

In 1962 Ulf Fernström of Uddevalla, Sweden began replacing damaged lumbar intervertebral discs with a mobile prosthesis now known as the Fernström ball.[12] The prosthesis consisted of a solid stainless steel sphere implanted via a posterior approach at the time of lumbar discectomy. In addition to the lumbar application, Fernström developed a smaller prosthesis for use in the cervical spine.[13]

Between 1962 and 1964 Fernström replaced 191 lumbar discs in 125 patients and 13 cervical discs in 8 patients. In 1966, he published his 6 to 30 month results on 105 lumbar cases.[10] Fernström compared his results of disc replace-

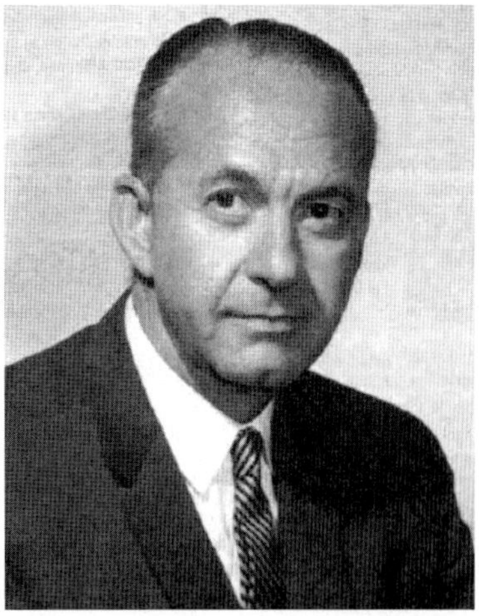

Fig. 2-2 Paul B. Harmon, MD.

ment with the steel ball prosthesis to a "control" group of 100 discectomy patients with follow-up of 5 to 8 years. He divided the patients into two groups: those with a herniated disc (HNP group), and those with disc degeneration (DDD group; i.e., positive discography and no root compression). At follow-up, 12% of patients in the HNP group treated with arthroplasty reported back pain, compared to 60% of those treated with discectomy alone. In the DDD group, 40% of the patients treated with arthroplasty reported back pain at follow-up, compared with 88% of those treated with discectomy alone (Table 2-1). In the HNP group, 14% of patients treated with arthroplasty reported sciatica, compared to 50% of patients treated with discectomy alone. In the DDD group, 47% of patients treated with arthroplasty reported sciatica, whereas 80% of patients treated with discectomy alone (Table 2-2).

Fernström reported complications in two patients, or 1.4% of the cases. He described one case of prosthesis displacement into the spinal canal and one case of temporary peroneal palsy. Total collapse occurred in 48% of the discectomy group and in 0% of the arthroplasty group. Fernström concluded that the results obtained after discectomy and arthroplasty are better than that of discectomy alone and similar to the results after discectomy and fusion. In 1972

TABLE 2-1 PERCENTAGE OF PATIENTS REPORTING BACK PAIN FOLLOWING ARTHROPLASTY OR DISCECTOMY*

Treatment	HNP Group (%)	DDD Group (%)
Discectomy	60	88
Arthroplasty	12	40

*In patients diagnosed with herniated disc or degenerative disc disease.

TABLE 2-2 PERCENTAGE OF PATIENTS REPORTING SCIATICA FOLLOWING ARTHROPLASTY OR DISCECTOMY*

Treatment	HNP Group (%)	DDD Group (%)
Discectomy	50	80
Arthroplasty	14	47

*In patients diagnosed with herniated disc or degenerative disc disease.

he published a series of 267 ball prostheses in 195 patients. In this article Fernström reported a "splendid result" in 34% of the disc degeneration group and 65% of the disc herniation group after a follow-up of 4 to 8 years.[11]

Alvin H. McKenzie (Fig. 2-3) of Edmonton, Canada reported on 60 prostheses implanted in 40 patients at the Royal Alexandra Hospital in Edmonton.[25] According to McKenzie, "It was initially feared that the steel ball might erode into the vertebral bodies or displace into the canal, but these complications have not materialized. The results to date were encouraging." In 1995 McKenzie published an article on 67 patients he performed disc replacement on with an average follow-up of 17 years. Similar to Fernström, McKenzie subdivided his patients into two groups: group I with disc herniations, and group II with disc degeneration. McKenzie reported good and excellent results in 83% of group I patients and 75% of group II patients. McKenzie also reported that 95% of the patients were able to return to work, and that removal of the prosthesis was required in only one of a total of 155 patients. Why this procedure did not gain wider acceptance and was discontinued remains the topic of speculation, but the author believes that political issues and jealousy played a major role.[24]

The first Fernström prosthesis was implanted in the late 1950s and early 1960s in Sweden. In 1964 Reitz, an orthopedic surgeon, and Joubert, a neurosurgeon, both from South Africa, following Fernström's initial work published a study on replacement of a cervical disc with a metal prosthesis for the treatment of intractable headaches and neck pain. The authors indicate that they both visited Fernström and were "favorably impressed by his results." Between November 1963 and June 1964, the authors implanted 75 cervical disc prostheses in 32 patients, and 19 lumbar disc prostheses in 12 patients. They concluded that

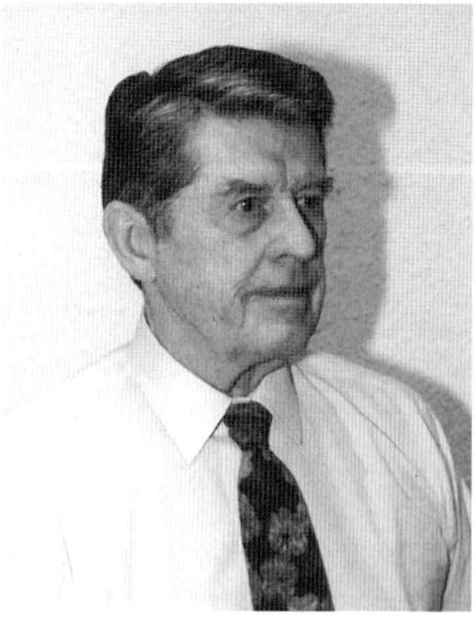

Fig. 2-3 Alvin H. McKenzie, MD.

"we can definitely state that the clinical results so far have been infinitely better than our past experiences over many years with spinal fusion procedures."[28]

In 1974 Schneider and Oyen from Germany reported their initial experience with a silicone rubber prosthesis. The authors injected fluid polysiloxan into the disc space after a typical discectomy, because they believed that a discectomy resulted in increased postoperative instability, and that injection of silicone into the disc space "restored residual disc stability and mobility in approximately normal fashion."[29]

In 1977 Schulmann reported his results after dorsally infusing rapid-setting polyurethane in 62 patients followed up for 5 years. The authors concluded that the implantation of the polyurethane allowed for correction of the statodynamic incompetence of the spine. They also concluded that the results were better in patients with a clinical pattern of radicular compression, and worse in patients with "caudal syndrome" caused by persistent gross neurologic deficits.[31]

In 1978 Fassio and Ginestie of France published their preliminary experience with replacing human lumbar discs with a silicone prosthesis.[9] Beginning in January 1976, the authors implanted a two-part prosthesis composed of a central silicone sphere 14 mm in height surrounded by a peripheral silicone plateau approximately 7 mm in height. The central core was deformable but incompressible. The authors indicated that single-level discopathy was their primary indication, and they recommended a posterior approach for application. The authors noted that their experience with their first three patients was "very encouraging," and indicated that they hoped to replace discectomy with arthroplasty.

In 1981 Edeland published an article on the subject of artificial lumbar discs. He described several "suggested implants" and made a number of important observations about approach, design, and materials but provided no biomechanical or clinical data. Edeland believes that although the article itself provided no clinical or laboratory data, it may have stimulated others to pay more attention to the concept of arthroplasty.[7]

Before 1984, all attempts at disc replacement were in fact attempts to replace the nucleus. The first attempt at total disc replacement was made by Drs. Karin Büttner-Janz and Kurt Schellnack of Berlin, Germany. After extensive biomechanical and biomaterial testing, Büttner-Janz and Schellnack developed a three-piece modular lumbar prosthesis consisting of two metal plates that attach to the adjacent endplates via multiple spikes, and a central plastic sliding core that articulates with the metal plates. The prosthesis was known as the SB Charité prosthesis, and it was first implanted in September 1984 at the Charité Hospital of the Humboldt University School of Medicine.

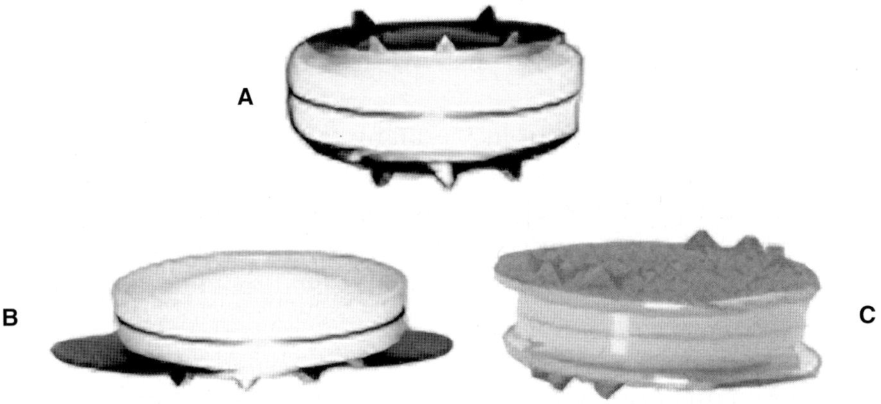

Fig. 2-4 The three designs of the SB Charité prosthesis. **A,** The SB I was introduced in 1982. **B,** SB II was introduced in 1985. **C,** Model III, which is known as the CHARITÉ Artificial Disc and remains in use today, was introduced in 1987.

The SB Charité prosthesis has evolved through three generations (Fig. 2-4). The first-generation prosthesis, or SB Charité I, was used between 1984 and 1985; SB Charité II was used between 1986 and 1987, and the SB Charité III was developed in 1987.

Büttner-Janz and Schellnack first published the results with their prosthesis in 1987. The authors reported on 16 patients with an average age of 42 years. After short follow-up of 1 to 13 months the authors concluded that "we can reorient ourselves with respect to surgical treatment of disk attrition damage, especially since, with problem cases, ventral fusion remains an available alternative."[3]

In 1988 Büttner-Janz et al published their experience with the Charité prosthesis on 62 patients. The mean follow-up period was 15 months, the maximum was 3 years. The authors reported that 54% of the patients were "highly satisfied" with the results, 29% felt "better than before the operation," and only 2% were "worse than before the operation."[4]

Since its introduction in 1987, more than 5000 SB Charité III prostheses have been implanted worldwide. There have been numerous reports on the short- and mid-term clinical results, but more recently Thierry David of France has reported his results after more than 10 years of follow-up.[6] The CHARITÉ Artificial Disc prosthesis has now been in clinical use since 1987 without substantial changes in its design.

Between 1988 and 1989, Enker et al[8] performed total lumbar disc replacement in six patients. In 1993, they reported the results of disc replacement on these six patients with a minimum follow-up of 3 years. The prosthesis used was the

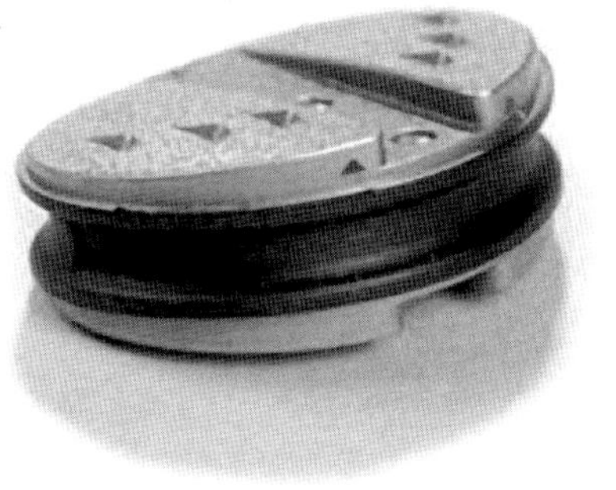

Fig. 2-5 The Acroflex disc prosthesis.

Acroflex disc, which consisted of a Bion rubber core vulcanized to two porous coated titanium endplates. The authors reported satisfactory results in four of the six patients. They also reported an average of 8 degrees of angular motion and 2 mm of translational movement, and porous ingrowth in all interfaces. However, one of the patients experienced a device failure when the core of the device ruptured. In addition, one of the chemicals used in the vulcanization process of the Bion rubber was found to be toxic in rat studies; use of the device was discontinued in 1990.

The second generation consisted of a high-performance silastic core bonded to two titanium endplates. The device was implanted in eight patients in Australia. The U.S. Food and Drug Administration (FDA) approved a feasibility study for a series of 13 patients. Six patients were implanted with the device. This device also produced unsatisfactory results, because the core was unable to withstand the loads of the lumbar spine.

The third generation (Fig. 2-5) of the device consists of a single piece of Bion rubber, with the toxic trace element removed through the vulcanization process. This device has been implanted in 14 patients in Australia.

In March 1990 Thierry Marnay of France first implanted a titanium and polyethylene modular prosthesis now known as the ProDisc. The prosthesis was originally composed of two titanium endplates and a polyethylene core. Between March 1990 and September 1993, Marnay and Louis Villete implanted 93 prostheses in 64 patients.[23]

At the 2001 Annual Meeting of the American Academy of Orthopedic Surgeons in New Orleans, Marnay presented a poster on his 8 to 10 year results of disc arthroplasty with the ProDisc prosthesis. The author indicated that between 1989 and 1992 he implanted 70 prostheses in 44 patients. The author reported 78% good and excellent results, four cases of poor results, and no explantations, or osteolysis.[22]

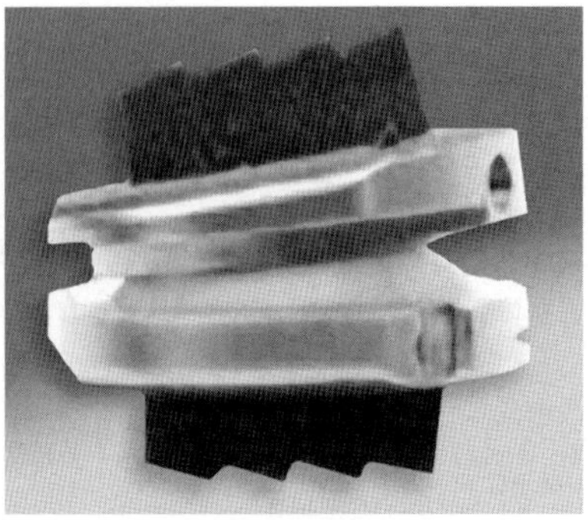

Fig. 2-6 The ProDisc prosthesis.

The ProDisc prosthesis (Fig. 2-6) has undergone some transformation from its original design. The metal plates of the original prosthesis were made of titanium whereas the current prosthesis uses cobalt chromium instead. In addition, the original design had two stabilizing keels, whereas the current design has a larger central keel.

In 1991 Chinese investigators published the results of replacing lumbar discs with silicone prostheses.[17] The authors first experimented with three different artificial disc models: a bag made of Dacron and filled with silicone, a silicone ball, and silicone prosthesis shaped like a horseshoe. After preliminary testing of material mechanics the authors settled on the horseshoe prosthesis. They performed biocompatibility studies on primates and biomechanical studies on fresh human lumbar spines, reporting good maintenance of disc height in the primate studies, and restoration of stability compared with postdiscectomy segments in mechanical testing.

In 1991 Lee et al[21] published a preliminary report on the development and mechanical testing of an elastomeric intervertebral disc prosthesis. The authors developed and tested two types of prosthesis, one with fiber reinforced polyurethane and the other made of multicomponent nonfiber reinforced polymers (C-flex). Although they did not test the implants in animals or humans, the authors concluded disc replacement may be an improved alternative to spinal fusion, and that preliminary results demonstrate that a disc prosthesis can be fabricated with mechanical properties similar to the natural disc.

John Kostuik[19] developed an all-metal "spring disc" (Fig. 2-7) that consists of an internal titanium spring between two cobalt chromium endplates. The endplates are plasma sprayed to induce osteointegration. The endplates have longitudinal extensions that allow for screw fixation into the vertebral bodies.

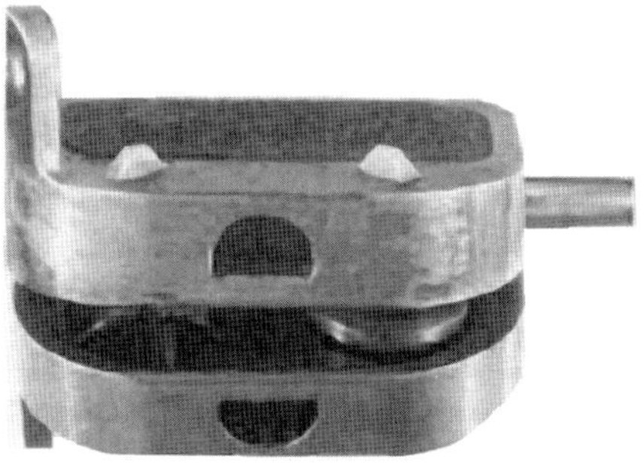

Fig. 2-7 The disc replacement designed by Kostuik incorporates a hinge design with two springs to provide motion.

Husson of France developed a nuclear prosthesis composed of polycarbonate urethane that takes the form of a memory coiling spiral. The product was implanted in 10 patients at the University of Rennes, France.[18]

In the early 1990s Charles Ray of Virginia developed an artificial nucleus pulposus called the prosthetic disc nucleus (PDN). The prosthesis consists of a hydrogel core surrounded by a tightly woven jacket of polyethylene. The hydrogel is a multiblock copolymer of polyacrylonitrile-polyacrylamide of approximately 65% to 85% water content by weight. The implant is compressed during manufacturing, is in a dehydrated state at the time of implantation, and begins to absorb fluid and expand upon implantation.[27]

In January 1996 Robert Schönmayr performed the first PDN implantation in Wiesbaden, Germany and subsequently completed the human pilot study for the PDN. Two prostheses were implanted at each level using a posterior approach at the time of unilateral laminotomy and microdiscectomy. Ten patients aged 29 to 52 were included in the study and were followed for 2 years. Initially the implants were placed longitudinally but after an implant migration on their third patient the authors changed their technique to transverse placement of the prosthesis. The patients were kept in the hospital for 6 to 7 days after the operation, and were allowed to return to work 6 to 12 weeks after surgery. The authors reported excellent results in eight (80%) patients; two patients (20%) had unsatisfactory results in the form of complications. One had implant migration requiring reoperation, and the other patient experienced a transient S2-5 sensory disturbance. The authors also reported loss of disc height correction in four patients in whom the implants seemed to "sink" into the endplates. Two patients required reoperation, one for implant migration and one for persistent low back pain requiring fusion. Three patients experienced implant migration.[30]

Conclusion

This book is a testament to the current interest in disc arthroplasty. The future of this field is very promising—the next wave of research will focus on defining the role of disc arthroplasty within the spectrum of surgical alternatives for the treatment of disc pathology, such as discectomy and fusion. Prospective randomized studies are currently under way comparing arthroplasty with arthrodesis and will prove pivotal in helping to define the role of disc arthroplasty. These studies will also force surgeons to reevaluate the way they currently diagnose, classify, and treat symptomatic disc pathology. Additionally, the most fascinating aspect of the future of disc replacement is that further research is likely to refine rather than expand indications for its use.

REFERENCES

1. Barr JS. Ruptured intervertebral disc and sciatic pain. J Bone Joint Surg 29:210-214, 1947.
2. Barr JS, Mixter WJ. Posterior protrusion of the lumbar intervertebral discs. J Bone Joint Surg 23:444-456, 1941.
3. Büttner-Janz K, Schellnack K, Zippel H. An alternative treatment strategy for lumbar disc damage using the SB Charité modular disc prosthesis. Z Orthop Ihre Grenzgeb 125:1-6, 1987.
4. Büttner-Janz K, Schellnack K, Zippel H, et al. Experience and results with the SB Charité lumbar intervertebral endoprosthesis. Zeitschrift fur Klinische Medizin 43:1785-1789, 1988.
5. Cleveland DA. The use of methylacrylic for spinal stabilization after disc operation. Marquette Med Rev 20:6, 1955.
6. David T. Long-term follow up. Lumbar disc prosthesis: An analysis of long-term complications of 272 SB Charité disc prostheses with minimum 10-year follow-up. Presented at the Annual Meeting of the North American Spine Society, Chicago, Oct 2004.
7. Edeland HG. Suggestions for a total elasto-dynamic intervertebral disc prosthesis. Biomat Med Dev Art Org 9:65-72, 1981.
8. Enker P, Steffee A, McMillin C, et al. Artificial disc replacement. A preliminary report with 3 year minimum follow-up. Spine 18:1061-1070, 1993.
9. Fassio B, Ginestie JF. Prosthese descale en silicone. Etude experimentale et premieres observations cliniques. Nouv Presse Med 7:207, 1978.
10. Fernström U. Arthroplasty with intercorporeal endoprosthesis in herniated disc and painful disc. Acta Chir Scand 70(Suppl):357, 1966.
11. Fernström U. Der Bandscheibenersatz mit Erhaltung der Beweglichkeit. Presented at the working session of the Association of Spiral Column Research, Bad Hamburg, Nov 5, 1971.
12. Fernström U. Diskprotes av metall vid lumbal diskruptur. Nord Med 71:160, 1964.
13. Fernström U. Intradiskal endoprotes av metall vid lumbala och cervicala diskrupturer. Nord Med 73:272, 1965.
14. Hamby WB, Glaser HT. Replacement of spinal intervertebral discs with locally polymerizing methyl methacrylate. J Neurosurg 16:311, 1959.
15. Harmon PB. Results from treatment of sciatica due to lumbar disc protrusion. Am J Surg 80:829-840, 1950.
16. Harmon PB. Personal communication, October 17, 1969, as cited by A. McKenzie.
17. Hou TS, Tu KY, Xu YK, et al. Lumbar intervertebral disc prosthesis. An experimental study. Chin Med J 104:381-386, 1991.

18. Korge A, Nydegger T, Polard JL, et al. A spiral implant as nuclear prosthesis in the lumbar spine. Eur Spine J 11(2):S149-S153, 2002.
19. Kostuik JP. Intervertebral disc replacement. Experimental study. Clin Orthop 337:27-41, 1997.
20. Lane JD, Moore ES. Transperitoneal approach to the intervertebral disc in the lumbar area. Ann Surg 127:537-551, 1948.
21. Lee CK, Langrana NA, Parsons JR, et al. Development of a prosthetic intervertebral disc. Spine 16(6):S253-S255, 1991.
22. Marnay T. Lumbar disc arthroplasty: 8-10 years' results using titanium plates with a polyethylene inlay component. Presented at the Annual Meeting of the American Academy of Orthopaedic Surgeons, San Francisco, 2001.
23. Marnay T. ProDisc. Retrospective Clinical Study: 7-11 year follow-up. New York: Spine Solutions, 2002.
24. McKenzie AH. Fernström intervertebral disc arthroplasty: A long-term evaluation. Orthop Internat 3:313-324, 1995.
25. McKenzie AH. Steel ball arthroplasty of lumbar intervertebral disc—a preliminary report. J Bone Joint Surg Br 54:766, 1972.
26. Mixter WJ, Barr JS. Rupture of the intervertebral disc with involvement of the spinal cord. N Engl J Med 211:210-214, 1934.
27. Ray CD, Schönmayr R, Kavanagh SA, et al. Prosthetic disc nucleus implants. Rivista di Neurorariologia 12:157-162, 1999.
28. Reitz H, Joubert MJ. Intractable headache and cervicobrachialgia treated by complete replacement of cervical intervertebral disc with a metal prosthesis. S Afr Med J 38:881-889, 1964.
29. Schneider PG, Oyen R. Surgical replacement of the intervertebral disc. First communication: Replacement of lumbar discs with silicon-rubber. Theoretical and experimental investigations. Z Orthop Ihre Grenzgeb 112:1078-1086, 1974.
30. Schönmayr R, Busch C, Lotz C, et al. Prosthetic disc nucleus implants: The Wiesbaden feasibility study. Two years follow-up in 10 patients. Rivista di Neuroradiologia 12(1): 163-170, 1999.
31. Schulmann CM. Metod kombinirowannogo chirurgitscheskogo letschenija kompressionnych form pojanitschnogo osteochondrosa alloprotesirowaniem porashennych meshposwonkowych discow. Z Vopr Neurokhir 2:17-23, 1977.

CHAPTER

3

Indications and Contraindications for Total Disc Replacement

Barton L. Sachs ▪ Junius Clawson

The possibility of progressing from offering spinal fusion to offering the use of motion-retaining implants to patients has generated great enthusiasm. However, as with any surgery, rigorous adherence to well-defined patient selection criteria remains the key to a successful outcome. Besides anatomic considerations, the patient's psychological status is also crucial. As with any surgical patient, a candidate for total disc replacement must have realistic expectations of the outcome. Although U.S. Food and Drug Administration (FDA)–approved trials for total disc replacements began in the United States in 2000, there is much to be learned from the European experience with total disc replacements, where the devices have prompted lawsuits since the 1980s. Although the European literature on artificial disc replacement in the lumbar spine is generally favorable, this enthusiasm must be tempered with careful training of surgeons in technique for the implantation of the devices as well as adherence to appropriate patient selection criteria. This chapter reviews general indications and contraindications for total disc replacements in the lumbar spine; specific indications may vary with the design of specific devices.

Before any operative intervention, the patient should have failed at least 6 months of nonoperative management, which should include medications, activity modification, active rehabilitation, and possibly epidural or facet injections. The patient must be informed of the potential risks of surgery and have realistic expectations concerning outcome. Patients should also be aware of the importance of their role in postoperative recovery. Surgery is sometimes viewed as the "big event" at the end of the treatment line; however, it is only one step in the treatment continuum. After surgery, patients need to be active in rehabilitation to recover from their period of reduced activity before and immediately after surgery.

Indications

The most common indication for total disc replacement is pain related to degenerative disc disease (DDD) at one or two lumbar intervertebral disc levels.

Diagnostic criteria for symptomatic DDD include back and/or leg radicular pain accompanied by correlative radiographic evidence of one of the following: instability (greater than 3 mm translation or more than 5 degrees of angulation), disc space height reduced by more than 2 mm, scarring or thickening of the anulus fibrosis, herniated nucleus pulposus, or vacuum phenomenon.

Typically, disc-related abnormalities can be identified from MRI. However, because of the high rate of false-positive findings on MRI,[4,5] this may not be reliable. In our clinic discography is generally used to confirm that the disc is indeed the pain generator. Also, patients who give what appear to be exaggerated pain responses may not be good candidates for surgery. In a few patients with equivocal clinical presentations and imaging findings, it is helpful to inject the disc with xylocaine to determine whether this relieves the patient's symptoms. If the patient has a mixed diagnostic picture and the xylocaine discogram does not relieve the patient's pain that was provoked by discography, the patient may not be a good surgical candidate. In published indications related to preoperative radiographic findings for total disc replacement, Bertagnoli and Kumar[1] described a "prime" candidate for disc replacement as one with single-level pathology, at least 4 mm of remaining disc height, no changes of the facet joints, no adjacent-level degeneration, and intact posterior elements.

Contraindications

Approach Considerations

The currently available total disc replacements are all implanted from an anterior approach to the lumbar spine so the patient must be screened concerning the number and types of previous abdominal surgeries. Depending on the type of previous surgery and the approach used, the patient may be excluded from receiving an artificial disc. Previous abdominal surgery makes it more difficult to access the spine. One must be particularly mindful of the scarring created from previous surgery and the increased risk of significant vascular injury given the possibility of scar adhesions on the great vessels.

Health Issues

Patients should not have any medical condition that could place them at unreasonable risk for complications related to surgery. As this procedure is elective, there is never an indication for total disc replacement (TDR) in pregnancy.

As it is in all joint replacement surgery, the presence of an active infection, systemic or local, is a clear contraindication. Any known allergy to the type of metal used in the implant disqualifies the patient from receiving a prosthesis. Also, if the implant has a polyethylene component, patients should be asked about allergies to this material.

Rheumatoid Arthritis or Other Autoimmune Diseases

The patient should be skeletally mature. An age range of 18 to 60 years has been specified in some of the investigational device exemption (IDE) studies for total disc replacements. Although there is no definitive method to determine exactly at what age a person should be ruled out as a candidate for disc replacement surgery, there are several factors to consider. Currently, total disc replacements are implanted using the same approach as for anterior lumbar interbody fusion. In older patients, there may be a greater risk of vessel injury because of calcification of these structures, as well as the fact that the retroperitoneal vascular structures in older patients tend to be more fragile and less mobile, which may increase the risk of significant vascular injury when the vessels are retracted to access the disc space. As will be discussed later in this chapter, osteoporosis and facet joint arthrosis are contraindications for total disc replacement; both of these conditions are more frequently encountered in older patients.

Osteoporosis

Osteoporosis is a contraindication for total disc replacement. Lack of structural integrity of the vertebral bodies can be a source for several possible complications. Osteoporotic bone may be more likely to fracture during the placement of the device. Fracture may also occur after surgery, particularly if the device is not ideally positioned. The thinner, osteoporotic bone may also set the stage for the device to subside into the vertebral endplates, which may lead to a poor result or the need for future surgical intervention. In addition, there may be an increased risk of vertebral body fracture in the context of a device that has subsided into already weakened bone. Another potential problem in patients with osteoporotic bone is that the process of bony ingrowth into the endplates of the device may be compromised, leading to increased risk of device displacement.

Metabolic bone diseases such as Paget's disease and osteomalacia are also exclusion criteria for total disc replacements. Like osteoporosis, these diseases may compromise the host bone and lead to subsidence of the implant. Bony ingrowth to anchor the device may be compromised as well. Particular care should also be taken with patients who are or have been on long-term treatment regimens involving steroids or other medications that are known to inhibit bone metabolism.

If a patient has risk factors for osteoporosis, a bone mineral density scan should be ordered. This screening step will help to reduce the number of patients who are likely to have complications related to poor bone quality. However, one must keep in mind that some patients who may not appear to be at risk for osteoporosis do in fact have osteoporosis or osteopenia.

Morbid Obesity

Morbid obesity is also a contraindication for total disc replacement in the FDA IDE studies. It is thought that excessive load on the bone-implant interface may lead to subsidence and subsequent failure. It may also be possible that the excessive load may contribute to displacement of the device, particularly at the L5-S1 level, where the disc space is generally highly angulated. As with any anterior spine procedure, accessing the spine in an obese patient is more difficult than in a thin patient. Although there is concern about using implants in obese patients, there are no data at present to determine whether obesity is related to a compromised clinical outcome.

Psychological Screening

As with any spine surgery, it is imperative to consider the psychosocial condition of the patient to optimize outcomes. Chronic pain is related to increased incidence of depression and other psychological problems. Psychological problems have been found to be highly related to surgical treatment outcome.[2,3,6,7] A study by Spengler et al found that psychological screening was more significantly related to clinical outcome than was MRI findings.[6]

Although some surgeons are aware of the important role of a patient's psychological makeup on treatment outcomes, they may not use a psychologist to perform a formal screening. However, it has been reported that physician's intuition about a patient has poor correlation to the results of formal psychological testing. At our clinic patients are screened for surgery using the psychosocial surgical screening instrument described by Block et al.[2,3] This instrument incorporates the Minnesota Multiphasic Personality Inventory (MMPI), medical history, personal history, and other items to generate a composite score from which the psychologist formulates a recommendation for the surgeon.

Number of Fusion Levels

With spinal fusion, the clinical outcome diminishes with the number of levels fused. Artificial discs are typically implanted at one or two lumbar spine segments; their use at three or more levels requires further investigation.

Nerve Root Compression

Pain related to a herniated disc is a contraindication for total disc replacement. Implanting a disc prosthesis does not solve the problem of a disc fragment compressing a nerve root. It is, however, viable for the treatment of a bulging disc, in which case the disc material is removed and the device generally increases the height of the disc space. In the FDA IDE studies, nerve root compression or a positive straight leg raise are exclusion criteria.

Previous Spine Surgery

One must carefully evaluate the patient who has had previous spine surgery. As with any failed back surgery patients, those being considered for total disc replacement generally require a more comprehensive evaluation than patients who have had no previous surgery. If the segment to be operated on has been accessed through a posterior surgery, one must carefully evaluate the condition of the posterior elements to determine whether there is enough structural stability. If the posterior elements are compromised, disc replacement is contraindicated. If the segment to be operated on is adjacent to a previously fused segment, one must carefully assess the condition of the posterior elements to confirm the absence of stenosis.

Spondylolisthesis

For total disc replacement to be successful, the posterior elements must be competent to maintain proper biomechanics and avoid excessive translation. It follows that degenerative spondylolisthesis of more than 3 mm or isthmic spondylolisthesis are contraindications for disc replacement. Also, device placement is likely to be difficult if the vertebral bodies are greatly out of alignment; this may also place undue and uneven loading on the implant, potentially leading to failure of the device or possible displacement.

Facet Joint Arthrosis

One must carefully evaluate the condition of the facet joints on the radiographic images because the facets are of particular concern for disc replacements. If a fusion is being undertaken, the goal is to eliminate motion of the segment, and thus the demands on the facets are significantly reduced. However, depending on the size and placement of the disc prosthesis, the load on the facets may not be reduced but may be increased. Also, the motion allowed by the prosthesis may further exacerbate any existing facet pathology.

Each level of the spine consists of a three-joint complex; the TDR replaces the anterior joint complex and may result in additional stress on the facet joints. If the facets are compromised, they may become a source of pain. This is particularly true if the load on these joints is increased because of TDR, as typically will occur if the prosthesis is placed anteriorly or is undersized. Thus it is recommended that any intervention be made before any degenerative changes of facet joints occur. Careful preoperative planning and precise intraoperative technique can minimize the likelihood of late facet syndrome.

TDR is designed to allow motion that may reproduce more normal spine mechanics. Because the TDR may be either semiconstrained or unconstrained, it is imperative that the posterior elements remain intact. Although load sharing by the facet joints (approximately 20%) is a theoretical advantage, their primary contribution to a successful TDR is restraint to translation.

Stenosis

Spinal stenosis is a contraindication for disc replacement in IDE studies. Replacement of a disc may not address narrowing of the spinal canal. Also, stenosis is usually related to degenerative changes of the facet joints, which is a contraindication for disc replacement.

Decreased Disc Space Height

With any TDR the metallic components have to have a certain distraction height for implantation. Additional height is required for those incorporating a polyethylene core. In some studies a disc space height of less than 4 mm has been used as an exclusion criterion. Severely narrowed disc space height may also be associated with increased changes of the facet joints, which are undesirable for total disc replacement.

Scoliosis

TDR is not indicated in patients with severe scoliosis. Minimal degenerative scoliosis, in one study defined as no more than 11 degrees, is acceptable. Greater degrees of scoliosis are considered contraindications for TDR for many of the same reasons that patients with spondylolisthesis are ruled out. Altered positioning of the spine may significantly alter the loading on the implant, possibly leading to its failure. Also, the risk of displacement may be greater if altered loading is present. The possible role of a disc implant in patients with previous scoliosis surgery and who now have a symptomatic degenerated disc at the level below the previous surgery has yet to be investigated.

Tumor, Infections, and Fracture

Tumors, infections, and vertebral body fracture are all considered contraindications for TDR because these conditions result in compromised vertebral bone quality. As with osteoporosis, this may result in device subsidence or fracture of the vertebral body.

Conclusion

This chapter has reviewed general indications and contraindications for total disc replacements in the lumbar spine; specific indications may vary with the design of specific devices. Before any surgical intervention, the patient should have failed at least 6 months of nonoperative management, which should include medications, activity modification, active rehabilitation, and local therapeutic spinal injections. The patient must be informed of potential risks of surgery and have realistic expectations of its outcome. Patients should also be aware of the importance of their role in postoperative recovery. Surgery is sometimes viewed as the "big event" at the end of the treatment line; however, it is only one step along the treatment continuum, and after surgery, patients must participate in an active rehabilitation program.

REFERENCES

1. Bertagnoli R, Kumar S. Indications for full prosthetic disc arthroplasty: A correlation of clinical outcome against a variety of indications. Euro Spine J 11:S131-S136, 2002.
2. Block AR, Gatchel RJ, Deardorff WW, et al. The psychology of spine surgery. In Block AR, ed. American Psychological Association, Washington, DC, 2003.
3. Block AR, Ohnmeiss DD, Guyer RD, et al. The use of presurgical psychological screening to predict the outcome of spine surgery. Spine J 1:274-282, 2001.
4. Boden SD, Davis DO, Dina TS, et al. Abnormal magnetic-resonance scans of the lumbar spine in asymptomatic subjects: A prospective investigation. J Bone Joint Surg Am 72:403-408, 1990.
5. Boos N, Rieder R, Schade V, et al. The diagnostic accuracy of magnetic resonance imaging, work perception, and psychological factors in identifying symptomatic disc herniations. Spine 20:2613-2625, 1995.
6. Spengler DM, Ouelette EA, Battie M, et al. Elective discectomy for herniation of a lumbar disc. J Bone Joint Surg Am 72:230-237, 1990.
7. Wiltse LL, Rocchio PH. Preoperative psychological tests as predictors of success of chemonucleolysis and treatment of low back syndrome. J Bone Joint Surg Am 57:478-483, 1975.

CHAPTER

4

Psychological Evaluation of Spinal Arthroplasty Patients

Andrew R. Block

A patient with intractable spine pain experiences many contradictory thoughts and emotions, often has had many months or years of uncertainty about what is causing the pain, and has been down many blind treatment alleys. The hope for a definitive diagnosis brings with it the promise of some sort of closure and a sense of vindication towards those who have told the patient that nothing is wrong. However, identifying a physiologic basis for the pain may lead to a recommendation for spine surgery, a procedure to be feared as much as desired. After all, it takes only a few mouse clicks on the Internet or a short stay in the waiting room of a busy orthopedic practice to hear surgical horror stories about patients with severe pain after surgery, patients dependent on strong doses of opioids, and patients in whom a "small" procedure, such as a microdiscectomy, has been followed by a much more invasive procedure such as a circumferential fusion. Thus, the patient's desperate desire for pain relief is contrasted with the personal stories of patients who have failed back surgery, as well as by research demonstrating that spine surgery's effectiveness is only around 70% to 80%.[27,56]

Of all the procedures in the surgeon's armamentarium, none is more capable of producing ambivalence than spinal fusion. Whether or not these fears are realistic, spinal fusion is often seen as a serious restriction of future mobility with the possibility of additional stress on discs adjacent to the surgical site. The possibility of future surgery is also a concern. Thus the prospect of spinal arthroplasty is appealing to the patient, offering the possibility of pain relief, correction of disease, and more rapid recovery without donor site pain and stiffness. Yet if many decades of experience with spine surgery have taught us anything, it is that there will always be surgical failures, patients who do not achieve pain relief or recovery of function despite excellent and complete surgical correction; patients need to be advised of this possibility.

Increasingly, there is a recognition that psychosocial factors may influence the outcome of spine surgery. Beginning with the pioneering work of Leon Wiltse,[59] factors such as pain sensitivity, depression, and substance abuse have been linked to poor surgical results. Indeed, even when perfect surgical correction is achieved, psychological factors can predispose patients towards continued pain, consumption of large doses of medication, and inability to work or enjoy recreational activity. Given that spinal arthroplasty draws from the same general population of patients as those seeking all types of spine surgery, it is likely that when spinal arthroplasty is unsuccessful in providing pain relief or recovery of functional ability, psychosocial factors will be at least partly to blame. In this chapter we discuss these emotional, behavioral, and social influences on the clinical outcome of spine surgery. Techniques for uncovering such factors are examined, and recommendations are made concerning surgical prognosis for patients with differing levels of psychosocial "risk."

Psychological Factors Associated With Poor Surgical Outcome

Even though spine surgery is conducted only on the basis of objectively identifiable disease or damage, the pain and distress arising from spinal pathology cannot be directly measured and are necessarily subjective. Patients hope that the surgery will reduce their pain, thereby improving their abilities and lifestyle; this creates a dilemma because psychosocial factors can undo the curative effects of spine surgery.

We have developed a procedure termed *presurgical psychological screening* (PPS) to objectively identify such psychosocial risk factors. PPS is a combination of a diagnostic interview and psychometric testing, which allows the psychologist to render a scientifically based determination of the patient's psychosocial prognosis, that is, the probability that the surgery will lead to positive clinical outcomes, such as reduction in pain and decreased use of narcotic medications as

Prognosis	Surgical Recommendation
Poor	• Avoid surgery if pain relief is the major goal; recommend discharge. • Avoid surgery if pain relief is the major goal; institute conservative care only.
Fair	• Hold on surgery, pending the outcome of psychological treatment of compliance measures.
Good	• Clear for surgery; postoperative psychological treatment recommended. • Clear for surgery; no psychological treatment necessary.

Fig. 4-1 Recommendations for Surgery and Conservative Care Resulting From Presurgical Psychological Screening

well as improvement in functional ability. The psychosocial factors that have been demonstrated to impact surgical outcome include (1) personality conditions and emotional states, (2) cognitive issues, and (3) environmental and historical factors. The determination of surgical prognosis is made by identifying, weighing, and combining the risk factors identified according to rules defined by previous research.[8] Using this system the PPS process culminates in a determination of whether the patient has a good, fair, or poor psychosocial prognosis (Fig. 4-1).

Personality and Emotional Factors

Personality characteristics are relatively stable aspects of an individual, and are defined as "deeply ingrained patterns of behaviors, which include the way one relates to, perceives, and thinks about the environment and oneself."[1] Emotions are relatively more volatile psychological states that combine with personality traits to influence each individual's behavior. It is this combination of personality trait and emotional state that is the key to understanding how spine surgery may be less than effective.

Each individual's behavior shows patterns that can occur in a wide range of situations. Individuals with type A behavior pattern, for example, show time urgency, competitiveness, cynicism, and hostility. Such behaviors are often seen across a number of situations, and have been shown to be associated with increased risk of coronary artery disease.[50] Other individuals may be passive and dependent, or histrionic, drawing attention to themselves on many occasions. Patients with back pain each have their own characteristic personality pattern, some of which may influence the ways that they perceive pain and how they deal with it. On top of longer-term personality traits are intense emotions such as depression, anger, and anxiety that often occur in response to an injury. In some cases, emotions may precede or even be a significant cause of an injury. For example, patients experiencing anger are likely to get into altercations in the course of which they may sustain a spine injury. These traits and emotions together can strongly influence the course of spine pain and of recovery from spine surgery.

Objective identification of long-standing personality traits, and more acute and changeable emotional reactions can be obtained through the use of psychometric testing. The results of such tests provide the strongest and most reliable evidence of the influence of psychosocial factors on the outcome of spine surgery. Further, psychometric testing is essential in documenting the psychosocial risks that predict poorer surgical outcome; without such tests the examiner has to base decisions about surgical prognosis primarily on a combination of clinical judgment and patient responses to the much less standardized interview. The Minnesota Multiphasic Personality Inventory (MMPI) is the most widely used tool to assess personality traits in studies of spinal surgery outcome, although other, more simple, instruments are also being used.

Pain Sensitivity

The strongest psychosocial risk factor involves a patient's tendency to experience pain in excess of that normally expected for a given level of physical pathology. Such "excessive pain sensitivity" is assessed on the MMPI by the Hysteria (Hy) and Hypochondriasis (Hs) scales. Elevations on these scales are the most common among patients with various chronic pain syndromes, although not necessarily in spine surgery candidates.[7,43] A study in our center demonstrates the manner in which pain sensitivity can influence a patient's perception of underlying tissue damage, and may confound medical evaluation.[9] In this study, the relation of MMPI score to discography results was examined in spine surgery candidates. All patients assessed had three-level discography. Patients with elevations of greater than 2.5 standard deviations (T score >75) on scales Hs and Hy were significantly more likely to report "discordant" pain (i.e., pain upon injection of normal, nondisrupted disc) than were patients whose scores on these scales were in the normal range. Significantly, many of the patients who reported discordant pain at one disc level had concordant pain reproduction at a different level (i.e., they experienced pain upon injection of disrupted disc). These results imply that it is difficult to determine whether a disrupted disc is the "pain generator" in patients with high levels of pain sensitivity, even if a concordant pain result is obtained at one level.

MMPI Hy and Hs scale elevations have been shown to be associated with poor spine surgery outcome in at least seven studies.[8,11,26,37] In some studies, the predictive value of these two MMPI scales may exceed the predictive value of medical test results. For example, Spengler et al, examining patients who underwent laminectomy/discectomy, found that MMPI-2 elevations on scales Hs and Hy contributed 26% to a multiple regression equation predicting clinical outcome in terms of pain reduction and improvement in functional activity, whereas imaging studies contributed only 10% and neurologic signs contributed only 3%.[52]

Depression

Depression is an emotion experienced by up to 85% of chronic pain patients,[34] and it can strongly affect the outcome of spine surgery. Individuals with depression tend to focus on negative events.[48] When receiving treatment for chronic pain, they are unlikely to recognize gains in functional abilities even though direct observation of their behavior demonstrates an increase in these capabilities.[33] Elevations on the Depression (D) scale of the MMPI are frequently associated with poor surgical outcome.[16,26,51] Studies that have used other psychometric tests such as the Beck Depression Inventory[32] and a modified version of the Zung depression scale[54] also confirm that depression is associated with poor results.

In the assessment of depression it is critical to determine whether this emotional condition is a reactive emotional response to the pain, or a relatively more stable personality trait. Depressive symptoms include: sleep disturbance, decreased appetite, withdrawal from and decreased pleasure in previously enjoyed activities, decreased concentration and memory, poor libido, foreshortened sense of the future, and, in severe cases, suicidal ideation. Some of these may be a direct result of the experience of continued pain and physical limitations; some, such as energy loss and cognitive difficulties, may result from medication taken to control pain. On the other hand, depression is frequently experienced before the onset of pain for many spine surgery candidates. Atkinson et al,[2] for example, in a systematic study of depressed male veterans with chronic pain found that 42% of patients experienced the onset of depression before the onset of the pain. Polatin et al[42] reported that 39% of the patients with chronic low back pain they evaluated had symptoms of depression that existed before the injury. Depression has been shown in a number of studies to be a risk factor for the development of back pain.[36] Such chronic depression is a strong risk factor for reduced surgical outcome when it has existed before the injury occurred, that is, when it is a personality trait. When depression exists as an emotional reaction to the injury, it is less of a risk factor, especially if the patient is treated with antidepressant medication.[4]

Anger

Anger can negatively impact pain and the outcome of spine surgery, in the same way that it impacts many other physical conditions.[58] Feelings of anger are common in patients who have back pain. Fernandez et al[17] reported a study in which chronic pain patients rated the frequency with which they had felt six different emotions in the preceding 30 days; these emotions were fear, guilt, shame, sadness, envy, and anger. Although all these emotions were felt commonly, anger was the most frequently experienced, at an average of 70% of the time.

The MMPI scale most closely associated with anger is the Psychopathic Deviant (Pd), with high scorers on this scale also tending to be aggressive, as well as rebellious toward authority figures.[21] Pd elevations have been found to be predictive of poor surgical outcome in several studies.[16,26,37] Trief et al[54] examined the relationship of spine surgery results to scores on the Cook-Medley Hostility subscale of the MMPI-2. In this study, patients who had high presurgical hostility scores reported less improvement in daily activities and were significantly less likely to be working 1 year after surgery than were patients who had scored low on this scale.

Anger can be destructive to the spine surgery patient because it can negatively impact the postoperative healing process by reducing immunosuppression.[31] Further, anger can lead to negative health-related behaviors, such as smoking, overeating, or alcohol consumption.[17] Such behaviors can work against postoperative rehabilitation, a process that requires dedication to improvement in general health and physical conditioning, as well as emotional stamina.

Anger may also negatively influence spine surgery results because it can alter the patient's goals. DeGood and Kiernan[14] found that chronic pain patients who were angry and blamed their employer for their injury reported higher levels of emotional distress and had poorer responses to treatment. For such patients, changes in pain status following surgery may have been more closely related to a need for vindication or revenge than to actual changes in the physical pathology.

Anxiety and Stress

Most patients being considered for spine surgery experience some levels of anxiety, stress, and fear. Such anxiety may result from loss of income, reduction in the quality of marital interaction, and uncertainty about future ability to work. Further, the anticipation of the surgery itself, anesthesia, postoperative pain, and an uncertain recovery can all make patients anxious. Unfortunately, several studies demonstrate that anxiety and stress can negatively influence spine surgery results.

On the MMPI, the scale that most closely assesses anxiety is the Psychasthenia scale (Pt), a scale that also measures the tendency toward excessive doubts, fears, obsessions, and compulsions. Poor response to spine surgery is associated with Pt elevations.[15,16,51] Additional studies have used different scales to assess the impact of stress and anxiety. Trief et al[54] found that elevated state anxiety scores on the State-Trait Anxiety Inventory (STAI)[53] were associated with reduced return to work, and less change in reported pain after spine surgery. Kjelby-Wendt et al[32] examined discectomy patients, dividing subjects into "discontented" and "contented" groups, based in large part on presurgical scores on the STAI. At follow-up, these researchers found that contented patients achieved better outcomes than did discontented patients, including greater lumbar range of motion, and less than one half the duration of postoperative sick leave. Schade et al,[46] again examining patients who underwent discectomy, found that "occupational mental stress" was significantly negatively correlated with return to work and had near significant negative correlations with improvement in activities of daily living, as well as reduction in pain. Thus anxiety is shown to reduce surgical effectiveness, regardless of whether it arises from the injury, from environmental conditions, or is a more stable personality trait.

Poor Pain Coping

Because pain is a totally subjective phenomenon, the patient's "coping strategies" (i.e., thoughts about the pain and its causes, and behavioral strategies for dealing with the pain) can significantly influence its overall impact.[10] Such pain-coping strategies affect both the patient's pain level as well as his or her ability to adjust to and overcome the pain.[55] A number of questionnaires have been developed to assess these coping thoughts and behaviors; the most widely used in the context of spine surgery is the Coping Strategies Questionnaire (CSQ).[45]

The CSQ consists of six cognitive and two behavioral coping scales. Cognitive strategies include diverting attention, ignoring pain sensations, praying or hoping, reinterpreting pain sensations, coping self-statements, and catastrophizing (i.e., making exaggerated negative self-statements). The two behavioral scales include increasing activity level and increasing pain behavior. In addition, the CSQ contains a measure of the patient's perception of his or her ability to control pain and reduce it. Some studies have combined scales using factorial analysis techniques.

Block et al[8] administered the CSQ preoperatively to 204 patients who underwent spine surgery (either laminectomy/discectomy or spinal fusion). A hierarchical regression analysis found that the CSQ Poor Self-Reliance (a combination of catastrophizing and lack of ability to increase activity level) was a significant contributor to the regression equation predicting overall surgical outcome. Gross[23] examined clinical outcome in 50 laminectomy patients who were given the CSQ before surgery. Patients who scored high on a factor termed *Loss of Control* (combining high scores on the catastrophizing scale and low scores on the pain control scale) had poorer surgical outcome than those who scored low on this scale and had greater postoperative pain. High scores on the Self-Reliance factor (combining high scores on the pain control scale and low scores on the praying/hoping scale) were positively associated with reported surgical outcome and negatively associated with postoperative pain and sleep disturbance. These two studies demonstrate that poor pain coping, especially "catastrophizing," can significantly reduce surgical effectiveness.

Pathological Distress

Thus far we have discussed personality and emotional issues as if each is experienced in isolation, that a patient who is depressed is not also angry. However, for most patients the sense of distress is multidimensional. When such distress is both broad-ranging and intense patients are particularly vulnerable to having poor clinical outcomes from spine surgery. For example, Riley et al[43] applied cluster analysis techniques to the MMPI profiles of 201 spine surgery candidates, obtaining a four-cluster solution. Surgical outcome 6 months postoperatively was analyzed by MMPI cluster type and the largest group, having all MMPI scales "within normal limits," obtained significant improvement. Similar but somewhat diminished results were obtained by the second group, which had elevations on scales Hs, D, and Hy (termed the *triad* group). A third cluster, which had elevations on scales Hs and Hy only (the *V* group), achieved poorer results than did the normal and triad groups. Finally, by far the worst results were seen in a group of patients having multiple elevations (the *depressed-pathological* group).

Research in our center has also applied cluster analytic techniques to the MMPI-2 profiles of spine surgery candidates, obtaining a three-cluster solution.[7] The clusters were a within-normal-limits group, a triad-type profile, and a depressed-pathological profile. We also examined outcome by MMPI profile type. Twenty-two patients (10% of the total population) were classified in the depressed-pathological group. This group obtained the least improvements in functional ability and pain reduction, with some patients experiencing a reported worsening of their condition. In fact, 82% of the depressed-pathological group reported poor outcome. The within-normal-limits group, comprising 115 patients, achieved the best surgery results. The remaining patients (N = 86), who had a triad-type profile showed similar improvement in functional ability but achieved less pain improvement when compared to the within-normal-limits group.

Behaviorial and Environmental Factors

Often the factors negatively impacting response to spine surgery lie not within the patient but in the patient's environment and include relationships, work, and legal factors. In order to probe for such factors, the evaluator must thoroughly question the patient during the interview portion of the PPS about the employment situation, the legal system, reactions of significant others, and even actions taken by health care providers; such responses may unwittingly reinforce the patient's pain and disability. In fact, such probing may reveal factors that may be acting against the patient's recovery. One of the major tenets of behavioral psychology is that behaviors increase in frequency when they are followed by rewarding consequences, and that they decrease in frequency when they are punished.[49] In some ways, pain behaviors can be considered like any other behaviors in that they occur increasingly when rewarded and decrease in frequency when either ignored or punished.[19] When individuals or factors in the patient's psychosocial environment reward pain or provide negative consequences for improvement, spine surgery is less likely to be effective. In the research on chronic pain, three primary sources of such reinforcement contingencies have been examined: spousal response to pain behavior, worker's compensation (including disability payments), and litigation.

Families and spouses may unconsciously provide rewards for pain behaviors. They may encourage rest, take over the patient's jobs or responsibilities, and provide more attention to the patient when they anticipate that the patient will experience pain; at the same time, they may ignore the patient when he or she appears to be in less pain or is engaging in alternative "well behaviors." Such a "solicitous" pattern of spousal response has been shown to increase the likelihood that patients will report high pain levels,[7] display a high level of pain behaviors,[30] and will show diminished physical exercise capabilities.[38]

Patients who were injured on the job tend to have a poorer response to spine surgery as compared to those who were injured in other locations.[13,22,25] Patients with job-related injuries not only obtain medical care under the worker's compensation system, they often receive temporary or even permanent disability payments if they are unable to work because of the injury. Such disability payments can be seen as a source of potential reward for pain behavior. However, purely economic considerations cannot fully explain the diminished response to spine surgery of patients with job-related injuries. Most patients qualifying for worker's compensation receive far less in disability payments than they received while working.[9] Further, patients with job injuries may experience job dissatisfaction,[3] heavy physical job demands,[13,28] or anger and/or blame towards the employer,[14] all of which are associated with high pain levels and poor treatment outcomes. Therefore, although reinforcement of pain behavior is one possible explanation for the poor results in patients with job-related injuries, many issues combine to make worker's compensation one of the strongest predictors of excessive disability among patients with back injury.[20]

Another possible factor that results in the reduced effectiveness of spine surgery is the financial gain that can come from the spine injury. Such gain can occur with litigation, or when patients are seeking permanent disability payments. Several studies have found that patients who have a history of previous medically related lawsuits and other litigation connected with spine injury tend to have poor outcome from spine surgery.[18,39] Additionally, Junge et al[28] found that patients who were applying for disability pension had poorer surgical outcomes than those who were not. This is not to say that patients with pending litigation or disability applications are malingering, since by definition a physical pathology underlies their pain complaints; instead it is likely that financial incentives may make certain patients more sensitive to pain.[12]

Historical Factors

In addition to investigating reinforcing factors in a patient's current situation, an examination of the patient's history and background can reveal much data that can improve the selection process for spine surgery candidates. One particularly important historical factor appears to be the existence of mental health problems that predate the development of spinal pain. It is clear that psychological problems can predispose patients to the development of chronic pain. In a classic study of Boeing employees, Bigos et al[3] found that employees with high scores on the MMPI Hs and Hy scales were at significant risk of developing occupational back pain complaints over a 4-year period, compared to those without such elevations. Furthermore, studies have shown that patients with preexisting psychological problems have reduced spine surgery outcome. In our study a history of prior psychological treatment contributed significantly to a regression equation of reduced surgical outcome[5] (see also the findings of Keel[29] and Manniche et al[39]). Such results imply that the more chronic the mental health problems are, the more they can be expected to have a substantial negative effect on surgical outcome.

Of the many horrific events that can happen in one's life, none has more devastating or long-lasting effects than abuse. Unfortunately, in the population of chronic pain patients, abuse is quite common. For example, evaluating patients for entrance into a multidisciplinary pain program, Haber and Roos[24] found that over half the patients they evaluated had been victims of physical or sexual abuse; in over 90% of subjects the abuse occurred in adulthood. In a general population study, Linton found that physical and sexual abuse greatly increased the likelihood that individuals would develop chronic pain.[35] Abuse may also predispose patients to have worse results after surgery. Schofferman et al[47] found that spine surgery candidates who reported at least three types of childhood abuse (i.e., either sexual, physical, emotional, parental substance abuse, or abandonment) had an 85% clinical failure rate after spine surgery, compared to a 5% failure rate among patients who reported no such trauma.

Even marital distress can influence the effectiveness of spine surgery. A number of studies have demonstrated that marital dissatisfaction and problems within a marriage are common in chronic pain patients.[44] Dissatisfied spouses have expectations for outcome that are more negative,[16] and tend to attribute the patient's pain to psychological rather than physical problems.[40] Schade et al[46] found that social support by the spouse was significantly associated with greater pain relief in patients undergoing lumbar discectomy. Thus the quality of the marital relationship should be given consideration, as it may negatively influence treatment outcome.

Finally, patients experiencing chronic pain typically are prescribed narcotic medication to help relieve the pain. However, some spine surgery candidates may become dependent on and addicted to this medication. Two of the studies that looked at the potential role of substance abuse or dependence on spine surgery outcomes found that abuse of medications and alcohol was associated with a high failure rate among patients undergoing spine surgery.[52,57] One must keep in mind, however, that drug addiction and abuse are not defined merely as the taking of large doses of narcotics; Merskey and Moulin[41] stated that drug addiction is "compulsive drug use despite harm, an overwhelming preoccupation with securing a good supply, and the tendency to relapse after withdrawal. Addiction is a behavioral pattern of drug use, in which medication is taken for its psychic effects rather than for its pain-relieving effects." Such a pattern has very strong implications for response to spine surgery, particularly if the PPS reveals a history of drug or alcohol abuse or dependence.

Determination of Surgical Prognosis

The studies reviewed in this chapter indicate that there are many psychological risk factors for poor surgical outcome. Several studies examined the effectiveness of combining such risk factors into a "scorecard" to sharpen predictive

Table 4-1 Psychosocial Risk Factors

Factor	Score	Data Source
Job dissatisfaction	2	Interview
Workers compensation	2	Interview
Litigation	2	Interview
Spousal solicitousness	1	Interview
No spousal support	1	Interview
Abuse and abandonment	1	Interview
Substance abuse	2	Interview
Psychiatric history	2	Interview
Pain sensitivity	2	Testing
Depression		
(Chronic)	2	Testing
(Reactive)	1	
Anger	2	Testing
Anxiety	2	Testing
Depressed-pathological profile	4	Testing

Scoring: 1 = medium risk, 2 = high risk, 4 = very high risk.

Table 4-2 Model for Determining Surgical Prognosis

		Psychological Risk Factors: LOW	Psychological Risk Factors: HIGH
Medical Risk Factors	LOW	Good outcome	Fair outcome
	HIGH	Fair outcome	Poor outcome

acumen.[18,39,52] In our center we created a scorecard to investigate the relationship of psychosocial factors to clinical outcome (pain, functional ability, and medication use), in 204 patients who underwent laminectomy/discectomy or spinal fusion.[5] In our scorecard psychological risk factors identified by a semistructured interview and by psychometric testing are each assigned a weight and are summed to obtain a total psychological risk score. Medical risk factors are also identified, weighted, and scored (Table 4-1).

We then used a 2 × 2 risk factor matrix to determine clinical outcome prognosis (Table 4-2). A high-risk threshold was defined for both the psychosocial risk factors and the medical risk factors. Outcome prognosis was a function of the quadrant into which the patient's combined scores fell. Patients whose scores fell above the high-risk threshold on both medical and psychological factors were determined to have a poor outcome prognosis; good outcome was projected for those whose scores fell below both risk thresholds. A fair prognosis was expected when the score fell above one risk threshold and below the other threshold. Results showed that the outcome was correctly projected for 82.8% of patients on whom this system was used. It was significant that 83% of patients with a poor outcome prognosis obtained such poor results. Examination of individual psychosocial risk factors revealed that the most significant outcome predictors were MMPI elevations on the scales indicating pain sensitivity (Scale Hy), depression (scale D), anger (scale Pd), and anxiety (scales Pt and Sc). Other important predictors were poor pain coping on the Coping Strategies Questionnaire,[45] spousal reinforcement of pain behavior, worker's compensation, preinjury psychological treatment history, and heavy job requirements (see Fig. 4-1 for a brief overview of the relationship between identified levels of psychosocial risk and recommendations for the surgery arising from PPS).

Clinical Implications

Presurgical psychological screening is demonstrated to accurately predict the outcome of spine surgery. Patients with a high level of psychosocial risk are likely to fare very poorly, even when the physical pathology responsible for the pain is effectively removed—a finding that has been obtained with many different types of surgeries including laminectomy/discectomy, spinal fusion, and chemonucleolysis. Thus, there is every reason to expect that the clinical results obtained from artificial disc implants would be similarly affected. Exhibit D is included in this chapter to help health care providers identify patients who may be experiencing emotional and psychosocial difficulties that could influence the results of medical treatments. Referral to a psychologist experienced in PPS should be considered when such problems are identified (Box 4-1).

This chapter has emphasized the prognostic use of PPS. However, PPS also helps surgeons and other health care providers to develop treatment plans in-

Box 4-1 Referral Criteria for Psychological Screening

- Excessive pain behavior
- Symptoms inconsistent with identified pathology
- High levels of depression or anxiety
- Sleep disturbance-insomnia or hypersomnia
- Excessively high or low expectations about treatment outcome
- Marital distress or sexual difficulties
- Negative attitude toward work or employer
- Emotional lability or mood swings
- Inability to work or greatly decreased functional ability (<3 mo)
- Escalating or large doses of narcotics or anxiolytics
- Litigation or continuing disability benefits resulting from spine injury

Referral Considerations

0-1 items	Not necessary to refer unless desired by patient
2-3 items	Consider referral
4+ items	Strongly consider referral

dividualized to a given patient. Such treatments may improve outcome even in candidates who have a good prognosis, they may test and improve motivation in marginal candidates, and they may point to noninvasive alternative therapies for patients who have a poor prognosis. The individualization of treatment is especially significant in patients with a moderate level of psychosocial risk (i.e., those whose surgical PPS prognosis is deemed to be "fair"). Treatments for these patients may be focused on augmenting the compliance with medical treatment recommendations in order to improve surgical outcome. Such treatments might include lowering narcotic medication use to a predetermined level, smoking cessation before surgery, or required weight loss. For such patients, noncompliance with or minimal effort expended in completion of such assigned tasks may be taken as a sign that surgical outcome is likely to be poor, and that surgery should be avoided.

Presurgical psychological screening may also allow for individualization of treatments for patients in the good prognosis category. Many of these patients have a tendency to expect very rapid recovery, and may increase activity during the postoperative period so quickly that they put the implant at risk. When PPS reveals such a tendency, patients may be appropriately counseled about recovery and healing periods. Further, PPS may reveal whether postsurgical treatments for pain control (e.g., biofeedback or hypnosis) may augment results.

Presurgical psychological screening may not only help to avoid a surgery that is highly likely to be clinically ineffective, but it may also suggest alternative, noninvasive treatments. Such patients may benefit by an intensive and coordinated treatment intervention, such as that provided by a multidisciplinary pain treatment center even when the underlying pathology remains uncorrected. Community pain management and support resources can be identified for the patient.

Conclusion

Disc replacement surgery offers new hope for relief from chronic back pain. Unfortunately, many decades of research and clinical experience demonstrate that even when spine surgery successfully corrects underlying pathology, many patients do not achieve pain reduction or recovery of function. Identifying patients who are most likely to have a poor surgical outcome can be a critical part of the evaluation of disc replacement candidates. The studies reviewed here demonstrate that about 80% to 85% of high psychosocial risk patients do not have good results from spine surgery. Thus, the inclusion of PPS within the diagnostic regimen of the spine surgery candidate, especially when the surgeon suspects the existence of several psychosocial risk factors, can significantly aid patient selection and prevent the worsening of problems for high-risk patients.

REFERENCES

1. American Psychiatric Association. Diagnostic and Statistical Manual of Mental Disorders, 4th ed. Washington DC: American Psychiatric Association, 1994.
2. Atkinson JH, Slater MA, Patterson TL, et al. Prevalence, onset and risk of psychiatric disorders in chronic pain patients: A controlled study. Pain 45:111-121, 1991.
3. Bigos SJ, Battie MC, Spengler DM, et al. A prospective study of work perceptions and psychosocial factors affecting the report of back injury. Spine 16:1-6, 1991.
4. Block AR, Gatchel R, Deardorff WW, et al. In Guyer RD. The Psychology of Spine Surgery. Washington, DC: American Psychological Association, 2003.
5. Block AR, Boyer SL, Silbert RV. Spouse's perception of the chronic pain patient: Estimates of exercise tolerance. In Fields HL, Dubner R, Cervero F, eds. Advances in Pain Research and Therapy, vol 9. New York: Raven Press, 1985.
6. Block AR, Kremer EF, Gaylor M. Behavioral treatment of chronic pain: The spouse as a discriminative cue for pain behavior. Pain 9:243-252, 1980.
7. Block AR, Ohnmeiss DD. MMPI profiles predict the outcome of spinal surgery. Presented at the Annual Meeting of the North American Spine Society, New Orleans, Oct 2000.
8. Block AR, Ohnmeiss DD, Guyer RD, et al. The use of presurgical psychological screening to predict the outcome of spine surgery. Spine J 1:274-282, 2001.
9. Block AR, Vanharanta H, Ohnmeiss DD, et al. Discographic pain report: Influence of psychological factors. Spine 21:334-338, 1996.
10. Brown GK, Nicassio PM. Development of a questionnaire for the assessment of active and passive coping strategies in chronic pain patients. Pain 31:53-64, 1987.
11. Cashion EL, Lynch WJ. Personality factors and results of lumbar disc surgery. Neurosurgery 4:151-155, 1979.
12. Chapman RC. Pain: The perception of noxious events. In Sternbach RA, ed. The Psychology of Pain. New York: Raven Press, 1978.
13. Davis RA. A long-term outcome analysis of 984 surgically treated herniated lumbar discs. J Neurosurg 80:515-521, 1994.
14. DeGood DE, Kiernan B. Perception of fault in patients with chronic pain. Pain 64:153-159, 1996.

15. Doxey NC, Dzioba RB, Mitson GL. Predictors of outcome in back surgery candidates. J Clin Psych 44:611-622, 1988.
16. Dvorak J, Valach L, Fuhrimann P, et al. The outcome of surgery for lumbar disc herniation. II. A 4-17 years' follow-up with emphasis on psychosocial aspects. Spine 13:1523-1527, 1988.
17. Fernandez E, Clark TS, Ruddick-Davis D. A framework for conceptualization and assessment of affective disturbance in pain. In Block AR, Kremer EF, Fernandez E, eds. Handbook of Pain Syndromes: Biopsychosocial Perspectives. Mahwah, NJ: Lawrence Erlbaum Associates, 1999.
18. Finneson BE, Cooper VR. A lumbar disc surgery predictive score card: A retrospective evaluation. Spine 4:151-154, 1979.
19. Fordyce WE. Behavioral Methods for Chronic Pain and Illness. St Louis: Mosby, 1976.
20. Frymoyer JW, Cats-Baril WL. An overview of the incidences and cost of low back pain. Orthop Clin North Am 22:263-271, 1987.
21. Graham JR. The MMPI-2: Assessing Personality and Psychopathology. New York: Oxford University Press, 1990.
22. Greenough CG, Fraser RD. The effects of compensation on recovery from low-back injury. Spine 15:947-955, 1989.
23. Gross AR. The effect of coping strategies on the relief of pain following surgical intervention for lower back pain. Psychosomat Med 48:229-238, 1986.
24. Haber J, Roos C. Effects of spouse abuse and/or sexual abuse in the development and maintenance of chronic pain in women. Adv Pain Res Ther 9:889-895, 1985.
25. Haddad GH. Analysis of 2932 workers' compensation back injury cases: The impact of the cost to the system. Spine 12:765-771, 1987.
26. Herron L, Turner JA, Ersek M, et al. Does the Millon Behavioral Health Inventory (MBHI) predict lumbar laminectomy outcome? A comparison with the Minnesota Multiphasic Personality Inventory (MMPI). J Spin Disord 5:188-192, 1992.
27. Hoffman RM, Wheeler KJ, Deyo RA. Surgery for herniated lumbar discs: A literature synthesis. J Gen Intern Med 8:487-496, 1993.
28. Junge A, Dvorak J, Ahrens S. Predictors of bad and good outcomes of lumbar disc surgery: A prospective clinical study with recommendations for screening to avoid bad outcomes. Spine 20:460-468, 1995.
29. Keel PJ. Psychosocial criteria for patient selection: Review of studies and concepts for understanding chronic back pain. Neurosurgery 15:935-941, 1984.
30. Kerns RD, Southwick S, Giller E, et al. The relationship between reports of pain-related social interactions and expressions of pain and affective distress. Behav Ther 22:101-111, 1991.
31. Kiecolt-Glaser J, Malarkey W, Chee M, et al. Negative behavior during marital conflict is associated with immunological down-regulation. Psychosomat Med 55:395-409, 1993.
32. Kjelby-Wendt G, Styf JR, Carlsson SG. The predictive value of psychometric analysis in patients treated by extirpation of lumbar intervertebral disc herniation. J Spin Disord 12:375-379, 1999.
33. Kremer EF, Block AR, Atkinson JJ. Assessment of pain behavior: Factors that distort self-report. In Melzack R, ed. Pain Management and Assessment. New York: Raven Press, 1983.
34. Lindsay P, Wyckoff M. The depression-pain and its response to antidepressants. Psychosomatics 22:571-577, 1981.
35. Linton SJ. A population-based study of the relationship between sexual abuse and back pain: Establishing a link. Pain 73:47-53, 1997.
36. Linton SJ. A review of psychological risk factors in back and neck pain. Spine 25:1148-1156, 2000.

37. Long C. The relationship between surgical outcome and MMPI profiles in chronic pain patients. J Clin Psychol 37:744-749, 1981.
38. Lousberg R, Schmidt AJ, Groenman NH. The relationship between spouse solicitousness and pain behavior: Searching for more evidence. Pain 51:75-79, 1992.
39. Manniche C, Asmussen KH, Vinterberg H, et al. Analysis of preoperative prognostic factors in first-time surgery for lumbar disc herniation, including Finneson's and modified Spengler's score systems. Danish Med Bull 41:110-115, 1994.
40. Maruta T, Osborne D. Sexual activity in chronic pain patients. Psychosomatics 19:531-537, 1976.
41. Merskey H, Moulin D. Pharmacological treatment in chronic pain. In Block AR, Kremer EF, Fernandez E, eds. Handbook of Pain Syndromes: Biopsychosocial Perspectives. Mahwah, NJ: Lawrence Erlbaum Associates, 1999.
42. Polatin PB, Kinney RK, Gatchel RJ, et al. Psychiatric illness and chronic low-back pain. The mind and the spine-which goes first? Spine 18:66-71, 1993.
43. Riley JL, Robinson ME, Geisser ME, et al. Relationship between MMPI-2 cluster profiles and surgical outcome in low-back pain patients. J Spin Disord 8:213-219, 1995.
44. Romano JM, Turner JA, Clancy SL. Sex differences in the relationship of pain patient dysfunction to spouse adjustment. Pain 39:289-296, 1989.
45. Rosensteil AK, Keefe FJ. The use of coping strategies in chronic low back pain patients: Relationship to patient characteristics and current adjustment. Pain 17:33-44, 1983.
46. Schade V, Semmer N, Main CJ, et al. The impact of clinical, morphological, psychosocial and work-related factors on the outcome of lumbar discectomy. Pain 80:239-249, 1999.
47. Schofferman J, Anderson D, Hinds R, et al. Childhood psychological trauma correlates with unsuccessful lumbar spine surgery. Spine 17(Suppl 6):S1380-S1384, 1992.
48. Seligman MEP. Learned helplessness and depression in animals and men. In Spence JT, Carson RC, Thibaut JW, eds. Behavioral Approaches to Therapy. Morristown, NJ: General Learning Press, 1976.
49. Skinner BF. About Behaviorism. New York: Knopf, 1974.
50. Smith TW, Gallo LC. Personality traits as risk factors for physical illness. In Baum A, Revenson TA, Singer JE, eds. Handbook of Health Psychology. Mahwah, NJ: Lawrence Erlbaum Associates, 2001.
51. Sorenson LV, Mors O. Presentation of a new MMPI scale to predict outcome after first lumbar diskectomy. Pain 34:191-194, 1988.
52. Spengler DM, Freeman C, Westbrook R, et al. Low-back pain following multiple lumbar spine procedures: Failure of initial selection? Spine 5:356-360, 1980.
53. Spielberger CD, Gorusch RI, Lushene R. Manual for the State-Trait Anxiety Inventory. Palo Alto, Calif: Consulting Psychology Press, 1983.
54. Trief PM, Grant W, Fredrickson B. A prospective study of psychological predictors of lumbar surgery outcome. Spine 25:2616-2621, 2000.
55. Turk DC, Rudy TE. Toward an empirically driven taxonomy of chronic pain patients: Integration of psychological assessment data. J Consult Clin Psychol 56:233-238, 1988.
56. Turner JA, Ersek M, Herron L, et al. Patient outcomes after lumbar spinal fusions. JAMA 268:907-911, 1992.
57. Uomoto JM, Turner JA, Herron LD. Use of the MMPI and MCMI in predicting outcome of lumbar laminectomy. J Clin Psychol 44:191-197, 1988.
58. Williams R, Williams V. Anger Kills. New York: Harper Perennial, 1993.
59. Wiltse LL, Rocchio PH. Pre-operative psychological tests as predictors of success of chemonucleolysis and treatment of low back syndrome. J Bone Joint Surg Am 57:478-483, 1975.

PART

II

BIOMECHANICS AND DEVELOPMENT

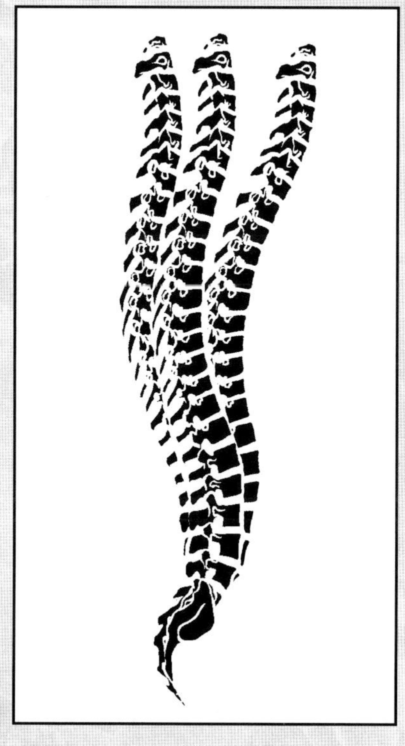

CHAPTER

5

Design Goals for an Intervertebral Prosthetic Disc

James Q. Spitler ▪ Barton L. Sachs ▪ Donna D. Ohnmeiss

For almost half a century, spine arthroplasty has been considered a viable alternative treatment to spinal arthrodesis or an adjunct to discectomy. Often, artificial discs are viewed as devices that primarily perform the opposite of a fusion-that is, to allow motion. During the middle to late 1980s, the technology matured with the introduction of a clinically viable total disc replacement, the SB Charité artificial disc; a few years later, the ProDisc was introduced. Both these devices allow motion through the articulation of concave and convex surfaces and are made of metallic endplates with a polyethylene core or spacer between the endplates. As more prospective randomized studies are reported, the clinical performance of these devices can be evaluated. These results will help to refine the design goals that should be incorporated in future implants.

Because pain associated with degenerative disc disease persists following nonoperative treatment, many patients undergo spinal fusion. However, ongoing development and evaluation of intervertebral prosthetic discs have the potential to widen the scope of available treatment options. Proponents of this technology believe an intervertebral prosthetic disc may reduce the potential for damage and degeneration to adjacent levels and permit a return to proper physiologic range of motion. It is also hypothesized that patients with prosthetic discs will demonstrate more rapid rehabilitation, which will translate to a more rapid return to work and normal daily activities. The intervertebral disc could also allow for less restricted activity. Finally, advocates of an intervertebral prosthetic disc surmise that fusion is always an option if disc arthroplasty fails. These potential advantages of arthroplasty can only be tested and verified with long-term follow-up data from clinical trials, but the possibility of a positive outcome begins when the proper design goals are addressed by the disc designer and manufacturer.

Intervertebral prosthetic discs for both lumbar and cervical regions are under development and clinical evaluation. The design goals for both are essentially the same, and therefore the design goals discussed here apply to both. The purpose of this chapter is to identify specific goals that should be considered in the design of a total disc replacement and to discuss how these goals have been addressed by various disc prosthetic designs so far.

Anatomy

In order to address the design of a total disc replacement, one must have a basic understanding of spinal anatomy and how the implant is expected to interface with the spinal structures. With spinal arthroplasty, the vertebral bodies and the endplates are of particular importance as the points of interface with the prosthesis. Ideally the prosthesis should "mate" on the harder cortical bone around the rim of the vertebral body to provide the most stability and reduce the potential for subsidence. Additional anatomic structures affecting load and motion of the spine include the anterior and posterior longitudinal ligaments and the facet joints. The relationship between these structures and the prosthesis should also be considered.

Design Goals

The following discussion of the design goals of an intervertebral prosthetic disc is not intended to consist of exact values for design variables, but is a compilation of design considerations to be taken into account when any prosthetic disc is being considered. Currently there is little literature available on the biomechanical testing of various disc prostheses. Whatever information is available about how various devices address particular goals has been included in the following discussion.

Motion

The primary function of an intervertebral prosthetic disc is to allow anatomically correct movement of the spinal motion segment while achieving adequate pain relief for the patient. To provide for this, two issues should be considered: the center of motion and the range of motion. The center of motion or center of rotation is the point about which the disc articulates in all three planes. The axis of rotation is the line going through the center of motion around which the disc rotates. There are three axes-one for each of the three planes. In a normal healthy disc, Gertzbein et al[5] and Seligman et al,[16] in a computer analysis, demonstrated that the center of motion of a lumbar disc was located in the posterior half of the disc space and was concentrated between the disc space and the bottom endplate. Although these studies identified a locus or centroid of instantaneous centers, an artificial prosthetic disc will most likely have a single center of motion. Any prosthetic disc design must consider where to locate the center of motion to maintain the existing biomechanical function of the motion segment.

The two most commonly used artificial discs, the CHARITÉ Artificial Disc and the ProDisc, allow motion through the articulation of concave and convex surfaces. For the sake of analysis, the convex surface can be viewed as the upper portion of a sphere. Articulation of the surfaces produces an arc of motion, and prosthetic motion is influenced by the height and diameter of the sphere. To maintain ideal biomechanical function of the spinal motion segment, the position of the vertebral body at each point along this arc and at the limits of motion should match that of a healthy normal disc as closely as possible. Otherwise, injury to other spinal elements and reduced range of motion may occur.

The range of motion is the extent to which the segment is allowed to move in any one of the three planes: flexion/extension, lateral bending, and rotation. The concept of constrained versus unconstrained motion has been the method of choice for describing the range of motion for total joint replacement, particularly in knee arthroplasty. By definition, unconstrained motion indicates that the disc can move through 360 degrees of motion on a particular axis. A totally constrained device allows no motion in the plane. Semiconstrained motion refers to motion ranging between 0 and 360 degrees. For the purposes of an intervertebral prosthetic disc, each of the three axes independently exhibits degrees of constraint so an intervertebral prosthetic disc can be semicon-

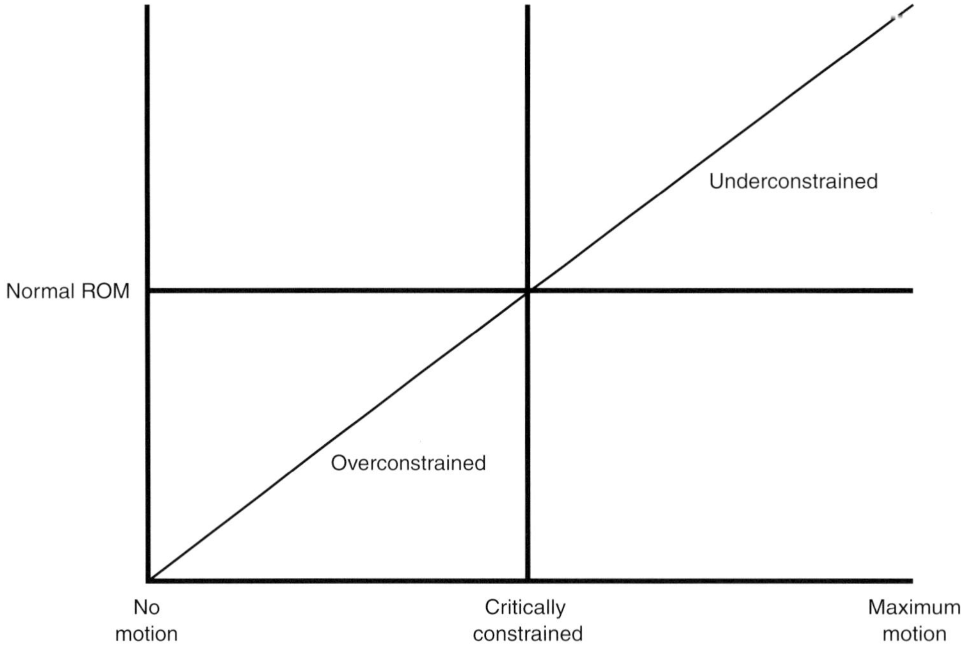

Fig. 5-1 Concept of overconstrained, underconstrained, and critically constrained characteristics for prosthetic discs in relation to the motion of a normal intervertebral disc.

strained in two planes and unconstrained in the third. A normal human disc is semiconstrained in all three planes of motion. An artificial disc can be described in terms of the motion it allows compared with the motion allowed by a normal disc. An artificial disc can be underconstrained, overconstrained, or critically constrained (Fig. 5-1). For example, if a device is overconstrained, its motion is less limited than that of a normal disc. An underconstrained device allows more motion than a normal disc does. When a disc is critically constrained, the range of motion of the prosthesis matches that of a normal healthy disc.

Several studies have been conducted in order to establish the biologic range of motion.[3,6,12,14,17] The center of motion and range of motion are two critical areas that must be defined on any disc design. There could be several combinations of the two that are acceptable as artificial prosthetic disc designs. It is most likely that no disc design will ever fully meet all anatomic and biomechanical needs perfectly, because there is simply too much variability in the population for one design to work perfectly for everyone.

The CHARITÉ Artificial Disc recently received FDA approval, and the ProDisc is currently under FDA IDE studies. Of the two, more information has been published about the CHARITÉ Artificial Disc. The CHARITÉ Artificial Disc actually has two centers of motion as it glides on a biconvex core.[1] The core is constrained physically by a flange circling its edge. Understanding the CHARITÉ Artificial Disc centers of motion is best accomplished by dividing the motion into two separate motions (Fig. 5-2).

The first motion occurs on a sphere from the bottom convex surface. This motion translates both the core and the top plate, and thus the vertebral level on the sphere having a center of rotation above the disc. The second motion occurs on a sphere from the top convex surface and has its center of rotation below the disc. This motion translates the top plate. These two motions obviously occur simultaneously, giving the perception of a single center of motion; however, there are two centers that generate a single effect, which sums the degrees of motion of the two arcs.

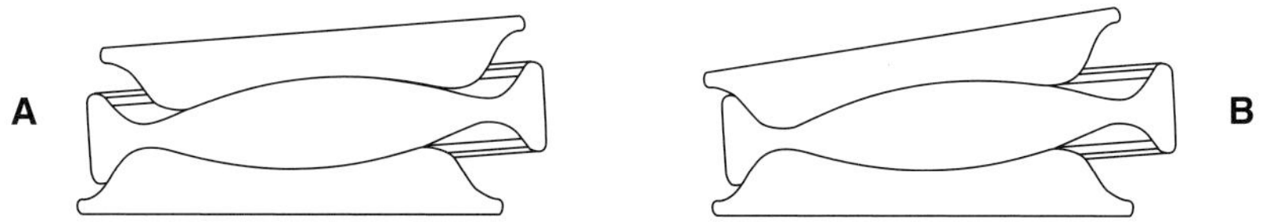

Fig. 5-2 **A** and **B,** The motion of the prosthesis is limited by the flange on the outer rim of the sliding core.

The CHARITÉ Artificial Disc allows identical amounts of flexion, extension, and lateral bending of 12 degrees in each direction.[1] Most data on range of motion categorize this disc as underconstrained in flexion/extension and lateral bending, and unconstrained in rotation.

Discs with a single center of motion include the ProDisc (Spine Solutions/Synthes, and MAVERICK (Medtronic Sofamor Danek, Memphis, TN). The ProDisc is near critically constrained in flexion/extension, overconstrained in lateral bending, and unconstrained in rotation. Very little information is available on the range of motion of the MAVERICK device. The overriding design element to note is whether the prosthetic disc itself or the anatomic structures of the motion segment limit motion.

Dimensions

Dimensional design goals relate to the size, shape, height, and geometry of the disc. This is relevant in that a primary function of any intervertebral prosthetic disc is maintaining or reestablishing proper disc height.

When considering size, a disc design must account for several factors including the actual disc height and the amount of lordosis. Lordosis designed into the disc should also be considered for each disc level. Rough data on lordosis by level have been published by Pearcy et al.[13] Multiple disc sizes may be needed to accommodate a large population of patients. Overall disc height at the installed position is important, because too little height will not adequately open up the degenerated disc space or the foramen, and a disc that is too tall increases the potential for nerve tissue stretching or overdistraction of the facet joints.

Intervertebral prosthetic disc shape must also be included in design goals, because the disc must anchor on the harder outer cortical bone of the vertebral body to reduce potential for subsidence. The original SB Charité I disc was revised to increase the contact surface between the prosthetic endplate and vertebral body. Additionally, subsidence has been documented with the SB Charité disc in patients who received undersized prostheses.[2]

Biocompatibility

As with any implant, a disc replacement must be made of biologically inert materials. Biosafe materials used in intervertebral prosthetic discs to date include titanium, cobalt chrome alloys, ultrahigh molecular weight polyethylene, and other various rubbers and polymers. If a new material is being considered, or if the material has been used elsewhere in the body but is new for spinal applications, sufficient testing is warranted to prove biocompatibility. This is of particular importance, considering the proximity of the device to major neural structures.

The initial design of the Acroflex disc incorporated two metal plates with a rubber core vulcanized between them.[4] A report of the preliminary results in six patients implanted with the device was published; however, the authors report that the use of the disc was stopped because a chemical used in the vulcanization process had been found to be possibly carcinogenic in rats. The manufacturers of the device acted responsibly and ceased using the initial materials, and the same basic disc design has been pursued with different materials. A polyolefin rubber compound and ultrahigh-molecular-weight polyethylene (UHMWPE) were tested for biocompatibility in sheep and rats.[11] This study found that the particles induced only a localized tissue response as with a normal foreign body reaction. Additional insight into material selection is seen with the SB Charité disc. The endplates were initially manufactured from stainless steel but were changed to the more biologically friendly cobalt chrome molybdenum alloy.

Load Bearing

Along with allowing motion, bearing the load of the body is a primary function of the intervertebral disc, so a prosthetic disc must be capable of handling loads transmitted through the spine. Peak loads in the lumbar spinal region have been measured at approximately 4000 N. Transmitting this load to the lower extremities must largely be addressed by the geometry of the disc design and the materials from which it is made. The geometry drives the load per unit area that must be transmitted through the disc. The optimal design maximizes the surface area so that any single unit area carries a smaller load.

The intervertebral prosthetic disc must transmit load between vertebral bodies without failure or permanent deformation. The ability to perform this function depends greatly on the materials selected. Sufficient testing should be conducted to ensure that maximum loads at failure are much higher than those encountered if the disc is placed in the human body. As an example, the SB Charité disc has undergone several loading tests to ensure that the materials are sufficient to handle the loads carried by the human disc.[1] This device underwent static and dynamic testing with two different core sizes and was found to perform within an acceptable range.

If using plastics, the possibility of cold flow must be considered. Developers of the SB Charité device addressed this concern about its polyethylene core by first performing calculations to allow for a sufficient safety margin under peak maximum loads, and then performing dynamic testing. The dynamic testing indicated a 0.403 mm permanent deformation for the 7.5 mm core, and a 0.738 mm permanent deformation for the 9.5 mm core.[15]

Another function of the intervertebral disc is to dampen the loads placed on the lumbar spine. In this way, the vertebral column functions as a shock absorber to reduce the loads transmitted to the sacroiliac joint. Ultrahigh molecular weight polyethylene has a considerable elastic range that provides some damping capability and is used in the core of the CHARITÉ Artificial Disc and the ProDisc. Other disc designers have attempted to incorporate mechanical springs to act as shock-absorbing dampeners.[7]

A further example of the use of unique materials to create a specific load capability is demonstrated by two intervertebral prosthetic discs developed by Lee et al.[8] The design of these discs was an attempt to mimic the physical and mechanical properties of the natural disc through the use of polymers to generate an outer annulus and an inner nucleus. Following testing, these discs were reported to have mechanical properties similar to those of a normal disc.

Creating a disc that has the load-bearing capabilities and shock-absorbing features of the natural disc is the key element of any design and should be considered as a design goal. The shock-absorbing features have been difficult to achieve, given the great number of bending cycles a prosthetic disc must endure.

Ease of Implantation

The implantation technique, approaches allowed, and ease of instrumentation are critical design goals for an intervertebral prosthetic disc. An element that is key to ease of implantation is to keep the number of disc components and implant steps to a minimum. Both the CHARITÉ Artificial and ProDisc devices have three components requiring a two-stage implant technique of the plates and then the core. The degree of distraction required to seat a core is a factor with a multicomponent disc. In addition to these issues, reducing the number of implant steps can reduce surgical time.

Each component of the disc should be intuitive, robust, and free of "fiddle factors." From a dimensional perspective, instrumentation entering the surgical site should ideally be no wider or taller than the intervertebral prosthetic disc itself so as to allow for the smallest possible approach site as well as maximum visibility. Retractors, distractors, and disc placement or alignment instruments should be as simple as possible with few moving parts and should mate to the disc for secure implantation. Further refinements in instrumentation should generate a more consistent placement in the disc space from physician to physician by reducing "eyeballing" and "float" of placing and cutting instruments.

The surgical approaches that can be used to implant the disc must also be considered. A direct anterior approach is generally preferred; however, a disc design that allows for more flexibility in surgical approaches when needed is appealing. The size of the devices may also be a limiting factor.

Finally, intervertebral disc prostheses should not preclude the use of pedicle screw fixation or other posterior fusion techniques as a salvage procedure for patients requiring revision surgery.

Reliability

Some estimates place the required life of an intervertebral prosthetic disc at 40 years. By various calculations, this equals up to 100 million cycles.[7] This number is far greater than the nearest orthopedic implant tested to date, and a reasonable goal has not been standardized yet. American Standard of Test and Measurement (ASTM) standards concerning spine fusion cages and pedicle screw systems are the best-documented numbers to date. The life of the product should be strongly considered when selecting materials. The materials should satisfy the high cycle wear demands that exist in all joint replacement implants. Specifically, the size and number of microscopic wear particles generated for the material must be evaluated. Published data on wear debris of the SB Charité disc are available. In addition to static and dynamic testing mentioned earlier, functional or simulated use testing was also performed.[9] The small size 2 implants together with the most common size 9.5 mm core were tested to 10 million cycles under a sinusoidal load function ranging from 0.5 kN to 2.5 kN. Motion of 4 degrees flexion, 2 degrees extension, 1 degree rotation, and 2 degrees lateral bending was used to simulate movement and stress the motion surfaces. Testing was conducted in calf serum diluted with deionized water maintained at 27° C. Evaluations under electron microscope evaluation found only minor scuffing of both the endplates and the core. No visible slide marks were detected, and no detectable wear particles were evident in the contact zone. This simulated use testing, combined with dynamic testing, is a required condition by the United States Food and Drug Administration (FDA) for an investigational device exemption to achieve premarket approval for the study now in progress. This represents the testing groundwork for future intervertebral prosthetic discs to build upon. Also included in reliability design goals is the need to eliminate catastrophic failures following extended life, which involves conducting a thorough failure mode and effect analysis.

Anchoring and Fixation

Consideration of fixation and anchoring is fundamental to the intervertebral prosthetic disc. Migration or instability of the device can give rise to autofusion, reduced range of motion, increased wear debris, premature failure, or catastrophic failure in the event of gross displacement. Anchoring features and/or bone ingrowth media should be added to the surfaces bordering bone to secure the implant in place. Several techniques have been used to achieve this goal. The ProDisc uses a midline keel fin with serrations as the primary means to secure the prosthetic endplates in the vertebral body. Additionally, a titanium spray is applied to the surfaces contacting the vertebral endplates to promote bone ingrowth into the prosthetic disc endplates. The CHARITÉ Artificial Disc incorporates six spikes to secure the prosthetic endplates. Endplates with a double-layer titanium coating to encourage bone ingrowth are available outside the Unites States. A recent study published by McAfee et al[10] tested the percentage of bone ingrowth in seven baboons implanted with the SB Charité device. Six months postoperatively, all 14 endplate prostheses were solidly fixed with no signs of loosening; bone ingrowth was measured at 47.9% of the total endplate area with a standard deviation of 8.12%. The authors reported that these values were significantly greater than those reported in studies evaluating bony ingrowth in other types of orthopedic prostheses.

Sterilization

Sterilization should not be overlooked as a design goal. The recommended sterilization technique must be compatible with the chosen materials. Ease of cleaning and sterilization should also be considered when designing implantation instrumentation to reduce the potential for contamination.

Manufacturing

Although not directly a clinical issue, manufacturing requirements and techniques should be used to reduce costs and allow for ease of manufacturing. As new materials are developed, certainly new manufacturing processes will follow. The manufacturing process required to produce a disc replacement should not introduce a new element of risk to the patient, such as wear debris generated from a rough surface or other possible problems.

Cost

The cost of a device and its implantation should be reasonable and not significantly greater than the current standard of care. This issue is particularly important when considering the current crisis in health care reimbursements.

Conclusion

Lumbar and cervical disc design goals vary in several ways. The range of motion in lumbar and cervical discs is different and may require different approaches to design. Implantation of the cervical disc is made more difficult because of the small size of the vertebral bodies and the small space in which to work. Another factor influencing the design of cervical disc replacements may be the opportunity to use a wider range of materials, because the loads on the cervical disc are much less than those encountered in the lumbar spine.

Maintaining the shock-absorbing nature of a normal disc has also proved difficult. Further developments in materials hope to achieve this goal. In addition, creating a design that lasts 40 years will be quite challenging as this goal approaches current material limitations.

Regarding the clinical elements, improvements in implantation techniques will prove helpful as this treatment option evolves. Most current designs favor a direct anterior approach. Greater flexibility in this area will certainly prove valuable in some cases; attention could also be paid to design and implant techniques that reduce the risk of selecting too small an implant and less than optimal positioning. Furthermore, a minimally invasive method of implantation has yet to be developed.

As with many other medical device implants, ASTM standards for testing these devices will ensure that all these devices are measured fairly; these standards are currently being developed.

The future of the intervertebral prosthetic disc is bright; some experts believe that this approach to the treatment of degenerative disc disease will revolutionize spine care. Certainly much clinical evaluation is warranted to prove these assumptions. As this technology moves forward, the best outcome for the patient will be from a device whose developers have thoroughly and diligently sought to meet well-defined design goals.

REFERENCES

1. Büttner-Janz K, Schellnack K, Zippel H. Biomechanics of the SB Charité lumbar intervertebral disc endoprosthesis. Int Orthop 13:173-176, 1989.
2. Cinotti G, David T, Postacchini F. Results of disc prosthesis after a minimum follow-up period of 2 years. Spine 21:995-1000, 1996.
3. Dvorak J, Panjabi MM, Chang DG, et al. Functional radiographic diagnosis of the lumbar spine: Flexion-extension and lateral bending. Spine 16:562-571, 1991.
4. Enker P, Steffee A, McMillin C, et al. Artificial disc replacement. Preliminary report with a 3-year minimum follow-up. Spine 18:1061-1070, 1993.
5. Gertzbein SD, Holtby R, Tile M, et al. Determination of a locus of instantaneous centers of rotation of the lumbar spine by Moiré fringes: A new technique. Spine 9:409-413, 1984.
6. Hayes MA, Howard TC, Gruel CR, et al. Roentgenographic evaluation of lumbar spine flexion-extension in asymptomatic individuals. Spine 14:327, 1989.
7. Hedman TP, Kostuik JP, Fernie GR, et al. Design of an intervertebral disc prosthesis. Spine 16(6):S256-S260, 1991.
8. Lee CK, Langrana NA, Parsons JR, et al. Development of a prosthetic intervertebral disc. Spine 16(Suppl 6):S253-S255, 1991.
9. Link HD, Keller A. Biomechanics of total disc replacement. In Hochschuler SH, Büttner-Janz K, McAfee PC, eds. The SB Charité Artificial Disc. Berlin: Springer-Verlag, 2003, pp 33-52.

10. McAfee PC, Cunningham BW, Shimamoto N, et al. Biological ingrowth using a non-human primate model. In Hochschuler SH, Büttner-Janz K, McAfee PC, eds. The SB Charité Artificial Disc. Berlin: Springer-Verlag, 2003, pp 63-72.
11. Moore RJ, Fraser RD, Vernon-Roberts B, et al. The biological response to particles from a lumbar disc prosthesis. Spine 27:2088-2094, 2002.
12. Pearcy M, Bogduk N. Instantaneous axes of rotation of the lumbar intervertebral joints. Spine 13:1033-1041, 1988.
13. Pearcy M, Protek I, Shepherd J. Three-dimensional x-ray analysis of normal movement in the lumbar spine. Spine 9:294-297, 1984.
14. Pearcy MJ, Tibrewal SB. Axial rotation and lateral bending in the normal lumbar spine measured by three-dimensional radiography. Spine 9:582-587, 1984.
15. Postak DP, 1999.
16. Seligman JV, Gertzbein SD, Tile M, et al. Computer analysis of spinal segment motion in degenerative disc disease with and without axial loading. Spine 9:566-573, 1984.
17. Yamamoto I, Panjabi M, Crisco J, et al. Three-dimensional movements of the whole lumbar spine and lumbosacral joints. Presented at the Annual Meeting of the International Society for the Study of the Lumbar Spine, Kyoto, Japan, May 1989.

CHAPTER

6

History and Development of the CHARITÉ Artificial Disc

Karin Büttner-Janz

The goal of the CHARITÉ Artificial Disc is to reconstruct degeneratively damaged intervertebral discs in the segments from L2-3 to the lumbosacral disc space. The prosthesis is implanted to restore the most important functions of the affected mobile segments, by just one operation. The specific construction of the CHARITÉ Artificial Disc and the use of materials that have been proven effective in extremity arthroplasty over the past several decades suggest the long-term functionality of the prosthesis. This chapter will discuss the historical evolution of the CHARITÉ Artificial Disc.

History

A new era in artificial intervertebral disc replacement and spine surgery began with the introduction of the SB Charité disc prosthesis, which in 1987 was developed further to become the CHARITÉ Artificial Disc.[5,6] In 1982 work began on developing a three-component low-friction artificial intervertebral disc at the Charité Hospital. In 1985, it was named after Dr. Kurt Schellnack and myself, its two inventors (SB is an acronym for Schellnack and Büttner-Janz), as well as the place of its development and first implantation.

Model I

Model I of the SB Charité prosthesis, which was first implanted in 1984, consisted of two symmetrical endplates made of 1 mm thick steel plate and an interpositioned polyethylene sliding core, which after the thirteenth implantation received a metal tagging ring for its radiographic identification. The round endplates (when viewed from above) were fixed to the vertebral bodies with anchoring teeth, which in the first eleven patients were eleven in number, and in the ensuing two patients were five in number. They were all 2 mm in height (Fig. 6-1). The endplates were 1 mm thicker ventrally than they were dorsally. In all, 14 implantations of the SB I prosthesis were carried out in 13 patients (one patient received implants at two levels).

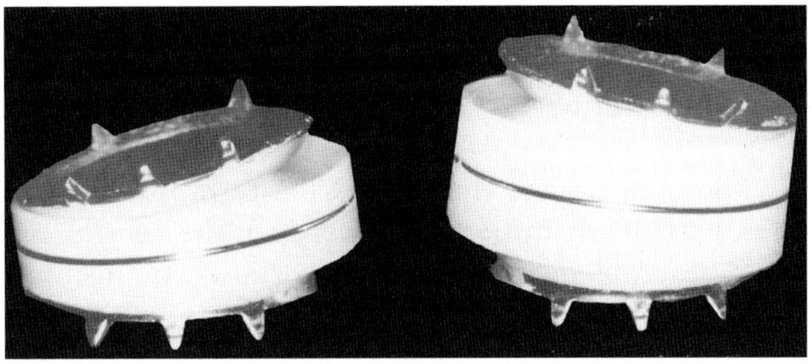

Fig. 6-1 Model I of the SB Charité Prosthesis. The endplates had five anchoring teeth. The sliding cores were of different heights and included an x-ray tagging ring.

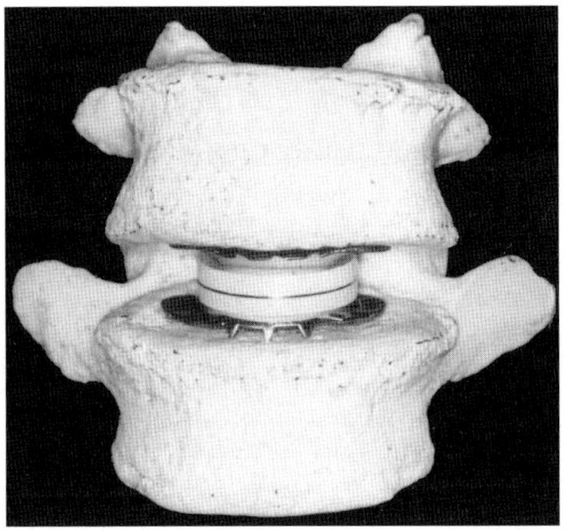

Fig. 6-2 Model II of the SB Charité Prosthesis positioned in the intervertebral space.

Model II

To achieve an improved intervertebral load transfer, the endplates of the SB Charité II prosthesis were made more oval in shape and had two lateral wings (Fig. 6-2). They were once again made of steel plate and were slightly convex with respect to the vertebral bodies. The three ventral and two dorsal anchoring teeth had an effective height of 1.5 mm. This design was monosegmentally or bisegmentally implanted 44 times in 36 patients.

Problems with Models I and II

In several of the 49 patients who underwent surgery, clinical problems arose initially with the model SB I and then with the model SB II, which made further implantation of either device impractical. The SB I Charité prosthesis proved to have too little surface area for an adequate intervertebral load transfer. Because the bottom of the steel endplates had indentations to accommodate the polyethylene sliding core, the surface area for load transfer to the vertebral body was reduced even more. Furthermore, the 11 anchoring teeth may have functioned like a punch, which could have contributed to subsidence of the prostheses into the vertebral bodies.

Postoperatively, the endplates of the SB II Charité prosthesis radiographically showed fractures, particularly in the region between the central aspects and the lateral wings. These problems may have been caused by insufficient mass or strength of the steel plate, with respect to the high intervertebral loads and the differently shaped bony vertebral endplates compared to the uniformly shaped endplates of the prostheses. No changes to the polyethylene sliding core were observed in either the model SB I or SB II; there were also no dislocations of the sliding cores observed from between the endplates.

As a result of these problems, and because of a few displacements of the complete SB II Charité prostheses ventrally resulting from the inadequate length of the anchoring teeth (mainly in patients with spondylolysis or spondylolisthesis), a few prostheses (both SB I and II) were removed and fusion of adjacent vertebral bodies was carried out instead. In some cases a posterior fusion was performed, leaving the anterior implant in place.

Development of the Charité Artificial Disc

After evaluating the problems that arose in the SB I and SB II prostheses, a revised third model of the prosthesis (the SB III Charité prosthesis) was developed in cooperation with Waldemar Link GmbH & Company, Hamburg, Germany. The material and shape of the endplates differed substantially from the previous models (Fig. 6-3). The functional principle of the prosthesis, however, stayed the same as in the first two models.

Design Rationale

Compared with other intervertebral disc replacements that have so far been implanted into human lumbar spines (ProDisc, MAVERICK, FlexiCore, Mobidisc, Kineflex), the SB Charité Intervertebral Prosthesis (hereafter referred to as the *CHARITÉ Artificial Disc,* Johnson & Johnson/DePuy Spine) exhibits unique characteristics. The CHARITÉ Artificial Disc is based on an unconstrained double joint prosthesis, a principle that is distantly related to mobile bearing knee replacements. It largely emulates physiologic biomechanics in terms of intervertebral motion, intervertebral load transfer, and function of the facet joints. This mechanism is what makes the CHARITÉ Artificial Disc principally different from prostheses that comprise two components or those that have binary functions. The basic functioning mechanism lies in the construction of the specially shaped surfaces of the endplates and the interposed polyethylene sliding core that is adapted to their shape. Segmental movements such as flexion, extension, and side bending occur as a result of transverse motion

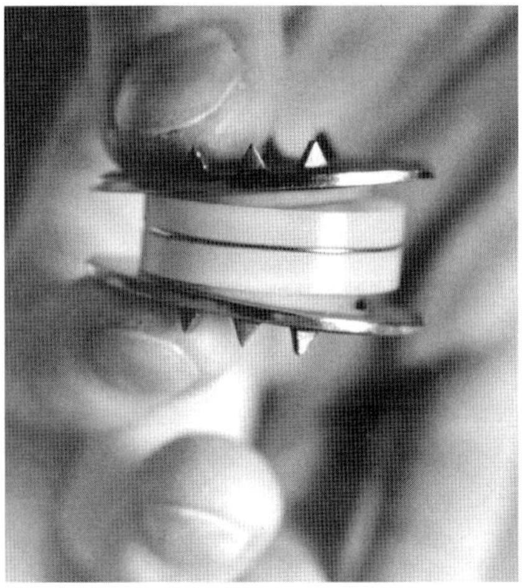

Fig. 6-3 CHARITÉ Artificial Disc in simulated bending.

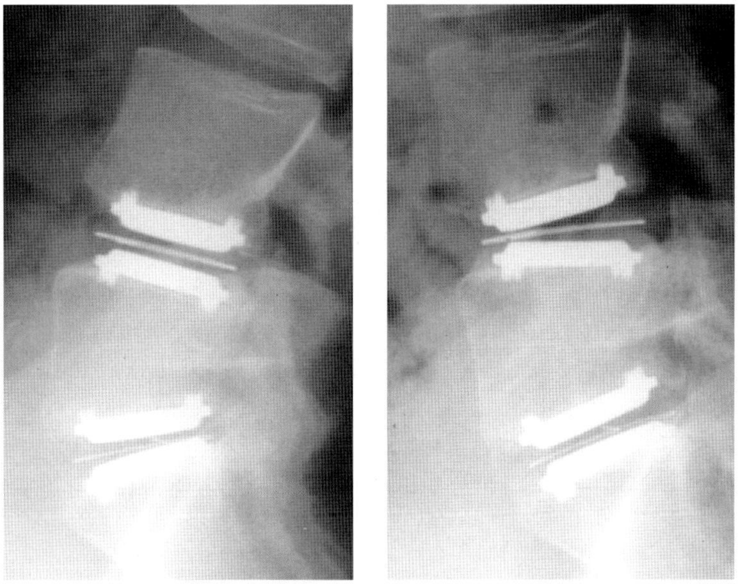

Fig. 6-4 CHARITÉ Artificial Disc in L4-5 and L5-S1 in extension and flexion 8 years postoperatively. The range of motion was 15 degrees at L4-5 and 11 degrees at L5-S1.

of the polyethylene sliding core. As these occur, the angles between the two endplates change with respect to each other (Fig. 6-4).

Endplates and Sliding Core

The two symmetrical endplates of the CHARITÉ Artificial Disc are made of a Vacucast molten alloy. They are in full contact with the vertebral bodies, free of any cavities, and adjusted to the concavity of the vertebral bodies by virtue of their slightly convex shape. Specially developed prosthetic endplates are available for patients with metal allergies. The sliding core, which moves transversely between the endplates, is made of ultrahigh-molecular-weight polyethylene (UHMWPE). The peripherally protective ring construction (collar) of the UHMWPE sliding core should prevent direct contact between the endplates, even in great ranges of motion or in cases where the CHARITÉ Artificial Disc has not been implanted optimally.

For radiographic identification, the sliding core is manufactured with a peripheral tagging ring.

The CHARITÉ Artificial Disc is fixed firmly to the vertebral body by three ventral and three dorsal anchoring teeth approximately 3 mm in height on each endplate for primary fixation. Further fixation is achieved through a bioactive coating (TiCaP, not available in the United States), which is slightly textured and achieves primary and secondary fixation. The elastic behavior of the UHMWPE sliding core is meant to partly counterbalance the disadvantages of the rigidity of the cobalt-chromium-molybdenum endplates with respect to the load transfer between implant and bone. Compared to one-component prostheses, no friction occurs between the endplates of the CHARITÉ Artificial Disc and the vertebral bodies and thus no wear particles are produced in the region bordering the body's own tissue. There is therefore a reduced risk of osteolysis of the vertebral bodies or of subsidence of the CHARITÉ Artificial Disc.

The three-component principle of the prosthesis with the constraining shape of the contacting surfaces of the endplates and the UHMWPE sliding core prevent excessive sagittal and frontal ranges of motion as well as translational instability of the adjoining vertebrae.[4] Because of the way the prosthesis is constructed, no dislocation of the sliding core should occur after it is correctly implanted.

Endplate and Sliding Core Sizes

The CHARITÉ Artificial Disc is available in five standard sizes of endplates whose width ranges from sizes 1 to 5: 28.5; 31.5; 35.5; 38.5, and 42 mm. The depth of the prosthesis ranges from sizes 1 to 5: 23, 25, 27, 29, and 31 mm. Five corresponding sizes are available for the sliding core (diameter: 23, 25, 27, 29, and 31 mm). (NOTE: The size 1 prosthesis is no longer available because of its small parameters.) To achieve a high surface area for intervertebral load transfer, the largest possible endplate size is selected; this should minimize the risk of the device endplate subsiding into the adjacent vertebral body. An adaptation to the lumbar lordosis and the anatomic angle of the intervertebral space can be achieved through the implantation of endplates with different sagittal angles, which are available at 0, 5, 7.5, and 10 degrees for each size.

Sliding cores are available in heights of 7.5, 8.5, 9.5, 10.5, and 11.5 mm for each prosthetic size (sizes 4 and 5 without 7.5 mm). The availability of five

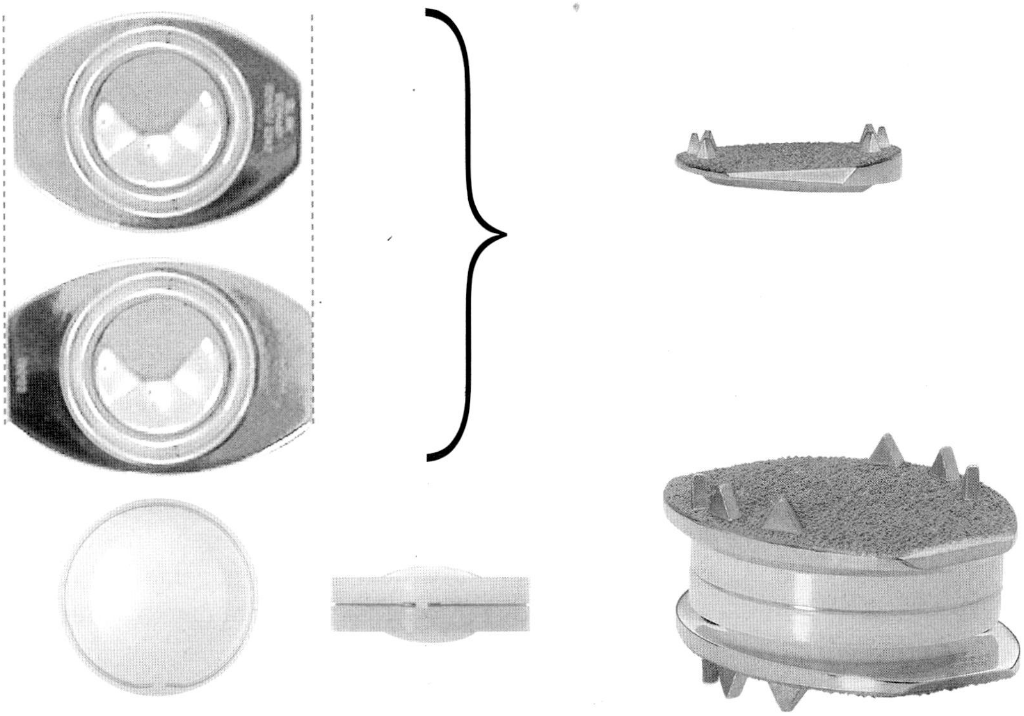

Fig. 6-5 Present product overview of the CHARITÉ Artificial Disc.

heights of the UHMWPE sliding core allows a well-directed reconstruction of the height of the intervertebral space. Because of the plastic-elastic behavior and the durability of the polyethylene, a not too small sliding core should be implanted.

To achieve an optimal relationship between the vertebral endplate and the implant, metal endplates are available in three additional intermediate coronal sizes. These endplates have the width of the next largest size and unchanged depth (size 3/2: 35.5 mm wide, 25 mm deep; size 4/3: 38.5 mm wide, 27 mm deep; size 5/4: 42 mm wide, 29 mm deep). Thus seven sizes of the CHARITÉ Artificial Disc are available (Fig. 6-5). This assortment also allows a physiologically adapted, slightly dorsal placement of the kinetic center of the prosthesis.

Biomechanics

The mechanical segmental stability of the prosthesis was evaluated by performing static range-of-motion testing in five fresh frozen cadaveric L4-5 segments, each with intact ligamentous and annulus structures before and after implantation of the CHARITÉ Artificial Disc.[1] Comparisons of ranges of motion in extension, flexion, bending to right and left, and in axial rotation with and without the CHARITÉ Artificial Disc showed a significantly greater range of motion in axial rotation with the prosthesis. The other ranges of motion were similar in the native and implanted specimens.

The load-dependent mechanical behavior of the implanted CHARITÉ Artificial Disc was tested under different conditions with static loads in neutral position, extension, and flexion positions to evaluate durability, changes to the implant surfaces, and retention of function.[3] Five prostheses in four different test conditions (straight and inclined endplates, sliding core heights 7.5 mm and 9.5 mm) were evaluated. All UHMWPE-sliding cores showed tolerable changes under maximal static compression in neutral and extension positions. However, the 7.5 mm sliding cores did demonstrate beyond-normal deformations under compression in maximal flexion. The study concluded that in vivo, even in these sliding cores, the mechanical integrity was retained. On the one hand, the ligamentous and anulus structures as well as the facet joints restrict the mobility in vivo; on the other hand, the polyethylene sliding cores showed no signs of delamination or breakage. Most of the sliding cores showed a regeneration of their shape of up to 50% compared with maximal deformation, so that despite strong deformation, their function was retained. In summary, the test results found that the CHARITÉ Artificial Disc is capable of fulfilling its mechanical functions under physiologic conditions without exceeding the boundaries of the viscoelastic behavior of the polyethylene.

Using dynamic compression tests, reversible and irreversible changes and deformations of the polyethylene sliding core were produced to show the functionality of the UHMWPE sliding cores after 5 and 10 simulated years of use.[2] Five size 2 prostheses with parallel endplates and 7.5 and 9.5 mm high sliding cores were tested with loads of 2.5 kN and 4.5 kN. Extensive calculations that took into account time-based parameters enabled predictions on the deformity of the sliding cores after periods of 5 and 10 years. The result showed retention of the articulation despite plastic deformation of the UHMWPE sliding cores. The extreme load of 4.5 kN showed a decrease of less than 8% in the height of the sliding cores after a period of 5 to 10 simulated years. There were no failures of the sliding cores caused by delamination or substantial cold flow. In summary, the dynamic tests showed that all tested sliding cores would "survive" in vivo. It is expected that in larger sizes that are more often clinically applied and that have a greater surface area (and thus a lower average load per square millimeter), fewer deformities will occur.

The range of motion required of the CHARITÉ Artificial Disc is much smaller than that of the peripheral joints. The demands made on the gliding characteristics of the polyethylene are thus greatly reduced, so there should be only minimal wear of the polyethylene in the intervertebral space if the prosthesis has been implanted correctly.

Factors Influencing Successful Implantation

A number of factors must work together to achieve the successful implantation of the CHARITÉ Artificial Disk (Box 6-1). As in any surgery, success in total

Box 6-1 Considerations for Successful Implantation

Implant

- Design
- Function/biomechanics
- Material(s)
- Sizes, angles, and their variability
- Anchoring (safety)

Indications

- Monosegmental/bisegmental disc degeneration resistant to conservative therapy
- Postdiscectomy syndrome
- Recurrent disc herniation
- Disc herniation with decreased height of the intervertebral space/instability
- Fusion adjacent disease (transitional level DDD)

Contraindications

- Osteopenia/metabolic disease/age limitation
- Destruction of the vertebral body
- (Prior) infection
- Narrowed (bony) spinal canal
- Arthritis of the facet joints with osteophytes
- Significant scoliosis
- Multisegmental, symptomatic disc degeneration
- Spondylolysis/spondylolisthesis
- Previous (hemi-) laminectomy
- Previous fusion of the same segment
- Radicular syndrome with significant disc herniation and neurocompression noted on MRI, disc decompression should be carried out

Patient Condition

- Constitution of patient (obesity)
- Previous abdominal/ventral spinal surgery
- Anatomy (of vessels)
- "Chronic pain disease"
- Psychosocial situation (e.g., unemployment)

Surgical Technique

- Experience of the surgeon and his or her team
- Suitable instruments
- Capability of surgeon to deal with problems
- Maintenance through the company

Follow-up Treatment

- No special treatment

In Cases With Complaints or Complications

- Ability for suitable salvage

disc replacement depends on meticulous attention to detail through the continuum of patient care:

1. The surgeon must choose the patient with the correct indication for disc replacement.
2. A properly sized and angled implant must be chosen.
3. The surgeon and the staff should be well trained. It is important to remember that implantation of the CHARITÉ Artificial Disc is more demanding than a simple ventral interbody fusion. A well-trained surgeon should not only have good surgical technique but also should understand the causes of complications and how to avoid them.

Present State of the CHARITÉ Artificial Disc

Implant Stability and Longevity

The prosthesis can last for years or decades only if implanted in sufficiently durable vertebral bone that is able to adapt to the device over time. According to Wolff's law of bony transformation, the adaptability of the patient's bone with respect to the implant is a limiting factor for the survival of the prosthesis in its intervertebral location.[9] Subsidence of the prosthesis into a vertebral body must be avoided. At the time of surgery, the biologic age more than the chronologic age of the patient determines the stability of the vertebral body and its ability to tolerate the implant. With the aid of the bioactive coating of the endplates, osteointegration of the prosthesis is achieved; this should minimize the potential for microdisplacements in the region between the implant and the vertebral bodies, thereby minimizing bone necrosis and device subsidence.

Indications

In selecting the correct patient for implantation of the CHARITÉ Artificial Disc, it is vitally important not to overextend the indications. Our evaluation has shown that patients with a postdiscectomy syndrome are especially suited for implantation of the prosthesis.[7] It was proved that after implantation of the prosthesis, leg pain disappeared in 83% of the patients, and in 93% the straight leg–raising test was negative. Furthermore, our experience has shown that even patients who had previously undergone discectomy, in some cases up to three times in the same segment, were rendered pain free after implantation of the CHARITÉ Artificial Disc. In patients with a recurrent herniated disc without cranial or caudal sequestration behind the vertebral body, the results of the physical examination and the findings on MRI are very important for differentiating indications for either a revision discectomy or an implantation of the prosthesis. If there are no neurologic deficits or only moderate ones, and if there are no positive tension signs or only moderate ones, we generally consider these to be indications for the implantation of the CHARITÉ Artificial Disc. This applies to patients with back pain, leg pain, or both. In patients who present with symptomatic degenerative disc disease adjacent to a fusion, the higher surgical risk associated with scar tissue in close proximity to blood vessels must be taken into account.

Contraindications

Arthritis of the facet joints is being discussed differently by different surgeons as a contraindication for the implantation of CHARITÉ Artificial Disc. In our experience, arthritis of the facet joints is only of special relevance when osteophytes are present. As a result of intervertebral distraction during implantation of the prosthesis, nerve roots may be damaged. If there are no osteophytes, the distraction and thus the relief of the facet joints is an advantageous basic principle for the treatment of the arthritis. However, postoperative decompensation of the facet joint arthritis is not to be ruled out. The unlimited rotation of the CHARITÉ Artificial Disc may be partly responsible for postoperative complaints caused by the facet joints. A theoretical concept for reduction of rotation based on a different design for an artificial disc replacement is available.[7]

Further medical scientific research on "chronic pain disease" needs to be conducted. It is not known why some patients continue to complain of pain postoperatively despite correct indications and correct surgery. We must continue to learn how these patients can be evaluated preoperatively and treated optimally postoperatively.

Instrumentation, Surgical Technique, and Disc Development

Further changes have been made to the surgical instruments used for implantation. These particularly simplify the final positioning of the operative approach for each segment (including bisegmental and trisegmental surgery) has been specified and the implantation technique facilitated thanks to the improved or new instrumentation.

The CHARITÉ Artificial Disc plays an important role in the surgical treatment of the intervertebral space, especially in a relatively young patient who is a less-than-ideal candidate for fusion. Such a patient needs a prosthesis that is well adapted to the physiologic biomechanical function of a natural intervertebral disc, which at the same time has long-term durability. A CHARITÉ Artificial Disc with a dorsal rotational center may be advantageous; this development could further minimize complications and improve mid- and long-term results.

Postoperative Care

The immediate postoperative treatment of the patient has also been modified in recent years, and patients are now able to stand on the day of surgery without any externally stabilizing braces. Also, often no physiotherapy is required after surgery.

CONCLUSION

More than 9000 CHARITÉ Artificial Discs have been implanted in more than 30 countries since 1987. Internationally published clinical findings and our own long-term experience show a broad applicability of the CHARITÉ Artificial Disc, which has become an accepted alternative to fusion. Developments regarding the fixation and the rotational center of the prosthesis could further minimize the complication rate and still improve mid- and long-term results.

In summary, biomechanical static and dynamic tests and clinical experience have shown that the CHARITÉ Artificial Disc is well suited to replace the lumbar intervertebral disc in several important functions. It can be implanted in patients with symptomatic degenerative intervertebral discs from segments L2-3 through to L5(6)-S1. The implant allows for long-term segmental motion in extension, flexion, side-bending, and rotation; stabilizes the surgical segment; and increases the height of the intervertebral space, which in turn leads to a clinically relevant relief of the facet joints and of the soft tissue structures within the spinal canal and the intervertebral foramina. Patients with CHARITÉ Artificial Disc do not require any specific postoperative physiotherapy and can be quickly reintegrated back into daily life and work.

REFERENCES

1. Ahrens JE. In vitro evaluation of the LINK SB Charité intervertebral prosthesis: Stability biomechanical testing (Project R). Institute for Spine & Biomedical Research, Plano, Texas, 1997.
2. Ahrens JE. Mechanical evaluation of the SB Charité artificial disc: Estimation of permanent deformation (project report). Texas Health Research Institute, Plano, Texas, 1999.
3. Ahrens JE, Phansalkar A. Mechanical evaluation of the SB Charité artificial disc: Static testing (project report). Texas Health Research Institute, Plano, Texas, 1998.
4. Bogduk N. Klinische Anatomie von Lendenwirbelsäule und Sakrum. Rehabilitation und Präventation. Heidelberg: Springer-Verlag, Band 57, 2000.
5. Büttner-Janz K. The Development of the Artificial Disc SB Charité. Dallas, Texas: Hundley & Assoc, 1992.
6. Büttner-Janz K. Die funktionelle Zwischenwirbelendoprothetik SB Charité—Implantatentwicklung, Biomechanik, Patientenanalyse, Perspektive. Doctoral dissertation. Berlin, 1989.
7. Büttner-Janz K, Hahn S, Schikora K, et al. Grundlagen einer erfolgreichen Anwendung der LINK® Zwischenwirbel-Endoprothese Modell SB Charité™. Orthopäde 31:441-453, 2002.
8. Büttner-Janz K, Keller A, Lemaire JP. Intervertebral disc endoprosthesis. US Patent No 5401269–28.03.95.
9. Wolff J. Das Gesetz der Transformation der Knochen. Berlin: Hirschwald, 1892.

CHAPTER

7

ProDisc: Design and Clinical Results

Jack E. Zigler

The ProDisc was designed in the late 1980s by the French orthopaedic spine surgeon Thierry Marnay. From March 1990 to February 1993, Marnay implanted this artificial disc into 64 patients.[2] In a situation somewhat unique in scientific endeavor, he resisted the impulse to accelerate the implantations, and instead allowed these 64 patients to "incubate" while he observed their progress. In 1999, these patients were studied to determine the long-term results of implantation, by which time three of these patients had died from unrelated causes, but 58 of the surviving 61 patients (95%) were found and studied extensively at 7- to 11-year follow-up. All implants were intact and functioning and there had been no implant removals, revisions, or failures. There was no evidence of subsidence on follow-up radiographs compared to the perioperative films, as reported by the operating surgeon as well as by an independent orthopaedic spine surgeon. A significant (p <0.001) reduction in patient-reported back and leg pain was identified; 92.7% of these patients were "satisfied" or "extremely satisfied" with the procedure. Two thirds of these patients had single-level implants whereas one third had two-level ProDiscs. There was no difference in outcome between the one- and two-level ProDisc implantations. What is most important, at this long-term follow-up no device-related safety issues, no untoward effects, no complications, and no adverse events were found.

Implant Design

The ProDisc (Spine Solutions/Synthes, New York, New York) is based on spherical articulations (Fig. 7-1) and has metal endplates made of a cobalt-chromium-molybdenum alloy (CoCrMo).

The convex bearing surface, which snap-fits into the inferior endplate, is made of ultrahigh-molecular-weight polyethylene (UHMWPE). It is anchored through a large central keel and two spikes on each endplate. Physiologically, the ProDisc matches normal ranges of motion in flexion, extension, axial rotation, and lateral bending. The device is modular, so the surgeon can customize

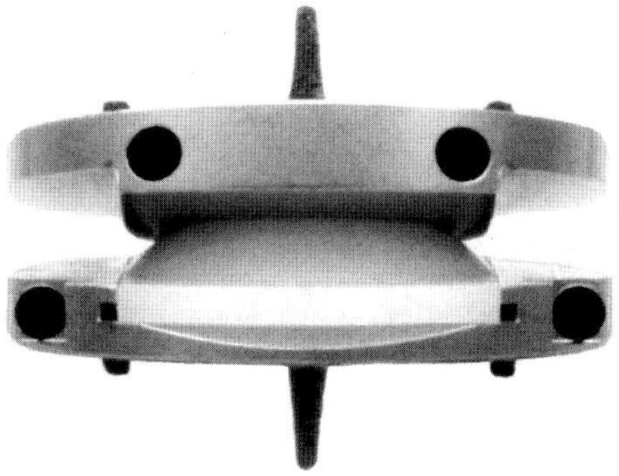

Fig. 7-1 The ProDisc device has two metal endplates and a polyethylene core.

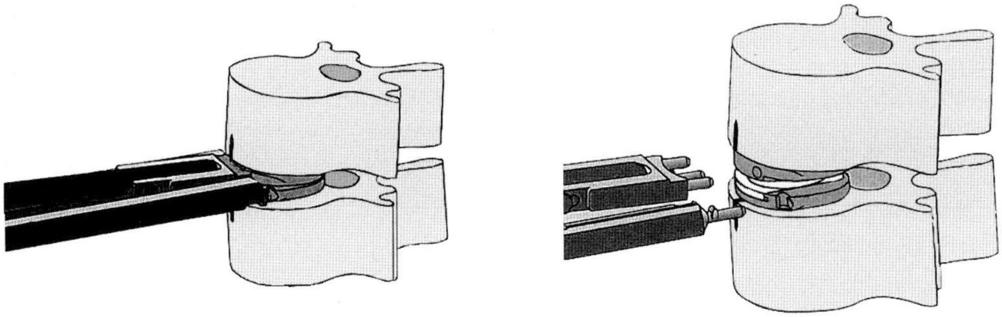

Fig. 7-2 The endplates of the devices are implanted, followed by insertion of the core, after which the insertion instrumentation is removed.

the device to each patient's unique anatomic and physiologic requirements. There are two endplate sizes (medium and large), three heights of the polyethylene component (10, 12, and 14 mm), and two lordosis angles (6 and 11 degrees).

The implantation instrumentation is very straightforward and user friendly. Minimal-access approaches to the lumbar spine are typically via a mini-retroperitoneal approach, and are possible given the streamlined design of the instrumentation. The endplates are inserted in a collapsed form so that overdistraction of the disc space is not required (Fig. 7-2). Only after the metal endplates are seated in the vertebral bodies is the disc space distracted. The surgeon can assess the soft tissue tension and insert an appropriately sized UHMWPE implant within the disc space, snap-fitting it into the lower metal endplate to complete the assembly process within the body.

Clinical Studies

The ProDisc has been implanted in over 1000 patients in Europe since December 1999. A multicenter FDA study was started in the United States in October 2001; the first ProDisc in the United States was implanted at the Texas Back Institute on October 3, 2001. Nineteen study centers will ultimately be

A

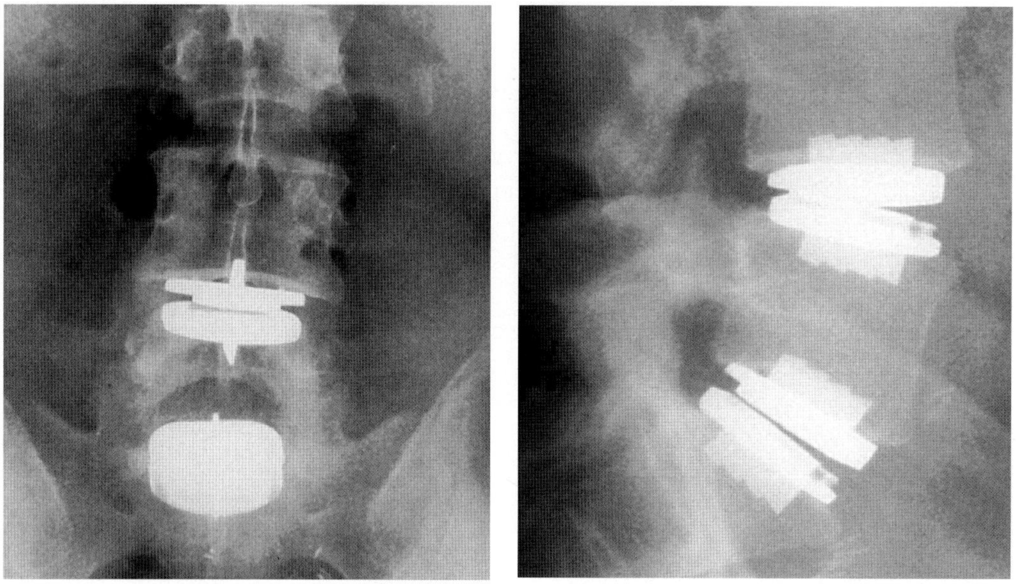

B

Fig. 7-3 **A,** Flexion and **B,** extension radiographs show segmental motion at each of the two replaced intervertebral segments.

participating in a prospective randomized study comparing the ProDisc with the gold standard of a 360-degree (front and back) fusion using allograft in the intervertebral space and pedicle screws with autograft posteriorly. Fig. 7-3 shows radiographs of a two-level disc replacement.

European Experience

Marnay reported his 7- to 11-year results in the initial implantation group.[2] From 1990 to 1993, 93 prostheses were implanted in 64 patients by the anterior approach at levels from L2 to S1. Of these, 39 cases were single-level, 21 cases required two levels, and 4 cases were three-level implants. The patients all had a history of chronic low back pain and had failed conservative therapy. Clinical evaluations, VAS, neurologic status, return to work, medication requirements, SF-36, Oswestry scales, and Beaujon scores were all recorded. Radiographic parameters including the height of the implant, motion, and any evidence of subsidence or resorption were also noted.

At average follow-up of 8.6 years after surgery, no ProDiscs had been explanted. Five patients with ongoing pain had undergone fusion by a posterior approach. Radiographically all implants are stable and show no migration or subsidence. Patients' back pain measured on VAS averaged 8.5 preoperatively and decreased to 3.0 at final evaluation; leg pain decreased to 1.9 from 7.1. At final follow-up, 65% of the patients reported that they were "entirely satisfied," 28%

were "satisfied," and only 7% were "not satisfied." These patient-reported outcomes were supported by Oswestry, SF-36, and Beaujon scores.

Mayer et al[3] in Munich, Germany reported preliminary results in 34 consecutive patients. Their follow-up was shorter, averaging 5.8 months on patients implanted between June 2000 and March 2002. In their patients VAS averaged 6.3 preoperatively and decreased by 3.9 points on average. Oswestry averaged 19.1 points before surgery and decreased postoperatively by an average of 11.5 points. Although all patients had back pain preoperatively, 76% reported no back pain when they were evaluated postoperatively. Subjectively, 82.6% of the patients were either "completely satisfied" or "satisfied."

Bertagnoli and Kumar[1] reported the results of 134 ProDiscs implanted in 108 patients in a prospectively designed study. Follow-up ranged from 3 months to 2 years in 58 male and 50 female patients with an average age of 41.5 years. Preoperative diagnoses included disc degeneration with vertical instability in 67, failed disc surgery syndrome in 35, and transition zone syndrome in six patients. All patients had been treated conservatively for at least 6 months, and all had positive discography at the operated levels. Overall clinical outcomes were excellent in 90.8%, good in 7.4%, and fair in 1.8% (two patients). There were no poor results. Nine patients had residual leg or facetogenic back pain after surgery. Of the 54 patients with greater than 1 year follow-up, 35 resumed their usual occupations, and 17 needed to go back to lighter duty; two patients were unable to return to work, and all patients had increased range of motion at the operated levels.

Bertagnoli and Kumar[1] correlated their surgical results with the preoperative findings (number of levels, amount of degenerative disc and facet disease, adjacent level disc height, and presence of instability), and were able to organize these indication complexes into predictive categories. They termed the *prime* indication as a single level disc of more than 4 mm in height with no osteoarthritic changes in the facets, no adjacent level degeneration, and intact posterior elements without instability.

Patients considered to be *good* candidates were similar to the prime group, but this group allowed patients with involvement of two disc levels and minimum changes of the adjacent disc segment, facet, and posterior segment instability. The *borderline* and *poor* groups permitted patients with up to three involved levels. The borderline group had patients with decreased disc space height and patients in the poor group had gross degenerative changes in the spine.

Average patient satisfaction levels were 98% in the *prime* category, 93% in the *good* category, and 83% in the *borderline* category. Bertagnoli and Kumar[1] noted that the overall outcome of disc replacement surgeries may be compromised by

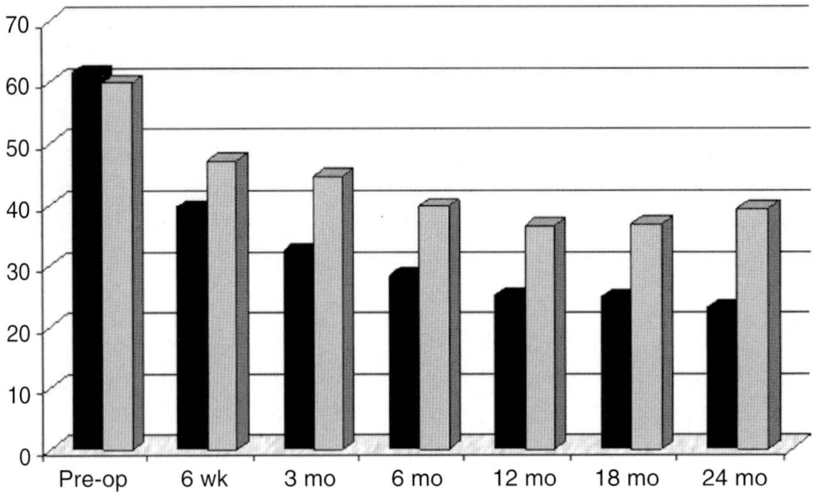

Fig. 7-4 The Oswestry scores improved in both surgical groups. At most of the follow-up periods, the total disc replacement (TDR) scores *(black columns)* were significantly lower than the 360-degree fusion scores *(gray columns)* ($p < 0.05$).

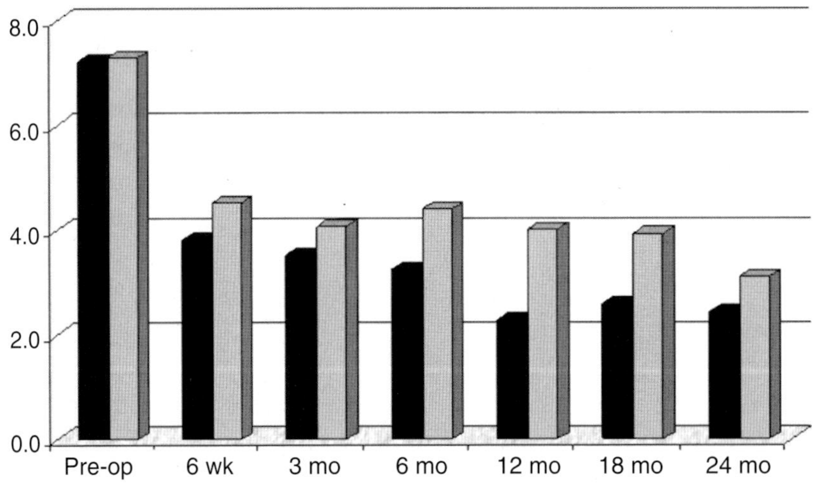

Fig. 7-5 The VAS scores assessing pain improved in both surgical groups. At most of the follow-up periods, the ProDisc scores *(black columns)* were significantly lower than the 360-degree fusion scores *(gray columns)* ($p < 0.05$).

the inclusion of patients with borderline and poor indications. They stressed that surgeons should place great emphasis on the appropriateness of the indications of these patients for arthroplasty.

Experience in the United States

On October 3, 2001, the first ProDisc was implanted in the United States to initiate an FDA IDE study comparing the efficacy of ProDisc with 360-degree lumbar fusion at one or two adjacent levels from L3 to S1.[4] In total, 19 centers participated in this study. More than 1000 ProDiscs have been implanted so far in the United States. Multicenter data will be collected and presented to the FDA at the completion of the study.

What follows is an overview of our experience with the first 100 patients who have reached a minimum of 12-month follow-up and 35 patients who have reached 24-month follow-up at our clinic. The class I data from this prospective randomized study allow comparison of the 12 to 24 month results of 72 patients receiving ProDisc (three were nonrandomized "teaching" cases at the beginning of the study) and 28 who received fusion. Data were collected preoperatively and at 6 weeks and 3, 6, 12, 18, and 24 months postoperatively. The ProDisc and fusion groups were similar in demographics, including gender, age, weight, smoking history, preoperative medication usage, nonoperative treatment, and prior surgeries.

Intraoperative data showed statistically significant differences in operative time and blood loss between the groups, favoring the ProDisc patients. The ProDisc patients left the hospital in 2.2. days, compared with 3.3 days for the fusion patients.

Presented in Fig. 7-4 are the mean Oswestry scores for the two surgical groups. In both groups, the scores were significantly improved at all follow-up periods compared to the preoperative value. Although the preoperative mean scores were similar, at most of the follow-up periods the ProDisc scores were significantly lower than the scores in the fusion group. The VAS scores assessing pain followed a similar pattern (Fig. 7-5). In both groups the outcome scores were significantly lower than the preoperative mean. At the 12-month follow-up, the scores for the TDR group score were significantly lower; complications in the two groups were similar.

CONCLUSION

The ProDisc has been used since the early 1990s and the results from Europe have been encouraging. Our center's short-term results from the FDA IDE study being conducted in the United States have also been encouraging and demonstrate that the device yields results as good as, or better than, those achieved with combined anterior/posterior lumbar fusion. Only long-term follow-up will determine whether TDR can prevent the potential problems related to adjacent segment breakdown that may occur with rigid fusion.

REFERENCES

1. Bertagnoli R, Kumar S. Indications for full prosthetic disc arthroplasty: A correlation of clinical outcome against a variety of indications. Eur Spine J 11(Suppl 2):S131-S136, 2002.
2. Marnay T. Lumbar disc replacement: 7- to 11-year results with ProDisc. Spine J 2:94S, 2002.
3. Mayer HM, Wiechert K, Korge A, et al. Minimally invasive total disc replacement: Surgical technique and preliminary clinical results. Eur Spine J 11(Suppl 2):S124-S130, 2002.
4. Zigler JE, Vialle EN, Burd TA, et al. Lumbar spine arthroplasty: Early results using the ProDisc II—a prospective randomized trial of arthroplasty versus fusion. J Spinal Disord Tech 16:352-361, 2003.

CHAPTER

8

Development of Disc Nucleus Replacement

Qi-Bin Bao ▪ Hansen A. Yuan

Although disc arthroplasty has been attempted since the early 1960s, with relatively less success than arthroplasty of knee and hip joints, the demand for better treatment of low back pain has accelerated the developmental activities of disc arthroplasty since the late 1980s. Because the intervertebral disc has a multicomponent structure, when disc arthroplasty is considered, either the entire disc or only part of the degenerative disc can be replaced. The majority of efforts in replacing part of the disc have been on the replacement of nucleus pulposus.

Rationale for a Nucleus Prosthesis

Discectomy remains the most common surgical treatment for degenerative disc disease, despite the introduction of interbody threaded metal cages. If the degenerative nucleus is not replaced with a nucleus prosthesis, the biologic and biomechanical function of the nucleus pulposus will be compromised after surgery. Biologically, the nucleus pulposus functions as a fluid pump that facilitates body fluid diffusion, carrying nutrients and removing metabolites for the avascular disc. Biomechanically, although the nucleus presents as loose gel and has little resistance to physiologic loads by itself, it inflates the anulus, shares a significant portion of compressive load with the anulus, and makes the disc construct more stable against physiologic loading. Unless these functions are restored after discectomy, the remaining nucleus and the inner layers of anulus will degenerate further and more compressive load will shift to the anulus, causing disc instability and disc height loss.[15,16,18] Many secondary complications associated with these functional changes can occur in discectomy patients.[18,27]

Therefore in considering disc arthroplasty it is logical to replace only the nucleus pulposus instead of replacing the entire disc for patients whose other disc tissues, such as anulus and endplate, are still functional. There are several obvious advantages of a nucleus prosthesis over a total disc prosthesis. Replacing only the nucleus preserves the remaining disc tissues, that is, the anulus and endplates and their functions. Because the nucleus has a much simpler structure and function than the anulus and endplates, a nucleus prosthesis is relatively easier to design than a total disc prosthesis.

Another major advantage of having a nucleus prosthesis is that because of its small size and the fact that it does not need to be attached to the endplate, this prosthesis can be implanted using minimally invasive surgery. Depending on the design and choice of material, the device can even be implanted percutaneously. For biomechanical reasons, almost all the artificial total discs attempted so far have required the removal of the entire disc. An implant with cross-sectional dimensions similar to that of the disc is then inserted by either an anterior or a lateral approach, both of which are more traumatic and carry a higher risk than the posterior approach. Although a nucleus prosthesis might be easy to extrude because it is not fixed to the vertebra, the severity of implant extrusion is worse with a total disc prosthesis than a nucleus prosthesis because of the bulkiness and rigidity of a total disc prosthesis. The salvage procedure, especially for levels L4-5 and above, is also much more difficult and riskier for a total disc prosthesis than for a nucleus prosthesis. Because of the relatively high risk and more difficult salvage procedure, it is difficult to justify using total disc prosthesis for patients with early stage disc degeneration or simple disc herniation, especially when less invasive and less riskier options, such as nucleus replacement, are available.

Design Requirements and Desirable Features for a Nucleus Prosthesis

There are several basic design requirements that a nucleus prosthesis has to meet. The device has to be biocompatible as a long-term implant; it should have sufficient static and fatigue strength; the wear on the implant should be minimal; and the wear particles generated from the implant should cause minimal adverse reactions to surrounding and systemic tissues. Finally, the device should be able to restore or maintain normal disc anatomy and function.

Because of the design difference, the actual benefits that a nucleus prosthesis offers can be quite different from device to device. The choice of both material and design can affect the final performance of the nucleus prosthesis. In addition to meeting the basic design requirements, such as biocompatibility and fatigue strength, the following are several desirable features of a nucleus prosthesis:

- Restores normal load distribution
- Avoids endplate abrasion
- Has a good implant-cavity conformity
- Allows proper disc distraction
- Maintains normal lordosis, especially for the L5-S1 disc
- Restores body fluid diffusion capability
- Implants through a small anular incision
- Implant bonds with and/or integrates into the surrounding tissues
- Is compatible with different discectomy techniques
- Is easy to implant

When designing a prosthesis, researchers often choose a material with mechanical properties similar to those of the targeted tissue. However, in replacing the nucleus pulposus, using a loose gel like the normal nucleus pulposus would not work, because such a material would readily herniate through the anular defect unless the anular defect is repaired. Currently there are no effective ways to seal the anular defect, so the nucleus prosthesis has to be firm enough and have adequate compressive and shear moduli and strengths, such that it will not easily extrude through the anular defect. Because of the high hoop tensile stiffness of the anulus, the nucleus is significantly "stiffened" in the disc construct; that is, the modulus of the nucleus (the ratio of stress to strain) in the disc construct is several orders of magnitude higher than the modulus of the nucleus material itself. Therefore the implanted disc could have virtually similar mechanical properties when materials with a wide range of modulus are used. Whereas conceptually the low modulus material might provide more even stress distribution on the implant, the low modulus material also presents a high risk of implant extrusion. Therefore the selection of material modulus for the nucleus prosthesis should be balanced between stress distribution and the risk of implant extrusion. The lower limit of material modulus for the nucleus implant is largely dictated by the risk of implant extrusion because of the anular defect. The upper limit of the material modulus for the nucleus application is dictated by the risk of stress shielding. A nucleus material that is too stiff might create an abnormally high contact stress against the endplate and might accelerate endplate wear, causing reactions to the endplate. The surface finishing of the implant could also affect the wear of both implant and endplate. In general, a material with a low coefficient of friction is desirable.

The peak contact stress on the implant/endplate interface also depends on the conformity of the implant with the cavity. Because the geometry and size of the disc cavity created in the discectomy are highly variable from patient to patient and also depend on surgical technique, it would be difficult to achieve good implant/cavity conformity when using a preformed nucleus implant. An undersized implant could be problematic in evenly distributing the stress on the endplate and cause high contact stress, especially when a high modulus nucleus implant is used and also could cause excessive movement within the disc and lead to high wear on the endplate and/or implant. An oversized implant could increase the chance of implant extrusion. Good implant/cavity conformity would also help to reduce the motion of the implant and evenly distribute the lateral bulge force to the surrounding anulus.

Because most patients with disc degeneration will have different degrees of disc height loss, a nucleus prosthesis should have the capability to distract the disc space so that normal disc height can be restored. Predistraction with ancillary instruments, such as an external distraction pin, internal distraction tamper, or balloon, might help to open the disc space. However, this adds to the complexity of the surgery, and the disc, which is elastic, is likely to lose most of the distraction as soon as the internal distraction is removed. Thus the nucleus prosthesis should be able to distract the disc space during implantation. Maintaining normal lordosis, especially for the L5-S1 disc, should also be taken into consideration. If a preformed implant with a high modulus material is being used, it may be necessary to design the implant in a wedge shape for the L5-S1 disc.

Although most nucleus prostheses might not need nutrients if the device does not contain living cells, it may still be beneficial if the device can restore normal body fluid pumping function. This function is likely to enhance nutrient diffusion for the remaining nucleus and inner anulus that are still avascular. Fluid diffusion can be enhanced via two mechanisms: by restoring the modulus elasticity of the disc so that the remaining nucleus and inner anulus can maximize the fluid pumping in the cyclic loading and by using materials such as hydrogel or another hydrophilic matrix with swelling pressure similar to that of the normal nucleus pulposus.

Because the nucleus prosthesis is designed to share the compressive load with the anulus, the nucleus prosthesis can be subject to high compressive stress, that is, over 2 MPa in daily life.[34,37] In addition, the anular defect, either preexisting or created during surgery to remove the nucleus and place the implant, will leave a weak area for implant extrusion. Preventing implant extrusion is just as important as dealing with disc reherniation after discectomy in determining the success of a nucleus replacement. In general, the nucleus prosthesis is not designed to be fixed into the vertebral bodies, so other measures have to be taken to address this issue. One of the most effective ways is to design the nucleus prosthesis so that it can be inserted into the disc space through a small anular incision. Many advances in minimally invasive surgery now allow the discectomy to be performed through a small anular opening; therefore the limiting factor is how big an anular incision is required for implant insertion. The smaller the anular incision, the less chance there is that the implant will extrude. Another way to reduce the likelihood of nucleus implant extrusion is to repair the anular defect. If the nucleus prosthesis can be bonded to the surrounding anulus or endplates, either by mechanical means or by tissue integration, the risk of implant extrusion can also be reduced.

Because the most popular technique for discectomy continues to be open or microdiscectomy using a posterior approach, it will be easy to gain acceptance if a nucleus device can be easily implanted through a posterior approach with minimal risk of implant extrusion. If a device has to be implanted via an anterior or lateral approach, the application is limited, even though it may be beneficial to some patients. With the development of many other less invasive techniques, such as arthroscopic microdiscectomy (AMD), automated percutaneous lumbar discectomy (APLD), and microendoscopic discectomy (MED), a device that can be implanted via these minimally invasive techniques would also capitalize on the benefits of minimally invasive surgery and of the nucleus prosthesis itself.

Preclinical Studies

Preclinical studies on the nucleus prosthesis should focus on three major areas: biomechanical testing, biocompatibility testing, and surgical technique evaluation. Biomechanical testing can be further divided into testing of the implant and testing of implanted cadaver discs. Implant testing should include mechanical property characterization, compressive strength, fatigue/wear test, and biodurability test if the biostability of the material has not been established. The average compressive strength for the lumbar functional spinal unit (FSU: two vertebrae and one intervertebral disc) has been reported in the range of about 1000 to 5300 N, and the common failure mode is vertebral fracture through the endplate.[7,19,36] The variation in compressive strength of the FSU is very high and depends largely on the patient's age and bone density. Although it has never been measured directly, the stress at failure in the nucleus area is likely to be close to the failure strength for the cancellous core of a vertebral body. The compressive strength of cancellous bone of vertebrae has been reported to average 1.55 to 4.6 MPa[31]; therefore it is important to design a nucleus prosthesis with at least as much compressive strength so that the implant would not fail before the fracture of vertebrae.

As yet, there are no well-defined and accepted standards for the fatigue and wear testing of nucleus prostheses. The fatigue test should mimic the load and motion of a lumbar disc under normal walking conditions, similar to what has been tested for hip and knee prostheses. Because the nucleus prosthesis is designed to replace only a part of the disc and to share the compressive load with the remaining anulus, the actual load on the implant depends on the size of the implant, so it would be better to set the stress range in the fatigue test instead of setting a load range that is commonly used to test interbody fusion devices and total disc prostheses. The peak compressive load on the lumbar discs is estimated to be 1000 N in normal walking.[32] Because the corresponding intradiscal pressure (or stress) for this load range is between 0.53 to 0.65 MPa,[34,37] the upper stress in the fatigue test of nucleus prostheses should be at least 0.7 MPa. Also, because the device is rigidly fixed onto the vertebral bodies, artificial total discs should include a shear component in the fatigue test so that the shear fatigue strength of a total disc prosthesis can be assessed. However, because the nucleus prosthesis typically is not fixed to the endplates and the shear resistance of the implanted disc should come primarily from the remaining anulus, the shear force on the nucleus implant might not be nearly as high as that on the artificial total disc. However, in normal walking, a human disc has about 3 degrees of flexion and extension,[35] and this range of flexion and extension movement should be included in the fatigue test. Most nucleus prostheses are made of viscoelastic materials, so the frequency of the fatigue test should not be much higher than the physiologic walking frequency. If a much higher frequency is to be used, justification should be provided to demonstrate that the increase in loading frequency will not affect the device fatigue strength. Although the implant is intended to be used in relatively young patients and has been proposed to have a fatigue life of at least 40 to 100 million loading cycles, at least 10 million cycles should be tested before a clinical trial.[12] Longer fatigue cycle testing is strongly recommended before the product is made commercially available.

Because the nucleus prosthesis is allowed to have some movements against the endplate, the implant should not be fixed into the upper and lower testing platens during fatigue tests, so that the relative movement between the implant and testing plates is permitted to occur and the wear between the interfaces can be assessed. The contacting plate material and surface finishing should be chosen to mimic the wear between the implant and cartilage endplate. The device should be tested in saline solution at 37° C. If evaluators are considering using more biologic fluids, such as animal serum, they must weigh the trade-off between ease of collection and analysis of wear particles and attempts to mimic the effect of the liquid medium on the wear of the implant. Another challenge in the nucleus prosthesis fatigue test is to mimic the anular constraint. If the implant has a much lower compressive modulus than that of a disc, it would not be possible to simulate physiologic stress and strain without a means to simulate the constraint of the anulus. One way to mimic this constraint is to design an artificial ring with tensile modulus similar to that of the anulus; the second option is to test the implant in a sealed liquid vessel that provides a compression modulus similar to a disc.[2]

The most direct way to demonstrate the effectiveness of a nucleus prosthesis in restoring disc height and biomechanical functions is to use a human cadaver model.[10,14,21,30] Although a calf cadaver model has been used to test fusion devices, its adequacy for nucleus prosthesis testing has yet to be established. Details on cadaver sample preparation, setup, and data analyses are described by Goel et al.[17] The common testing procedure is to test human cadaver functional spinal units (FSUs) in three different stages: when intact, at discectomy, and at the time of implantation. The test should cover all major loading modes: compression, flexion, extension, lateral bending, and torsion, to a physiologic load of 800 to 1000 N for compression and of at least 6 Nm for rotational loading. Because of the viscoelastic nature of human disc, the stiffness from the first loading cycle could be fairly variable depending on the recovery time between loadings. Therefore it is recommended to load at least three consecutive cycles and use the last cycle data for the calculation of disc height, stiffness, and range of motion (ROM). Disc height and load Vs displacement curves should be recorded so that the ROM and stiffness of a disc can be calculated and compared for a FSU at different stages. Discectomy should be performed in accordance to clinical practice; typically, there will be a decrease in the disc height and an increase in ROM after discectomy. The nucleus implant should demonstrate the restoration of normal disc height and normal ROM without significantly increasing the stiffness for the implanted disc. Because of the high variability of disc height, ROM, and stiffness between the different FSUs, it is preferable to use each individual FSU as its own control and compare the changes for each FSU at the three different stages: intact, after discectomy, and at implantation.

Implant extrusion should be assessed in the preclinical study; because implant extrusion is largely dependent on the actual constraint from the anulus and on the surgical technique used, it should be assessed with human cadaver discs using the actual surgical technique to remove the nucleus and to implant the device. If the implanted cadaver discs show a high rate of implant extrusion under physiologic loading conditions, the implant might not be stable enough for clinical use. To further assess the potential risks of implant extrusion and other failure mechanisms, discs with nucleus implant should be compressed to failure. The failure modes should be assessed and it should be ascertained that the implant does not cause premature failure of the endplate or the vertebral body and that there is no implant extrusion. The failure load for the implanted disc should be equal to or larger than the average failure load for intact lumbar discs reported in the literature. However, the maximum strength of an intact FSU is highly variable and depends largely on the bone density and the degenerative status of the specimen. Also, although cadaver testing can provide valuable information before clinical trials, it has its limitations, one of which is that it is difficult to find human cadaver discs with disc herniation, which could significantly increase the implant extrusion rate.

For general biocompatibility testing, ISO 10993 has provided good guidelines for a long-term implant. The main issue in the biocompatibility study is whether an animal disc implant study needs to be conducted. This issue has been debated for many years in the literature and it is generally agreed that there is no good animal model to assess the efficacy of a disc implant because of the mechanical loading differences between quadrupedal animals and bipedal humans.[8,28] In any animal disc implant study, the implant should be used to replace only the disc nucleus with most of the anulus and endplate preserved, so the implant is exposed to a similar biologic environment to that in the human application. The assessment should focus on the necropsy and histologic examination of surrounding disc tissues and local nerve tissue. Some radiographic examinations might help to evaluate the disc height change and potential osteophyte formation. Because of the difficulty in conducting a discectomy and placing the implant in small animals, small animal models, such as rabbit and mice, cannot be used. Even some large animals, such as sheep, dogs, and goats, which have been widely used for many fusion devices, might not be the right models for a nucleus prosthesis because the lumbar disc of these animals may be too small for a complete discectomy and/or a nucleus implant. Thus we are left with only a few animal models to choose from. Mini-pigs, with weight near 100 kg, have a relatively good size disc; however, it was found that disc surgery of this model leads to severe disc degeneration and significant increase in disc stiffness.[23,24] The most suitable animal model for nucleus prosthesis found so far is the baboon. The anatomy and structure of the baboon lumbar disc are similar to that of humans, and the disc has a height in the range of 4 to 6 mm, which is large enough to perform a discectomy without significantly damaging the endplate. However, even in this model some degenerative changes and autofusion were found to occur at both implanted discs and sham-operated discs.[1] Because it is rare to see disc autofusion in humans after a discectomy, it indicates that some animals might react very differently to disc surgery than humans. Although an animal study is often used also to evaluate surgical technique and implant extrusion, the chance of implant extrusion in an animal model could be higher than in a human because of the difference in disc size. The dimension ratio of the implant to anular incision hole for an animal is generally much smaller than that for a human.

Surgical technique of device implantation should also be evaluated before clinical trials. Because human cadaver is probably the best model for this evaluation, the surgical technique evaluation is best when combined with human cadaver biomechanical testing. Intended surgical approach and technique should be used to remove the nucleus and implant the nucleus device. In this way, the biomechanical behavior of the implanted discs is more likely to reflect the real range found in clinical use.

Historic and Current Development of Nucleus Replacement

Historically, the first human implanted nucleus prosthesis, developed by Fernström in 1964, was a spherical endoprosthesis made of a stainless steel ball.[13] This solid ball device was meant to serve as a spacer that allows movement of adjacent vertebrae. It did not, for obvious reasons, restore the normal load distribution of the disc. Although this device is no longer used and has been considered a failure by the public, the only published research with long-term follow-up on a fairly large number of patients in whom this device was used showed reasonably good results in pain relief and return to work for these patients.[26]

Because solid metals are too stiff for nucleus devices, most nucleus prostheses use various elastomers or designs with viscoelastic properties. These elastic nucleus prostheses can be further divided by their design difference into nucleus prostheses that are preformed and those that are formed in situ.

Since the first attempt by Nachemson in 1960,[29] many nucleus prostheses formed in situ have been proposed and studied.[11,14,33] The most common design concept in this category is to inject an in situ curable polymer into the disc space and cure the polymer in situ to form a nucleus prosthesis. Materials proposed include silicone and polyurethane, the two most widely used medical elastomers. Several other in situ curable hydrogel elastomers have also been proposed recently.[6,25] The main advantage of this design is that a large implant can be formed by injecting the in situ curable material through a small anular window; this reduces the risk of implant extrusion and can be used in percutaneous surgeries. This design also has the advantages of better implant/cavity conformity and better stress distribution and implant stability. However, this design also presents several challenges. First, although many polymers might be able to cure in situ, it is not easy to design a polymer system that can be cured in situ and yet has enough mechanical strength to withstand the load with required fatigue life. The effect of curing conditions on the polymer mechanical property has to be taken into consideration. Second, the in situ cured polymer should be biocompatible. Because most monomers are toxic, it is critical that the polymerization be completed with minimal leaching. Third, the polymerization should be done within a reasonable amount of time. A long reaction time will not only lengthen the surgical time, but also may cause incomplete polymerization. Finally, during injection it is important to prevent the flowable polymer from coming out through the anular incision or other existing anular defects.

Recently, in an effort to address these challenges, Disc Dynamics, Inc, of Minneapolis developed an in situ formed nucleus device, DASCOR, which is formed by placing a folded expandable balloon into disc space after discectomy and then inflating the balloon by injecting an in situ curable polymer through the delivery catheter that is attached to the balloon to a predetermined endpoint (Table 8-1). The company has conducted extensive in vivo and in vitro studies to demonstrate the biocompatibility of the in situ cured polymer. The extractable study showed that the monomer leachables are minimal.[20] The balloon is made of a compliant yet very robust material, which allows significant expansion during polymer injection to fill and conform with the cavity. Because of these characteristics, the surgeon can distract the disc space under controlled pressure. The biomechanical study using a human cadaveric disc model showed that this device is able to restore both the disc height and the normal function of the disc.[9] The fatigue test of this device also demonstrated adequate mechanical fatigue strength for nucleus replacement application.[22]

An alternative to in situ cured polymer for nucleus replacement is to use precured polymer for nucleus implant. The advantages of this approach include more consistent implant properties and less concern about biocompatibility. The disadvantages include the difficulty in matching the implant size and shape with the cavity and the need for a big incision in the anulus for implant insertion. After some biomechanical, biocompatibility, and animal studies,[21] Hou probably was the first one who had the experience of implanting a preformed horseshoe-shaped silicone nucleus into over 30 patients with maximum follow-up of 4 years. The details of this study, unfortunately, have not yet been published.

In between these two markedly different design features, there is another design concept in which the size or shape of the nucleus prosthesis can be significantly reduced or altered during implantation, and regained or restored after the implantation. This can be achieved either by inserting a collapsible balloon into the disc and then inflating it with incompressible liquid or by implanting a

TABLE 8-1 DESIGN FEATURES

Device Name	Company	Material	Design
Prosthetic disc nucleus (PDN)	RayMedica	Polyacrylonitrile-polyacrylamide (HYPAN) hydrogel core enveloped by polyethylene (PE) jacket	A pair of pillow-shaped implants with a preformed and dehydrated hydrogel pellet encased in a flexible but inelastic PE jacket. Implants become hydrated in the disc.
Aquarelle	Stryker/ Howmedica	Polyvinyl alcohol (PVA) hydrogel	Preformed bullet-shaped implant injected in a semidehydrated state into disc space with an injection device. Implant adjusts its water content based on the intradiscal pressure.
DASCOR	Disc Dynamics	Polyurethane elastomer	In situ curable polyurethane is injected into a polyurethane balloon via a catheter and sets in the disc in minutes. The catheter is then removed.
Newcleus	Sulzer Spine-Tech	Polyurethane elastomer	A preformed, curled, spiral-shaped implant is straightened and inserted into disc space with an applicator device. The device is curled back to a spiral coil in the disc.
BioDisc	Cryolife	Protein hydrogel, similar to BioGlue	An in situ curable protein hydrogel is injected into disc space and sets in the disc in minutes.
Injectable disc nucleus (IDN)	SpineWave	In situ curable recombinant protein copolymer	Injected directly into disc space and cures in the body.
NeuDisc	Replication Medical	Hydrogel	Insert a dry hydrogel in rolled-up wafer form and hydrate in the body.

dehydrated hydrogel nucleus prosthesis that rehydrates in the disc. The preformed spiral-shaped nucleus implant belongs to this category.

In an attempt to restore the biologic function of the nucleus, in 1990 the concept of using hydrogel material for intervertebral nucleus replacement was developed.[4,5] It was demonstrated that the hydrogel nucleus implant can mimic the water imbibe-and-release capability of the nucleus tissue under cyclic loading.[3] Biomechanical studies have confirmed restoration of the disc anatomy and function after a hydrogel nucleus is implanted.[30] A fairly large animal study using a baboon model showed no evidence of local or systemic toxicity.[1] Since then, several other hydrogel nucleus replacement devices have been proposed and are currently under development.

Conclusion

Currently there are several nucleus prosthesis designs with active development activities, most of which are preclinical, and more are expected in the near future. Only very few nucleus prosthesis designs have been used clinically, and none of them is commercially available in the United States yet. Although the progress of disc arthroplasty has been slow compared with the progress of arthroplasty of other joints, and the development cycle is long and costly, the future of nucleus prostheses is bright because of the unparalleled benefits this device can provide for the treatment of low back pain.

REFERENCES

1. Allen MJ, Schoonmaker JE, Ordway NR, et al. Preclinical testing of a poly(vinyl alcohol) hydrogel nucleus in baboons. Presented at the Annual Meeting of the North American Spine Society, New Orleans, Oct 2000.
2. Bagga CS, Williams P, Higham PA, et al. Development of fatigue test model for a spinal nucleus prosthesis with preliminary results for a hydrogel spinal prosthetic nucleus. ASME/AICheE/ASCE Summer Bioengineering Conference, Sunriver, Ore, 1997.
3. Bao QB, Bagga CS, Higham PA. Swelling pressure of hydrogel: A perceived benefit for a spinal prosthetic nucleus. Transactions of the Tenth Annual Meeting of the International Intradiscal Therapy Society, Naples, Fla, 1997.
4. Bao QB, Higham PA. Hydrogel intervertebral disc nucleus. US Patent No 5,047,055, Sept 10, 1991.
5. Bao QB, Higham PA. Hydrogel intervertebral disc nucleus. US Patent No 5,192,326, March 9, 1993.
6. Benton PG, Yuksel KU, Cash A, et al. Use of a polymerized protein hydrogel for post-discectomy nucleus augmentation. Transactions of the Spine Arthroplasty Society, Scottsdale, Ariz, 2003.
7. Brown T, Hanson R, Yorra A. Some mechanical tests on the lumbo-sacral spine with particular reference to the intervertebral disc. J Bone Joint Surg Am 39:1135, 1957.
8. Brown M, Ray CD, Frymoyer JW, et al. Discussion of the artificial disc. In Weinstein JN, ed. Clinical Efficacy and Outcome in the Diagnosis and Treatment of Low Back Pain. New York: Raven Press, 1992.

9. Dooris A, Hudgins G, Goel V, et al. A nucleus replacement may restore normal multisegment biomechanics after discectomy. Presented at the Annual Meeting of the Orthopaedic Research Society, Feb 2002.
10. Eysel P, Rompe JD, Schoeymaye R, et al. Biomechanical behaviour of a prosthetic lumbar nucleus. Act Neurochir (Wien) 141:1083-1087, 1999.
11. Fassio B, Ginestie JF. Disc prosthesis made of silicone. Experimental study and first clinical cases. Nouv Presse Med 2:207, 1978.
12. FDA Guidance Document for the Preparation of IDEs for Spinal Systems. Jan 13, 2000. http://www.fda.gov/cdrh/ode/87.html.
13. Fernström U. Metallic disk prosthesis for lumbar disc rupture. Nord Med 71:160, 1964.
14. Garcia A, Lavignolle B, Morlier P, et al. Intradiscal polymerization: preliminary results of chemical and biomechanical studies. In Brock M, Mayer HM, Weigel J, eds. The Artificial Disc. Berlin: Springer-Verlag, 1991, pp 39-43.
15. Goel VK, Goyal S, Clark C, et al. Kinematics of the whole lumbar spine—effect of discectomy. Spine 10:543-554, 1985.
16. Goel VK, Nishiyama K, Weinstein JN, et al. Mechanical properties of lumbar spinal motion segments as affected by partial disc removal. Spine 11:1008-1012, 1986.
17. Goel VK, Weinstein JN, Patwardhan AG. Biomechanics of intact ligamenous spine. In Goel VK, Weinstein JN, eds. Biomechanics of Spine: Clinical and Surgical Perspective. Boca Raton, Fla: CRC Press, 1990, pp 97-156.
18. Hanley EN, Shapiro DE. The development of low-back pain after excision of lumbar disc. J Bone Joint Surg Am 71:719-721, 1989.
19. Hirsch C, Nachemson A. A new observation on the mechanical behavior of lumbar discs. Acta Orthop Scand 23:254, 1954.
20. Ho J, Bao QB, Arsenyev A, et al. HPLC analysis of methylene dianiline from extracts of an in-situ joint restorative polymer. Presented at the Meeting of the Sixth World Biomaterials Congress, Kamuela, Hawaii, May 2000.
21. Hou TS, Tu KY, Xu YK, et al. Lumbar intervertebral disc prosthesis. Chin Med J (Engl) 104:381-386, 1991.
22. Hudgins RG, Bao QB. Durability test method for a prosthetic nucleus (PN). In Melkerson MN, Griffith SL, Kirkpatrick JS, eds. Spinal Implants: Are We Evaluating Them Appropriately? ASTM STP 1431. West Conshohocken, Penn, ASTM International, 2002.
23. Kaapa E, Holm S, Inkinen R, et al. Proteoglycan chemistry in experimentally injured porcine intervertebral disc. J Spinal Disord 7:296-306, 1994.
24. Kaigle A, Ekstrom L, Holm S, et al. In vivo dynamic stiffness of the porcine lumbar spine exposed to cyclic loading: Influence of load and degeneration. J Spinal Disord 11:65-70, 1998.
25. Kitchel A, Gappello J. Injectable biomaterials for augmentation of the nucleus pulposus. Presented at the Annual Meeting of the Spinal Arthroplasty Society, Scottsdale, Ariz, May 2003.
26. McKenzie AH. Fernström intervertebral disc arthroplasty: A long-term evaluation. Orthop Internat 3:313-324, 1995.
27. Manniche C, Asmussen KH, Vinterberg H, et al. Back pain, sciatica and disability following first-time conventional haemilaminectomy for lumbar disc herniation. Use of "Low Back Pain Rating Scale" as a postal questionnaire. Dan Med Bull 41:103-106, 1994.
28. Matsuzaki H, Wakabayashi K. Animal models for reconstruction of vertebral column and intervertebral disc. In Animal Models in Orthopedic Research. Boca Raton, Fla: CRC Press, 1999.
29. Nachemson A. Some mechanical properties of the lumbar intervertebral disc. Bull Hosp Joint Dis (NY) 23:130-132, 1962.

30. Ordway NR, Zheng YG, McCullen GM, et al. Biomechanical evaluation of the functional spine unit with a hydrogel implant. Presented at the Annual Meeting of the North American Spine Society, Vancouver, Canada, Oct 1996.
31. Panjabi MM. A study of the compressive properties of lumbar vertebral trabeculae: Effect of tissue characteristics. Spine 12:56, 1987.
32. Patwardhan AG, Havey RM, Meade KP, et al. A follower load increases the load-carrying capacity of the lumbar spine in compression. Spine 24:1003-1009, 1999.
33. Roy-Camille R, Saillant G, Lavaste F. Experimental study of lumbar disc replacement. Rev Chir Orthop Reparatr Appar Mot (Suppl II)1 64:106-107, 1978.
34. Sato K, Kikuchi S, Yonezawa T. In vivo intradiscal pressure measurements in healthy individuals and in patients with ongoing back problems. Spine 24:2468-2474, 1999.
35. Thurston AJ. Repeatability studies of a television/computer system for measuring spinal and pelvic movements. J Biomed Eng 4:129-132, 1982.
36. Virgin W. Experimental investigations into physical properties of intervertebral disc. J Bone Joint Surg Br 33:607, 1951.
37. Wilke H-J, Neef P, Caimi M, et al. New in vivo measurements of pressures in the intervertebral disc in daily life. Spine 24:755-762, 1999.

PART III

TECHNIQUES AND TECHNOLOGIES

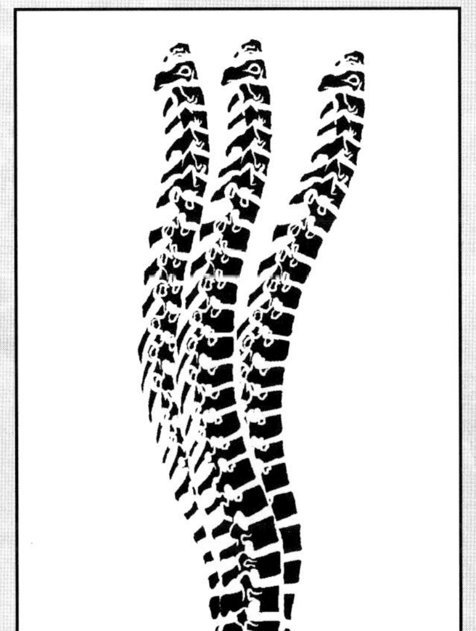

CHAPTER

9

Anterior Approach to the Lumbar Spine

Salvador A. Brau

Spinal arthroplasty presents new challenges for access surgeons because this technique requires a safe and fast approach to the lumbar spine through a relatively small incision. Mini-open approaches for surgery of the anterior lumbar region have been described[1,5,6]; however, total disc replacement (TDR) requires wider mobilization of the vessels because of the increased width of the prosthesis when compared with threaded cages. This requirement may result in a higher complication rate, especially at L4-5, where more than 90% of vascular injuries occur.[3]

In this chapter we will address the anterior approach for general and vascular surgeons who would like to enhance their knowledge of the minimally invasive open approach for single-level and two-level TDRs.

General Considerations

As a rule, a small transverse incision is preferable, because the disc is a transverse midline structure. A wider exposure is obtained with this incision than with a similar sized vertical paramedian incision, particularly in obese patients. In addition, the transverse incision allows for easier mobilization of the left rectus muscle along its lateral edge without denervating it, thus facilitating access to the retroperitoneal space. Intercostal nerves 7 to 11 innervate the rectus muscle with segmental overlap; therefore damage to one or two of these nerves is of no clinical consequence. These nerves enter the muscle after perforating the posterior rectus sheath near its lateral edge and can be injured when dividing the posterior rectus sheath from the medial side as well. Lateral mobilization of this muscle helps to avoid injury to the peritoneum, which is thicker and more easily dissected from the posterior rectus sheath laterally. Furthermore, because of the size of the incision, it is easier to perform the initial retroperitoneal dissection if this muscle is retracted medially. The muscle is also mobilized along the midline and retracted to the left to keep it from acting as a resistance when the final table-held retractor is used. For two-level approaches, the incision is slightly oblique. For surgery involving more than two levels, the approach can no longer be considered mini-open. This larger incision requires mobilization of only the left rectus muscle from the midline to access the posterior rectus sheath and proceed into the retroperitoneal space.

Lacerations to the peritoneum can be repaired more conveniently during closure, because they can probably be incorporated to the repair of the posterior rectus sheath. However, when to repair peritoneal defects is based on the surgeon's judgment and depends on the size and location of the defects.

The incision for lumbar arthroplasty is small, measuring 5 to 6 cm for a single level and 6 to 8 cm for two levels, depending on the size of the patient. Therefore it is extremely important to localize the disc spaces for proper placement of the incision. For surgeons with experience, localization can be achieved by looking at the lateral plain film of the lumbar spine, which shows the location and angle of L4-5 and L5-S1 in relation to the iliac crest, and palpating the iliac crest. The surgeon can judge how far caudad or cephalad to place the incision, based on the radiographic location and angle of the disc spaces. Fluoroscopy can be helpful, using pins or other markers to localize the incision. Although this method is more time consuming, it may be appropriate for surgeons with minimal experience with access surgery. For these surgeons it may also be beneficial to make larger incisions to avoid struggling through a small one. It is also more forgiving to err by placing the incision slightly more caudad than cephalad, because of the usual lordotic angle at L4-5 and L5-S1.

The lateral plain film of the lumbar spine can also be used to identify calcifications of the iliac vessels and aorta and the degree of osteophytic activity in the area. Both of these findings are predictive of increased risks. Calcified arteries are more difficult to mobilize and may be more prone to intimal tearing or cracking, which may lead to thrombosis. A heavily calcified left iliac artery or aorta may be a contraindication to TDR, especially at L4-5. Osteophytes are indicative of increased inflammatory reaction in the area with scarring and fibrosis, which may make dissection and mobilization of the left common iliac vein much more difficult and more prone to laceration. All surgeons should be keenly aware of these conditions before surgery. Therefore critical preoperative evaluation of the lateral x-ray of the lumbar spine by both the spine surgeon and the access surgeon is mandatory.

In most cases, L5-S1 is approached between the iliac vessels. L4-5 is exposed by mobilizing these vessels to the right. Therefore it is frequently necessary to transect the ileolumbar vein. This vein must be ligated and not just clipped, at least on the side that joins the common iliac vein. Failure to properly control this vessel has led to catastrophic events, including death. With a very high bifurcation, L4-5 can sometimes be approached between the iliac vessels. If the bifurcation is very low, L5-S1 can sometimes be approached by going lateral to these vessels. Vascular imaging studies are not routinely necessary because the location of these vessels in relation to the disc being approached becomes obvious when they are exposed. Occasionally it may be helpful to evaluate the magnetic resonance imaging study to determine the location of the vessels and the degree of inflammatory reaction present at the target level. However, appropriate placement of the incision relative to the disc is more important than the location of the vessels relative to the disc.

It is important to minimize the occurrence of left iliac artery thrombosis while approaching L4-5. This goal is achieved by mobilizing this vessel as far toward the femoral canal as possible to allow retraction far to the right without undue stretch. This maneuver is easy to perform with blunt dissection using a Kittner or peanut sponge, because the internal iliac artery is the only branch of the left iliac artery. The lymphatics will be disrupted and there may be minor oozing. Mobilizing this artery distally also allows excellent access to the left common iliac vein and easier identification of the ileolumbar vein (or veins). Although the left iliac artery tolerates compression very well for close to an hour, it does not do well when stretched to the right.[4] This distal mobilization minimizes the stretch, which can result in small intimal tears that can lead to a thrombogenic situation. A study has shown that at L4-5 the left iliac artery is occluded by compression of the retractors in the majority of the cases.[4] Some surgeons recommend that a pulse oximeter be used on one of the toes of the patient's left foot to monitor this event. If the oxygen saturation, which goes to 0% with this compression, does not return to normal quickly upon removal of the retractors, left iliac artery thrombosis should be strongly suspected and either promptly ruled out in the operating room by segmental arterial Doppler studies or treated by immediate thrombectomy.[2,4]

Retrograde ejaculation is uncommon and almost exclusively related to L5-S1 approaches. The superior hypogastric plexus (Fig. 9-1) travels with the peritoneum and the retroperitoneal fat, coursing over the bifurcation of the aorta down the midline over the promontory. Although this plexus is a midline structure, it is slightly closer to the left than to the right iliac artery. However, this proximity to the left iliac artery is not very significant. To avoid damaging this structure, dissection should be started bluntly at the anterior wall of the left iliac artery, just lateral to the ureter. The ureter and peritoneum are then lifted away. The nerve fibers are lifted with the peritoneum. This blunt finger or Kittner dissection is then carried superiorly and far to the right while hugging the promontory. When the middle sacral vessels are clearly seen, the nerve fibers should be out of harm's way and cautery or clips can be used to control these small vessels. In thinner patients, these fibers can be clearly seen and avoided. There is no real advantage to approaching L5-S1 with a retroperitoneal approach from the right simply to avoid damaging this nerve plexus. In a transperitoneal approach, in which a higher incidence of retrograde ejaculation

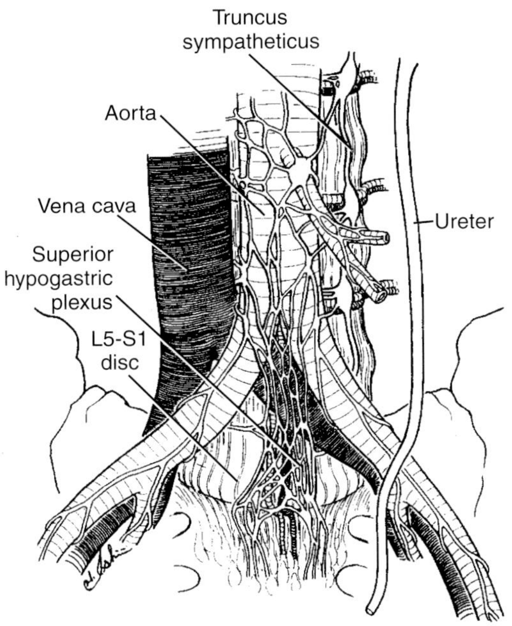

Fig. 9-1 The superior hypogastric plexus travels with the peritoneum and the retroperitoneal fat over the bifurcation of the aorta, down the midline over the promontory.

occurs, it may be wise to incise the retroperitoneum close to the right iliac artery, then sweep to the left to avoid injuring the neural plexus.

The retroperitoneal route should be used routinely. There is no added benefit to the transperitoneal approach, which should be reserved for patients who have undergone prior retroperitoneal surgery or who have retroperitoneal pathologies that may have obliterated the usual anatomic planes. These procedures include radiation to the pelvis and radical prostatectomy or hysterectomy with lymph node dissection. Patients with prior retroperitoneal sarcoma and cases of discitis, infection of the vertebral body, or psoas abscess formation are not likely to be candidates for TDR. A previous Pfannenstiel incision, low cervical C-section, or lower midline incisions for intraperitoneal pelvic surgery should not be a deterrent to the retroperitoneal approach through a separate, small transverse incision. The true Pfannenstiel incision is actually too low to use to approach L5-S1 with a very small size incision, except on patients with the steepest angles at that disc space. This incision should seldom be reincised. The transperitoneal route is also less desirable because of the potential for unsuspected damage to the small bowel, which can be catastrophic, and the increased incidence of ileus resulting from bowel manipulation. The right-sided approach to L5-S1 should be reserved for reoperative cases and for patients with prior multiple operations or devices present in the left lower quadrant. Because all the other levels are approached from the left, it is probably more comfortable to approach L5-S1 from that side as well.

As for the upper levels, L3-4 is easier to expose than L4-5 because there is no need to mobilize the iliac vessels and transect the ileolumbar vein (or veins) unless the bifurcation is very high. Taking the segmental vessels over the bodies of L3 and L4 is sufficient to provide adequate exposure, again using a small transverse incision with circumferential mobilization of the left rectus muscle. L2-3 can only be exposed with the patient in the neutral supine position when patients are not more than 20% to 25% above the ideal body weight with an ectodermic body habitus. This approach to L2-3 may be too difficult to perform on obese patients with short and wide abdomens.

Conventional knowledge has been that one anterior retroperitoneal approach precludes additional such surgeries.[7,8] However, with the use of the mini-open technique in recent years, it has become possible to go back a second time for adjacent level disease. In fact, TDR at L3-4 has been performed through a mini-open retroperitoneal approach in a patient with a prior L4-5, L5-S1 interbody fusion done with a similar mini-open approach. With the number of anterior fusions having been performed over the past decade, this is a scenario that is likely to be repeated in the future and may expand the indications for TDR.

Although ureteral injuries are rare, they do occur. To avoid them, the left ureter should be lifted anteriorly and toward the right with the peritoneum. Separating the left ureter from the peritoneum and keeping it on the left is likely to cause segmental devascularization, which can lead to necrosis of that particular segment. This is true for all levels, including L5-S1, where it is sometimes tempting to dissect the ureter away from the peritoneum and keep it retracted to the left of the disc space. When using cautery in the depths of the incision, the tip of the device should be shielded, exposing only the most distal 2 to 3 mm. Failure to do this may allow arcing of the current, causing thermal injury to structures such as the ureter and the vessels that may not be physically close to the area being cauterized.

Other minor problems associated with this approach include injury to the left sympathetic trunk, which will cause the left leg to be warmer than the right. This complication is usually unavoidable and likely to be temporary, yet the patient should be warned in advance so that he or she does not become anxious about this. Mild lymphedema can result from the necessary wide mobilization of the iliac vessels, which inevitably disrupts the lymph nodes in the area. This problem is temporary and usually goes unnoticed; however, the patient must be informed of this potential complication, because there have been cases in which the severity and permanence of this created a significant clinical problem. Damage to the lumbosacral plexus is possible and can be prevented by avoiding deep penetration or dissection of the psoas muscle. If the psoas needs to be retracted, usually at the higher levels, the disc should be identified and the muscle carefully dissected away from it with a blunt Cobb elevator.

Surgical Technique

The patient is placed in a supine position on a Jackson or other radiolucent table with an inflatable bag under the affected disc. Discretionary inflation of the bag allows for extension of the spine at the time of discectomy and artificial disc placement. Some artificial discs require this increased lordosis for proper placement. The approach surgeon should be familiar with the requirements of the device being used.

The approach surgeon stands to the patient's left and the assistant to the right. The level of the transverse incision in the craniocaudad plane depends on the level of the spine to be approached. Fig. 9-2 shows the typical location of these incisions, which are subject to variation depending on the evaluation of the lateral film of the lumbar spine. Proper placement of this small incision is crucial for alignment of the templates, spacers, distractors, inserters, and artificial discs at the proper angle, parallel to the vertebral endplates in a straight anteroposterior (AP) plane.

For a single-level TDR, the incision begins at the midline and extends transversely for 5 to 6 cm, depending on the size of the patient. For two-level exposure, the incision should be more oblique. The incision should start at the midline at the level of the lower disc and end at the level of the upper disc, approaching the lateral edge of the rectus muscle for 6 to 8 cm. For three levels, the obliquity increases; however, the incision is never paramedian, although a vertical midline incision is acceptable.

The incision is carried to the anterior rectus sheath using electrocautery. The subcutaneous portion of the incision extends beyond the ends of the skin incision, with undermining both medially and laterally. This dissection should expose the anterior rectus fascia from beyond the midline to the lateral edge of

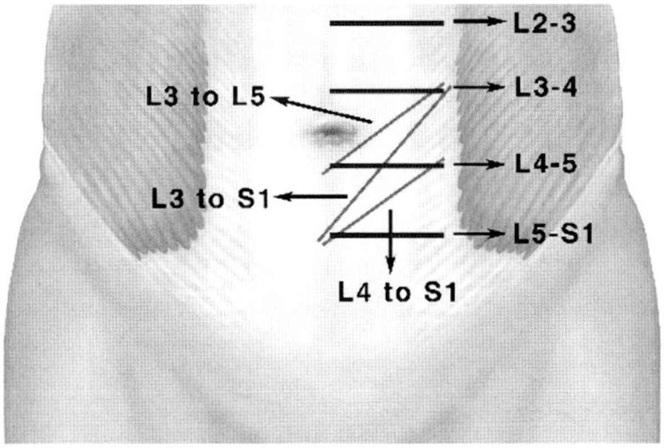

Fig. 9-2 Common incision locations.

the left rectus muscle. The rectus fascia is incised beginning 1 cm to the right of the midline, just enough to see a little of the right rectus muscle, and extending to the edge of the rectus muscle laterally. The anterior rectus sheath is then elevated anteriorly away from the muscle belly for 4 to 6 cm. The sheath is elevated both superiorly and inferiorly to allow full mobilization of the rectus muscle (Fig. 9-3, *A*). Medial, lateral, and posterior dissection of the muscle is then carried out. Great care must be taken to avoid injury to the inferior epigastric vessels coursing along the undersurface of the muscle. These vessels must be elevated and retracted with the muscle. The rectus muscle is now mobilized circumferentially and can be easily retracted both medially and laterally (Fig. 9-3, *B*).

With the rectus muscle initially retracted toward the midline, the posterior sheath or transversalis fascia is carefully incised 4 to 5 mm until the peritoneum is seen to shine through. The edges are grasped with a hemostat, then lifted away and very carefully dissected from the peritoneum and incised as far inferiorly and superiorly as possible. This layer can be quite tenuous and care must be exercised to prevent peritoneal lacerations. The peritoneum will now bulge upward (Fig. 9-4, *A*). Using an index finger, the surgeon carefully pushes the peritoneum posteriorly at the edge of the fascial incision as a plane is slowly developed between it and the undersurface of the internal oblique and transversus muscles and fascia. This dissection leads to the retroperitoneal space (Fig 9-4, *B*)

Blunt finger dissection proceeds posteriorly and then medially, elevating the peritoneum away from the psoas muscle. Care must be taken to avoid entering the retropsoas space at this point, which causes unnecessary bleeding in a blind pouch. The genitofemoral nerve can be easily identified over the psoas muscle. The ureter can usually be identified as the peritoneum is lifted away from the psoas muscle. Both of these structures should be preserved from injury.

Once the psoas muscle is identified, the disc, vertebral body, and iliac artery can be palpated medially. If the size of the incision allows, the surgeon's entire hand is inserted as a closed fist in the retroperitoneal area. The fist is swept up and down, then the surgeon's fingers are opened to elevate the peritoneum away in all directions. A Harrington retractor is used to keep the peritoneal contents away from the vessels and to allow further dissection. A dry lap sponge is tucked superiorly to keep the retroperitoneal fat and peritoneal contents from creeping down and obscuring the field. A Balfour retractor with appropriately deep blades is inserted to keep the incision open in the craniocaudad plane (Fig. 9-5).

For operations on only L4-5 or for operations that combine L4-5 with either L3-4 or L5-S1, the ileolumbar vein (or veins) must be ligated and cut. These vessels serve as a tether preventing mobilization of the iliac vein away from the

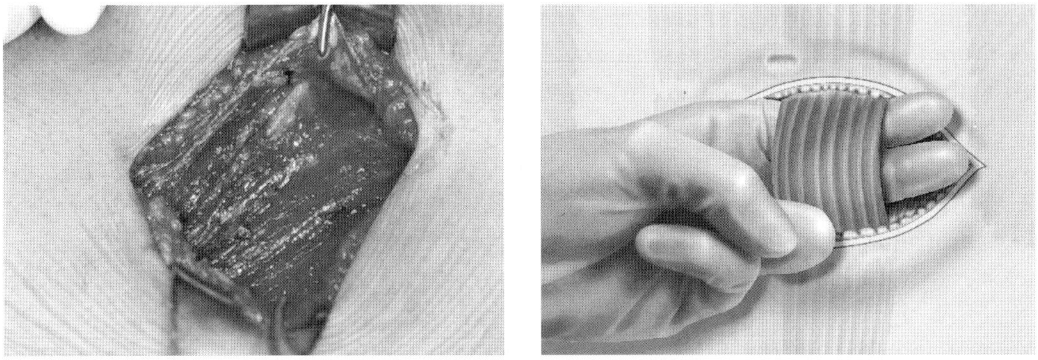

Fig. 9-3 **A,** Elevation of the rectus anterior sheath 4 to 6 cm. **B,** Circumferential mobilization of the rectus muscle. Note the easy retraction both medially and laterally.

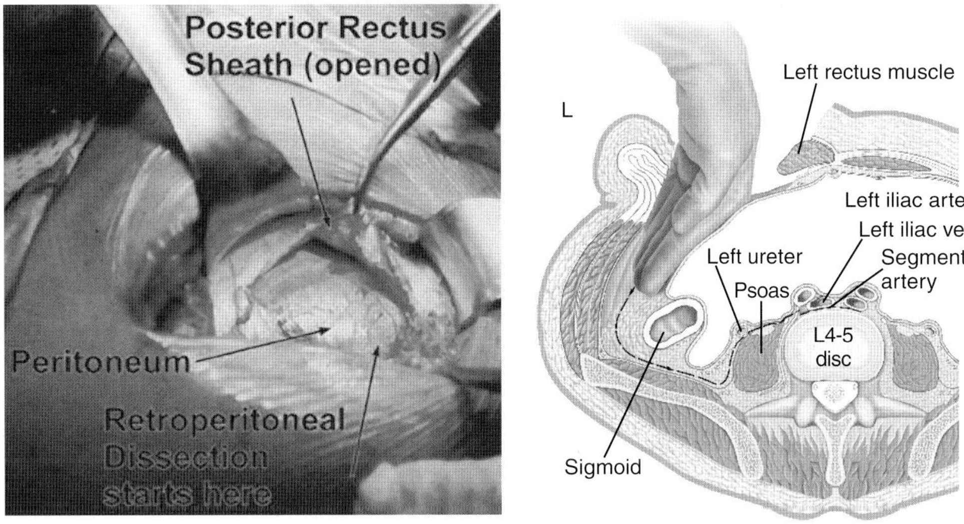

Fig. 9-4 **A,** After incising the posterior rectus sheath and dissecting the retroperiteum, the peritoneum will bulge upward. **B,** The retroperitoneal space is entered by pushing the peritoneum posteriorly at the edge of the fascial incision.

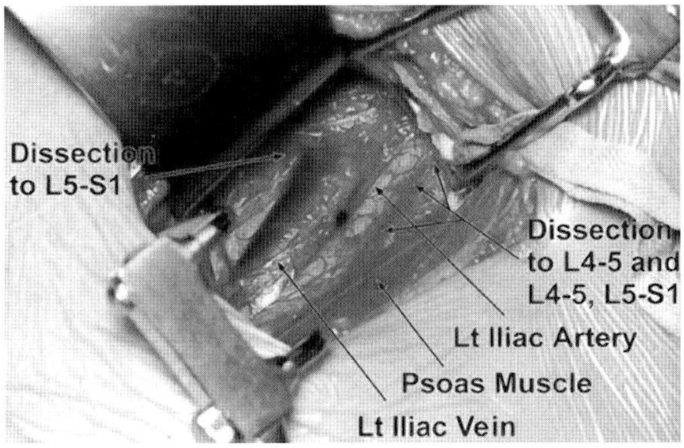

Fig. 9-5 The incision opening is maintained by placing a Balfour retractor in the craniocaudad plane.

anterior surface of the spine, thus preventing proper exposure. The peritoneal contents are elevated away with the Harrington retractor and dissected bluntly just above the left iliac artery to move the retroperitoneal tissues away from it. The entire length of the common and external iliac arteries are exposed as far distally as possible, and then careful blunt dissection is started along the lateral edge of the artery. Lymphatics will inevitably be disrupted, exposing the left common iliac vein just underneath the artery (Fig. 9-6, *A*). Dissection proceeds posteriorly to identify the ileolumbar vein (or veins), which cross the body of L5 and dive into the left paraspinous area. Variations in the formation of the common iliac vein and the lumbar veins are common. Great care must be exercised to identify, ligate, and transect these veins and avoid avulsion. Ligation should be carried out in place by placing a right angle clamp around the vessel and tying with a silk ligature before transection. Clips may be used to control the distal vein. For any operation that involves L4-5, these maneuvers are imperative.

The left iliac vein and artery can now be separated away from the spine using gentle dissection with a peanut sponge and fingertips (Fig. 9-6, *B*). The large, metal Yankauer-type suction tip can be effectively used as a pusher in this area. In most patients, the vein peels away from the anterior surface of the spine easily. However, in some patients there is an inflammatory reaction in the plane between the vein and the anterior longitudinal ligament, especially when osteophytes are present. In these patients dissection can be quite difficult and tedious.

All the vascular structures are thus swept from left to right providing adequate visualization of the disc or discs and vertebral bodies involved. Segmental vessels running across the valleys on the anterior surface of the bodies can be transected between clips and swept to the sides with blunt dissection. The surgeon must be able to insert at least one finger between the vein and the ligament to palpate the right lateral edge of the spine with the iliac vessels above the fingers (Fig. 9-7). The fingers must be kept on the disc, which is easily distinguished by palpation from the vertebral body, while pushing toward the right to prevent injury to the lumbar veins coming in from that side (Fig. 9-8). Great care must be taken to avoid tearing tissues that do not give way easily, or lumbar veins may be injured. If these vessels are torn, bleeding can usually be controlled with hemostatic agents without the need for suture repair. When this part of the exposure is completed (Fig. 9-9, *A*), the Balfour and Harrington retractors are removed.

The table-held retractor post and arms (or ring) are then set up. The surgeon's left hand finds its way into the retroperitoneal space, medial to the rectus muscle and with the muscle now retracted laterally. In a blind but safe maneuver, the fingers find their way to the right side of the spine following the planes previously dissected. An ALAS radiolucent, 1-inch-wide blade with a small reverse lip (Thompson Surgical Instuments, Traverse City, MI.) is placed blindly

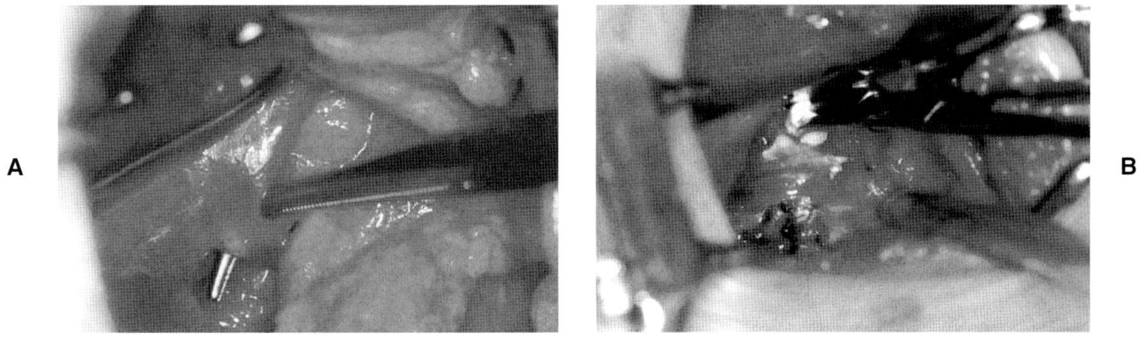

Fig. 9-6 **A,** Identification of the left common iliac vein. Great care must be exercised to identify, ligate, and transect the veins to avoid avulsion. **B,** Peanut sponge dissection.

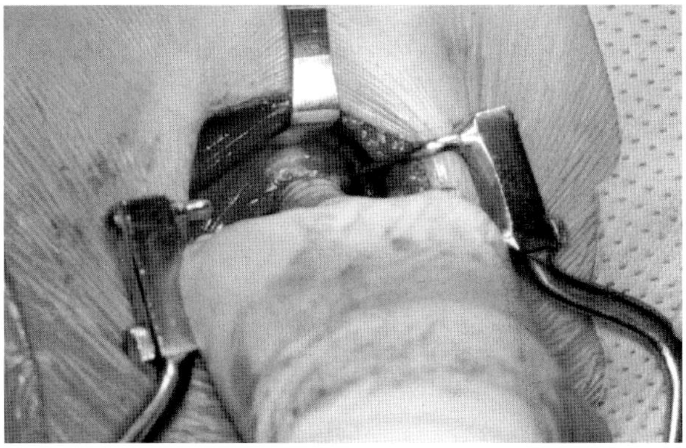

Fig. 9-7 Separating the left iliac vein and artery from the spine with fingertip dissection.

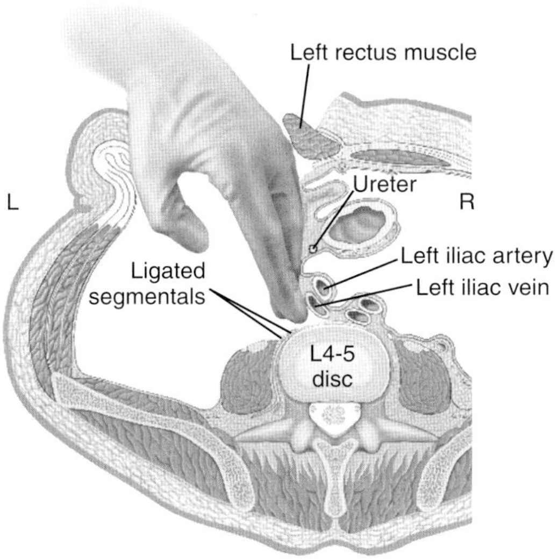

Fig. 9-8 Palpation of the right lateral edge of the spine. At least one finger should be placed between the vein and the ligament when performing the palpation, and the iliac vessels should be above your finger(s).

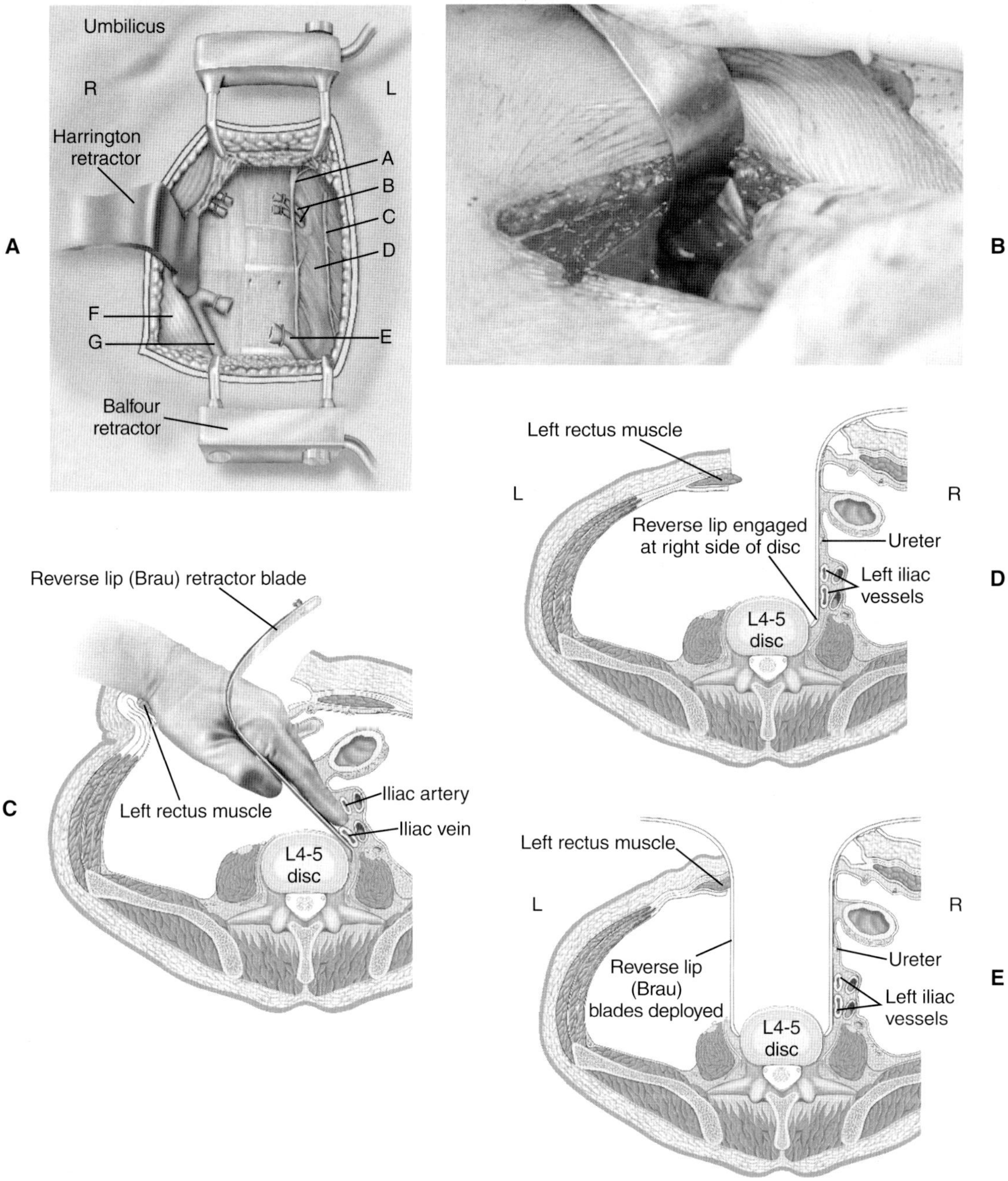

Fig. 9-9 A, Anatomic landmarks: *A,* sympathetic trunk; *B,* segmental vessels; *C,* genitofemoral vein; *D,* psoas muscle; *E,* iliolumbar vein; *F,* left rectus muscle; *G,* left iliac vein. **B,** Placement of an ALAS retractor. This retractor has a small reverse lip and is attached to a table-held retractor system. **C,** Elevation of the vascular structures and exposure of the anterior surface of the spine. **D,** When secured to the table-held retractor, the reverse-lipped blade will not move. **E,** Placement of a second ALAS retractor to complete spine exposure.

onto the right side of the spine, level with the disc space, using the fingers as a guide (Figs. 9-9, *B*). This blade is attached to the table-held retractor system, then pushed to the right to elevate the vascular structures and expose the anterior surface of the spine (Fig. 9-9, *C*).

Once secured to the table-held retractor, the reverse-lipped blade will not move. The reverse lip keeps the blade anchored to the edge of the spine, at the level of the disc, and prevents it from slipping anteriorly when tension is applied. Without this reverse lip, the retractor blade will not work effectively (Fig. 9-9, *D*).

With the rectus muscle now retracted laterally, there will be much less resistance when pushing the retractor blade to the right to expose the spine in a direct AP view, allowing placement of the instruments for insertion of the artificial disc. A second blade is placed on the left side of the spine, again at the level of the disc, and attached to the table-held system to complete the exposure (Fig. 9-9, *E*). Commonly, additional retractor blades need to be placed superiorly or inferiorly (Fig. 9-10). Radiographs should be taken to determine the midline after the first two blades are placed to avoid obscuring the field with too much hardware. With these blades well anchored to the lateral wall of the vertebral column, the spine surgeon and the assistant can now work on the disc without other hands or retractors being in the way and with relative security that vessels will not slip around the retractors and become injured. The utmost care must still be exercised to prevent such injuries.

For operations on L5-S1, the dissection is carried anterior and medial to the left iliac artery with the Harrington-Balfour retractor combination placed into that plane to elevate the peritoneal contents. The disc is palpated and dissection is carried toward it with blunt dissection between the iliac vessels and below the aortic bifurcation (Fig. 9-11). The middle sacral vessels may be taken between clips, ligatures, or cauterized. Cautery is kept to a minimum in males to avoid injury to the superior hypogastric plexus fibers. The left iliac vein

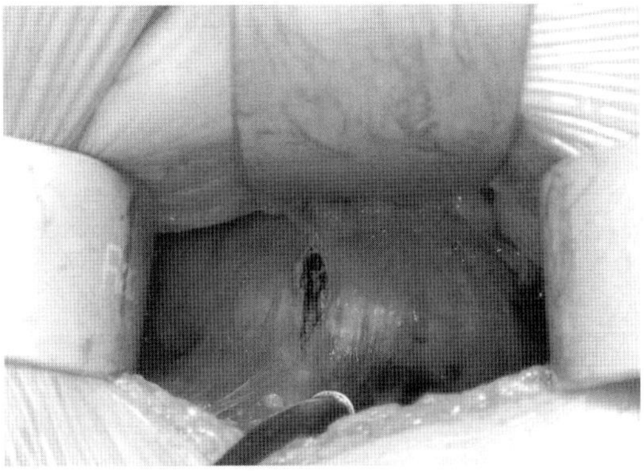

Fig. 9-10 Final exposure at L4-5.

sometimes needs to be widely mobilized to allow placement of the reverse-lipped retractor against the left lateral edge of the spine. This vein is seen deep to the artery and is swept toward the left with a peanut sponge to expose that side of the disc. Dissection toward the right exposes that side of the disc and a reverse-lipped retractor can be used to maintain exposure there by anchoring the lip onto the lateral aspect of the spine. The iliac vessels are not usually visualized on the right side. The table-held retractor is used to keep the two reverse-lipped blades in place with the left rectus muscle mobilized laterally.

For operations of L3-4 and L2-3, mobilization of the iliac vessels is usually not necessary. It is only occasionally necessary to transect the ileolumbar vein (or veins) to obtain adequate mobilization. Thus approaching these two levels is somewhat easier, with the exception that L2-3 is extremely difficult to expose in more obese patients and should only be used in patients as described in the General Considerations section at the beginning of this chapter.

Discectomy and instrumentation are then performed (Fig. 9-11, *B*). On completion, the retractor blades are sequentially removed, with the blade on the right side being removed last. Vascular integrity is thoroughly assessed, looking closely for arterial thrombosis or injury caused by stretching. Lap sponges are removed and the tissues are allowed to fall back together anatomically.

The individual fascial layers are closed separately with running absorbable sutures, making sure that the anterior rectus sheath is well approximated. The posterior sheath need not be closed if it is tenuous and does not offer any sig-

A

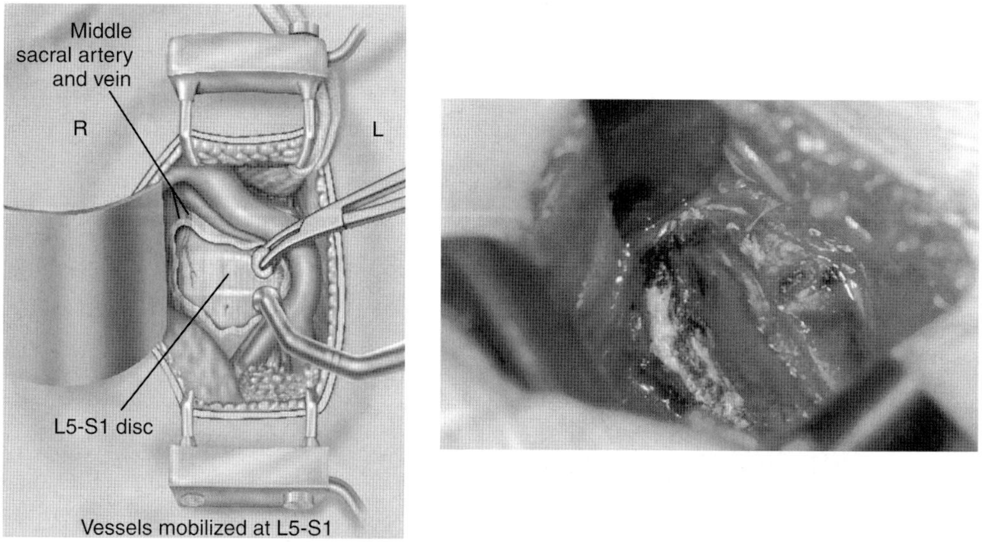

B

Fig. 9-11 A, With the Harrington-Balfour retractor in place, dissection is performed anterior and medial to the left iliac artery. **B,** Postdiscectomy at L5-S1.

nificant strength to the closure. However, a thick, substantial posterior rectus sheath should be closed. Subcutaneous tissues and skin are then closed as per the surgeon's preference.

Retrograde ejaculation is uncommon and almost exclusively related to L5-S1 approaches.

Conclusion

The techniques described here have been used in more than 1500 patients undergoing anterior lumbar surgery, including TDR, since 1997 and have proved safe and efficient. With practice, the incision can be made very small, and the time to exposure should average about 20 minutes for a single level. The complication rate has been very low despite the obesity seen in the majority of these patients and remains at 0.4% for arterial injury and 0.8% for venous laceration, with only one case of retrograde ejaculation and two cases of ureteral injury.

Of the many surgeons who have come to train in this approach at our institution, some have shown skepticism because it does not appear to allow sufficient room to practice the fundamental principle of vascular surgery: to always have proximal and distal control available. However, they soon learn that exposure of the iliac vessels can be quite adequate through this small incision. Bleeding during anterior lumbar surgery is almost always from the common iliac vein. In most cases bleeding can be controlled by applying pressure with sponge sticks and then repairing the laceration, without the need to extend the incision. Lacerations as large as 4 to 5 mm may be treated with hemostatic agents and may not require suture repair, especially if the arthroplasty has already been completed. Left iliac artery thrombosis, if detected before closure, can be easily treated via iliac arteriotomy without enlarging the incision.

Once trained, these access surgeons report that it may take as many as 20 to 30 cases before they feel comfortable enough to start reducing the size of the incision and the time needed to complete the exposure. However, when this comfort level is reached, the approach has proved reliable, safe, and fast. The spine surgeons with whom they work have been very satisfied. This experience has been true even for surgeons who had already been performing access procedures using other approaches and who have now adopted some of the techniques described here.

REFERENCES

1. Brau SA. Mini-open approach to the lumbar spine for anterior lumbar interbody fusion: Description of the procedure, results and complications. Spine J 2:216-223, 2002.
2. Brau SA, Delamarter RB, Schiffman ML, et al. Left iliac artery thrombosis during anterior lumbar surgery. Ann Vasc Surg 18:48-51, 2004.

3. Brau SA, Delamarter RB, Schiffman ML, et al. Vascular injury during anterior lumbar surgery. Spine J 4:409-412, 2004.
4. Brau SA, Spoonamore MJ, Snyder L, et al. Nerve monitoring changes related to iliac artery compression during anterior lumbar spine surgery. Spine J 3:351-355, 2003.
5. Buttner-Janz K. Surgical approach. In Buttner-Janz K, Hochschuler SH, McAfee PC, eds. The Artificial Disc. Berlin: Springer-Verlag, 2003, pp 103-114.
6. Mayer HM. Minimally Invasive Spine Surgery—A Surgical Manual. Munich: Springer-Verlag, 2000.
7. Selby DK, Henderson RJ, Blumenthal S, et al. Anterior lumbar fusion. In Cauthen J, ed. Lumbar Spine Surgery: Indications, Techniques, Failures and Alternatives, 2nd ed. Baltimore: Williams & Wilkins, 1988.
8. Watkins RG. Anterior lumbar interbody fusion surgical complications. Clin Orthop 284:47-53, 1992.

CHAPTER

10

Dynamic Stabilization Devices for Treatment of Low Back Pain

Dilip K. Sengupta ▪ Robert C. Mulholland

The traditional surgical treatment for chronic low back pain caused by degenerative disc disorders in the lumbar spine is spinal fusion. This treatment is comparable to arthrodesis of the hip or knee for the treatment of osteoarthritis. Because hip and knee fusion leads to major disability of locomotor function and gait, arthrodesis is no longer regularly recommended as treatment. On the other hand, spinal fusion has been practiced for over several decades; fusion of the spine is more successful than hip and knee fusion because the overall movement of the trunk and gait is only minimally affected following fusion of one or two segments in the lumbar spine. With the recent developments in fusion techniques, the rate of successful fusions has approached nearly 100%, but this number fails to reflect a comparable increase in successful clinical outcomes.[4] Several studies in the recent literature question the efficacy of spinal fusion for the treatment of low back pain.[17] In addition, spinal surgeons have always feared the development of adjacent segment disease in the long-term follow-up after spinal fusion, despite the lack of any clinical evidence.[7,10,11,28,32,38]

Stabilization of the lumbar spine without fusion has been sporadically performed since the early 1990s in Europe and the East.[18,39] These techniques are ideal for young, active patients with multisegment disc degeneration for which fusion has obvious disadvantages. Recently, there has been an upsurge in the interest in dynamic stabilization with further extension of indications like topping off an adjacent segment or stabilizing a segment following discectomy. Unfortunately, neither of these procedures has a sound biomechanical basis for action, nor is either procedure of any clinically proven efficacy.

Following the success of hip and knee replacement prostheses, disc replacement devices have been developed to treat degenerative disc disease. Several devices have undergone more than a decade of testing and over 5 years of clinical follow-up. The overall success rate, however, is no match to that of hip or knee fusion, or even of traditional spinal fusion. One basic difference between prosthetic hip or knee replacement and the intervertebral disc prosthesis is that the latter is only a partial rather than a total joint replacement. Like other dynamic stabilization devices, the disc prosthesis has to share the kinematics of the remaining joints of the spinal motion segment. The only difference is that the disc prosthesis is a load-bearing structure, not a load-sharing structure like the dynamic stabilization devices. Much attention has also been paid to the wear properties of the available disc prosthesis, while their effect on the remaining structure of the motion segment and kinematics has been largely ignored.

Dynamic stabilization can play an important role in the treatment of degenerative disc disease by favorably altering the movement and load transmission of the spinal motion segment without fusing the segment. In the first part of this chapter we will discuss the pathology and mechanism of chronic low back pain and how spinal biomechanics affect low back pain. Dynamic stabilization technology and the devices that are currently in development will be discussed in the second part.

Pathology and the Mechanism of Chronic Low Back Pain: Movement or Load

Mechanical Back Pain

Traditionally chronic axial pain in the low back that is caused by degenerative diseases of the lumbar spine and that is aggravated by activities of daily living is described as *mechanical back pain*. This was thought to be caused by instability of the lumbar motion segment, unlike leg pain, which is described as radicular pain or neurogenic claudication, and is caused by compression of the neural elements.

Spinal Instability

Instability in the lumbar spine as a cause of mechanical back pain is poorly understood. The term *instability* implies an abnormal motion under physiologic load. It is generally accepted that disc degeneration reduces the movement of the lumbar spine, except in the very early stages.[14,15] Despite considerable research over several years, no clear relationship has been established between low back pain and abnormal movement.[12,43,44,50,56,59] Most authors have related abnormal translation to the mechanical back pain (Fig. 10-1).[14,15,56,59] A degree

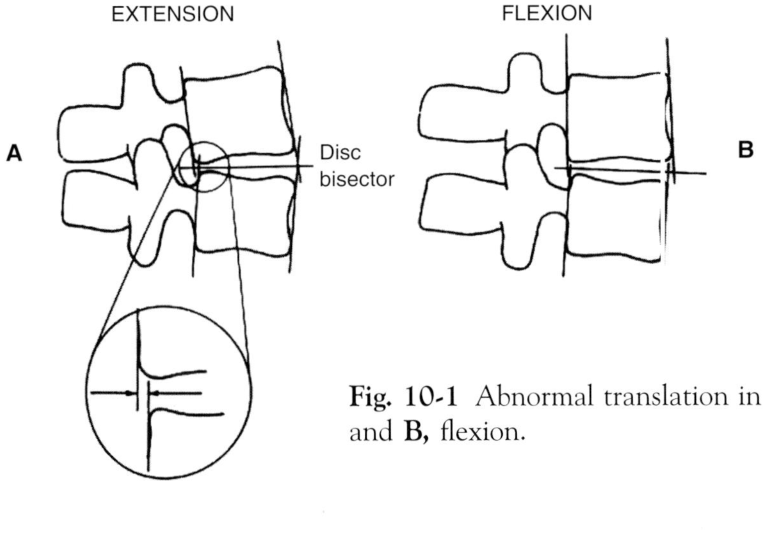

Fig. 10-1 Abnormal translation in **A,** extension and **B,** flexion.

of translation motion is normally associated with flexion-extension caused by the composite nature of spinal motion.[45,46] Although some investigators found excessive translation to be associated with disc degeneration,[59] others observed a reduced shear-flexion ratio at the symptomatic levels of disc degeneration.[56] It is generally accepted that disc degeneration reduces, not increases, movement, as the term *instability* implies.[14,15,41]

Although abnormal translation is seen radiologically in many cases of disc degeneration with spondylolisthesis, it is not always present in symptomatic disc degeneration. Even when pain is present, the patient may not experience continuous pain. Although the abnormal movement may be present continuously in this group of patients, their pain is not continuous. It is thus difficult to find any basis for the theory of abnormal movement or instability being a cause of back pain. *Instability* is a term that clinicians have used since the mid-1950s to refer to some nonspecific mechanical failure of the spine causing back pain, as opposed to infection or arthritis. Bioengineers define instability in a purely literal bioengineering sense as abnormal movement at the joint surface, and this definition indicates that fusion is an appropriate solution.[41]

Load Transmission Through the Normal Disc

The second important role of a motion segment in the lumbar spine is load transmission. Under normal circumstances load transmission is painless and its magnitude through the lumbar motion segment varies with change of posture and activities. This has been very well documented by the earlier work of Nachemson.[42] A volunteer study by Wilke et al on in vivo intradiscal pressure found a good correlation with Nachemson's data.[61]

The normal intervertebral disc is an isotropic structure.[22] The nucleus acts like a fluid-filled bag, distributing load uniformly across the endplate. This has been convincingly demonstrated by McNally and colleagues by stress profilometry in normal cadaver lumbar disc.[34,36] The nucleus also transmits the load in a lateral direction to the anulus, producing tension in the anulus like in an inflated car tire; this converts the anulus into a uniform load-bearing structure.[41]

Disc degeneration alters the isotropic nature of the disc.[27] In vivo stress profilometry studies also confirm that load distribution across endplates becomes uneven after disc degeneration, with areas of high spot loading, particularly associated with certain positions. McNally et al[37] found such irregular load distribution to be a strong predictor of pain reproduction by provocative discography (Fig. 10-2, *A-D*).

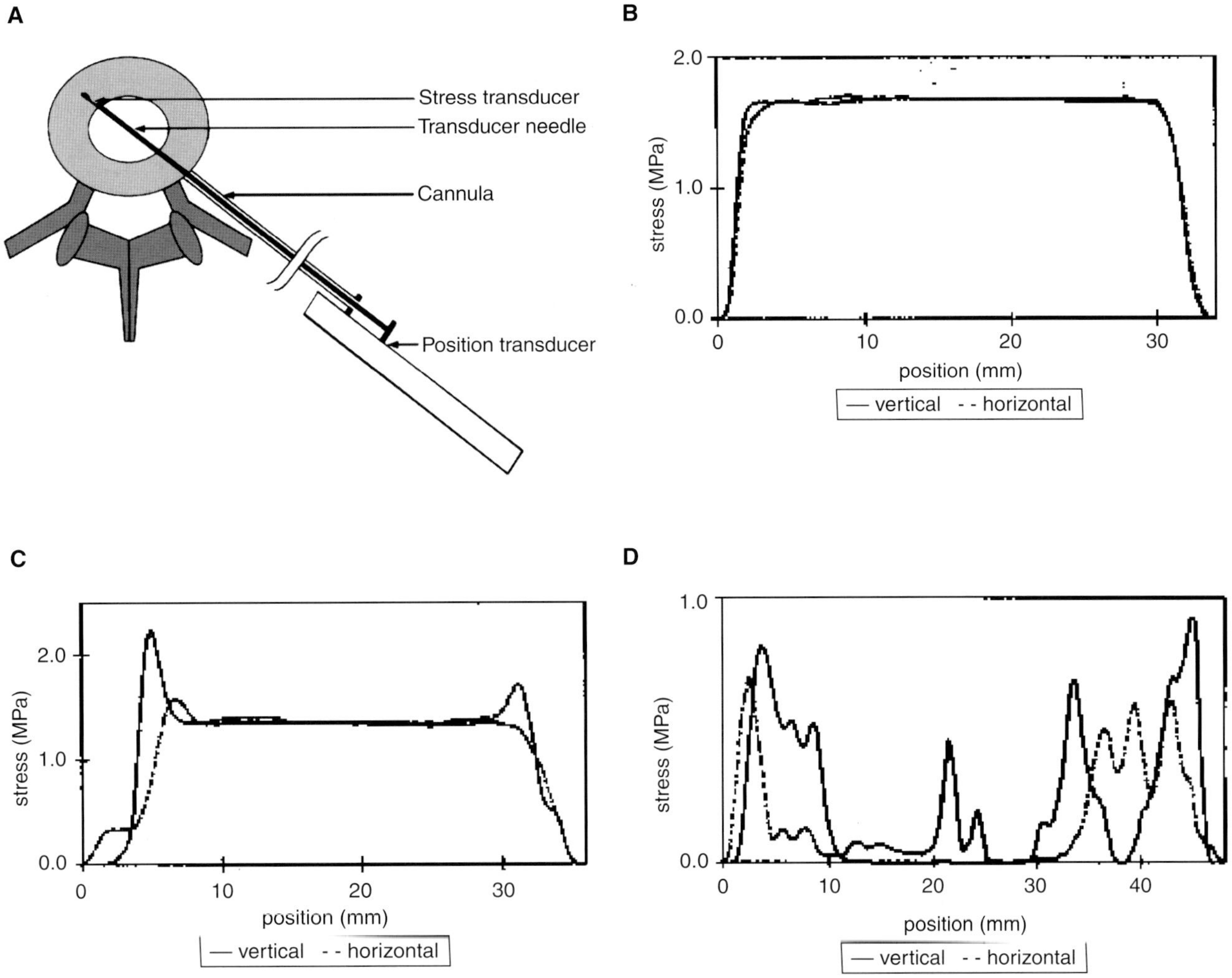

Fig. 10-2 A, Schematic diagram of the equipment and approach used in the in vivo stress measurements. **B,** A pair of stress profiles recorded in a healthy L4-5 disc in vitro showing a uniform, isotropic distribution of compressive stress within the nucleus and a rapid fall off in the peripheral anulus. **C,** A pair of stress profiles recorded in a degenerate L2-3 disc in vitro showing anisotropic concentrations of stress in the anulus. **D,** A pair of stress profiles recorded in an L5-S1 disc in vivo showing multiple stress concentrations in the posterolateral anulus and in the otherwise depressurized nucleus. (**A-D** from McNally DS, Shackleford IM, Goodship AE, et al. In vivo stress measurement can predict pain on discography. Spine 21:2580-2587, 1996.)

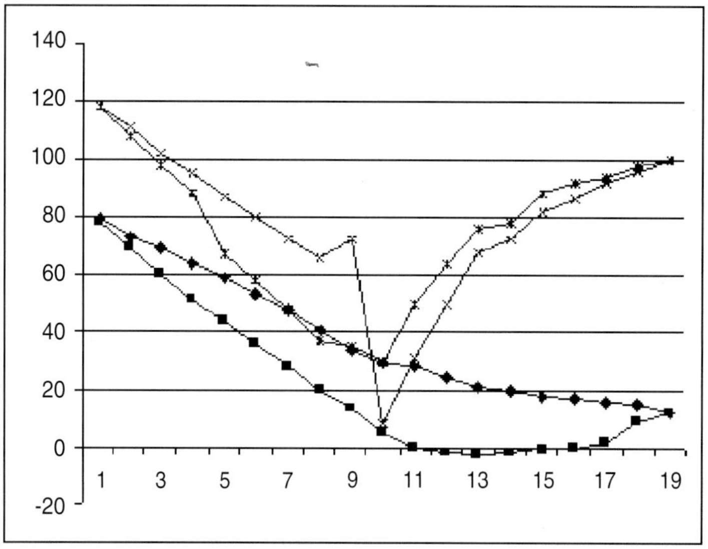

Fig. 10-3 In an unconstrained specimen, the pressure *(X)* rises both in flexion and extension. Following application of a soft stabilization system (Dynamic Stabilization Systems, DSS-I), the pressure in the disc *(dark rectangles on lower curve)* was lowered during flexion proportionately because of the load-sharing property of the soft stabilization device. However, during extension the disc pressure continued to be lowered, except at the end of extension, indicating that the soft stabilization device became more and more of a load-bearing structure toward the end of the extension.

Fig. 10-3 shows continuous pressure measurement from the center of the disc at the L4-5 segment in a cadaveric lumbar spine during flexion and extension motion.

The irregular load distribution across the joint surface is a well-recognized cause of pain in diarthrodial joints such as the hip and knee joint. High spot loading in varus or valgus deformity of the knee joint may lead to pain, and this may be relieved by corrective osteotomy, which redistributes the load transmission. Similarly, high spot loading in a subluxating hip may cause pain, which may be relieved by osteotomy and redistribution of load transmission. Although the intervertebral disc is not a diarthrodial joint, the endplates are rich in nerve supply, and it may be reasonable to believe that abnormal high spot loading may be a cause of pain in degenerative disc disease.

Load Transmission Through the Degenerated Disc

Normal nucleus consists of a homogeneous gel of collagen and proteoglycan. In a degenerated disc, the gel changes to a nonhomogeneous mixture of fragmented and condensed collagen, areas of fluid, and even areas of gas on occasion. Less commonly, isolated fragments of anulus or endplate may add to the loose fragment inside the disc.[40] In a degenerated disc the nucleus becomes depressurized, and an increasingly larger load is transmitted through the anulus.

Corresponding endplate changes, apoptosis of cells,[2] and destruction and thinning of the trabeculae in the central areas,[25] and thinning of the subchondral cartilaginous endplate[54] have been demonstrated by various observers. Loading the anulus, unprotected by the supporting pressure of the nucleus, can lead to splitting and inward folding of the anulus.[35] The principal areas of load transmission across the disc now become dependent on the posture: in flexion the anterior anulus, in extension the posterior anulus. The abnormal high load transmission through the different areas of the anulus with change of posture may explain the activity- and posture-related mechanical back pain that occurs in the presence of degenerated disc.

The "Stone in the Shoe" Hypothesis of Back Pain

In clinical settings of mechanical back pain, two commonly observed facts remain unexplained by the theory of instability. First, patients with disc degeneration almost always have a mild to moderate degree of baseline symptoms, superimposed with periods of acute exacerbations of back pain; patients are relatively asymptomatic between the acute episodes. If there is any abnormal translation or instability in that segment, it is present continuously. However, if instability or abnormal movement is the cause of pain, it is not clear why the acute pain is only periodic. Second, it is well recognized that manipulation of the lumbar spine, as performed by chiropractors, often results in dramatic relief of an acute episode of low back pain. Once again, the instability theory fails to explain why this should occur.

As described earlier, in a degenerated disc the nucleus loses its water content, becomes depressurized, and the opposing endplate cartilage and the supporting trabeculae thin out. However, the fragments of nucleus or endplate cartilage or the anulus in a degenerated disc may on occasion become areas of high spot loading, depending on their position within the disc. It is tempting to hypothesize that these abnormal loose fragments within the disc space act like a stone in the shoe, causing high spot loading and pain at the time of acute exacerbation. Manipulation of the lumbar spine by a chiropractor may on occasion dislodge the fragment from its weight-bearing position, bringing immediate relief of acute pain.[41]

This hypothesis, that the actual arrangement of tissues within the disc affects the load transmission, also explains why there is no clear correlation between degree of disc degeneration and pain.

Spinal Fusion and Low Back Pain

It is true that in many cases spinal fusion successfully relieves back pain. Following spinal fusion the load transmission across the motion segment becomes direct from bone to bone. However, if instability or an abnormal movement is the main cause of back pain, spinal fusion should always be successful in relieving back pain, but this has not been the clinical experience. Introduction of pedicle instrumentation in the 1980s, and of cage devices in the 1990s, and frequent use of circumferential fusion have increased the successful fusion rate to almost 98%, but has failed to improve the overall clinical success rate.[4] A recent review of the Cochrane database of the prospective randomized controlled trials fails to establish that spinal fusion significantly improves the natural history of low back pain.[17] A subsequent multicenter prospective randomized controlled trial in Sweden suggests better outcome with fusion compared with conservative treatment, but no difference in outcome between the different fusion techniques.[13]

The debate continues and fusion remains the seriously challenged standard surgical treatment of back pain. Most reported studies suggest 30% to 50% excellent to good clinical outcome, and 30% failure of improvement of back pain,[*] but no correlation between fusion success and clinical outcome. Not all cases of pseudarthrosis are painful, nor are all successful fusions painless.

Many suggestions have been put forward to explain the failure of good clinical outcome in the presence of a successful fusion. These include failure to recognize pseudarthrosis,[33] abnormal sagittal balance,[29] and abnormal load transmission through the metal-bone interface in cage fusion.[47] The load over the narrow footprint of the metallic cage on the endplate may be 500% higher than the rest of the endplate, even after successful fusion.[47] McAfee pointed out that clinical success was associated with the development of the bone around the cage, which inevitably increased the area of load transmission and reduced the load over the footprint of the cage.[33]

It may therefore be reasonable to conclude that stopping movement is not advisable to achieve relief of back pain. Creating a normal loading pattern is more important for clinical success, which heralds a new era in the problem of mechanical low back pain, one in which "stabilize but do not fuse" may be advisable.

Dynamic Stabilization

Dynamic stabilization of the lumbar spine may be defined as a system that would favorably alter the movement and load transmission of a spinal motion segment without fusion of the segment. This definition must be carefully differentiated from semirigid fixation of the spine where fusion is intended. It is often argued that a rigid fixation may discourage formation of a strong fusion mass because of load-sharing by the rigid implant, and that semirigid instrumentation may overcome this disadvantage. A dynamic stabilization, also known as *soft stabilization* or *flexible stabilization,* leaves the motion segment mobile, and seeks to alter the load-bearing pattern of the motion segment and to control any abnormal motion of the segment.

*References 1, 2, 8, 9, 24, 26, 31, 58, 60.

Principles of Dynamic Stabilization

The rationale underlying dynamic stabilization is that control of abnormal movement and more normal load transmission will relieve pain and also prevent adjacent segment degeneration. A remote expectation is that once abnormal motion and load transmission is fixed, the damaged disc may repair itself unless the degeneration is too advanced. Therefore the pertinent questions in dynamic stabilization are (1) how much control of motion is desirable, and (2) how much load should be shared by the system to unload the damaged disc? The long-term concern is about preventing implant failure in view of the constant movement of the stabilized segment. Fatigue failure of a rigid fixation implant is often caused by pseudarthrosis, because the rigidity of the implant does not permit accommodation of any motion originating at the pseudarthrosis. Flexible stabilization has an advantage in that it may accommodate the movement and therefore should avoid fatigue failure. Before this can be taken as granted, however, the kinematics of dynamic stabilization devices must be observed before their fatigue life can be determined.

As mentioned earlier, the dynamic stabilization system has to permit motion and also share load. It is expected that load-sharing by the implant would be more or less uniform during the entire range of motion, which is determined by the relative location of the optimal instant axis of rotation (IAR) of the system versus that of the motion segment. Any discrepancy in the kinematics between the dynamic stabilization system and the motion segment will lead to variability of load-sharing property. Normally the disc is loaded during flexion and extension. The average disc pressure rises during flexion and also during extension, and is lowest during the early phase of extension.[61] For example, if a dynamic stabilization system shares 30% of the load during flexion, it allows only 70% of the load to pass through the damaged disc. During extension, if the system forces the IAR to shift posterior to the disc, the disc will be distracted more and more towards the end of extension. This will be evident by a progressive lowering of the disc pressure towards the end of extension, which indicates that the dynamic stabilization system becomes an increasingly load-bearing structure in extension; this may lead to fatigue failure of the implant or the implant-bone junction (see Fig. 10-3). The relatively rigid dynamic stabilization devices like DSS, Dynesis, and Interspinous Spacers may have this disadvantage. Conversely, the ligament-based dynamic stabilization systems (Graf ligament) may load-share during flexion, but they become lax during extension and may not unload the disc at all during extension. This explains the fact that screw loosening has not been a problem with Graf ligament stabilization.[19]

In summary, dynamic stabilization devices must obey the biomechanical principles for uniform load transmission and preservation of the motion segment movement. Dynamic stabilization does not replace a component of the motion segment unlike disc prosthesis or nucleus prosthesis, and therefore its kinematic property should be complementary to that of the motion segment.

Box 10-1 Dynamic Stabilization Systems in Clinical Use

Interspinous Distraction Devices

Minn's silicone distraction device
Wallis system
X STOP

Interspinous Compression Devices

Elastic ligament (Bronsard's ligament across the spinous processes)
Loop system

Ligaments Across Pedicle Screws

Graf ligament
Dynesis device

Semirigid Devices Across the Pedicle Screws

FASS system
DSS system
AccuFlex system

Dynamic Stabilization Devices

The dynamic stabilization devices that are used clinically may be classified into four categories, outlined in Box 10-1.

Interspinous Distraction Devices

Minn's Silicone Distraction Device

The interspinous distraction devices are floating devices (i.e., not rigidly connected to the vertebrae), which avoids the possibility of loosening, a major concern with any implant that has to survive against motion. These devices work by distraction of the spinous processes. These silicone interspinous spacers on biomechanical testing in cadaver spine showed unloading of the disc and correction of sagittal plane imbalance of the spine. No clinical application of this system has since been described by the authors.[38]

Wallis System

Senegas et al[51] described a similar interspinous spacer in 1988 made of titanium and held between the spinous processes with a Dacron tape. After initial success in over 300 patients, the authors improved the system in the second generation, which is known as the *Wallis implant* (Fig. 10-4), which uses polyetheretherketone (PEEK) material instead of titanium. The clinical trials of the first-generation implant provided evidence that the interspinous system of dynamic stabilization is efficacious against low back pain caused by degenerative

A

B

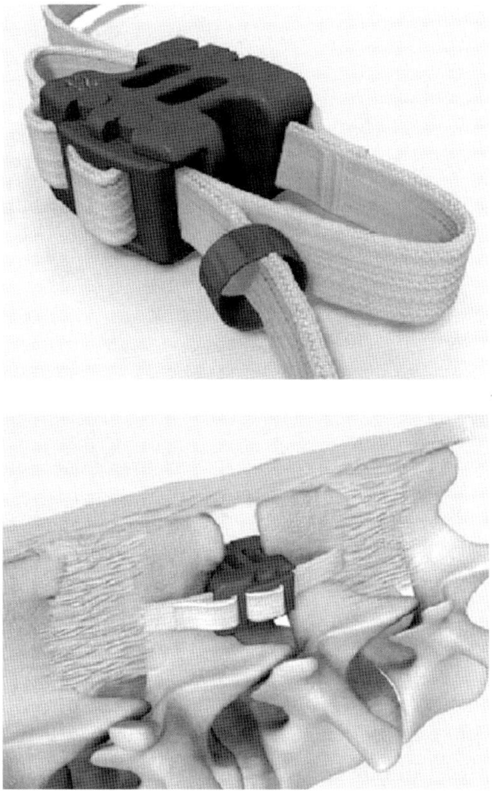

Fig. 10-4 The Wallis implant. (From Senegas J, Etchevers JP, Vital JM, et al. [Recalibration of the lumbar canal, an alternative to laminectomy in the treatment of lumbar canal stenosis. French.] Rev Chir Orthop Reparatrice Appar Mot 74:15-22, 1988.)

instability and free of serious complications. A randomized clinical trial and an observational study of the new implant are currently under way by the same authors. The authors recommend the Wallis system for lumbar disc disease in the following indications:

1. Discectomy for massive herniated disc leading to substantial loss of disc material
2. A second discectomy for recurrence of herniated disc
3. Discectomy for herniation of a transitional disc with sacralization of L5
4. Degenerative disc disease at a level adjacent to a previous fusion
5. An isolated Modic I lesion leading to chronic low back pain

X STOP

Another titanium interspinous distraction device, the X STOP, has been described by St. Francis Medical Technologies[55] and has completed FDA clinical trials and is awaiting FDA approval.[62] The implant has been described for use in patients with spinal stenosis, in whom the interspinous distraction holds the

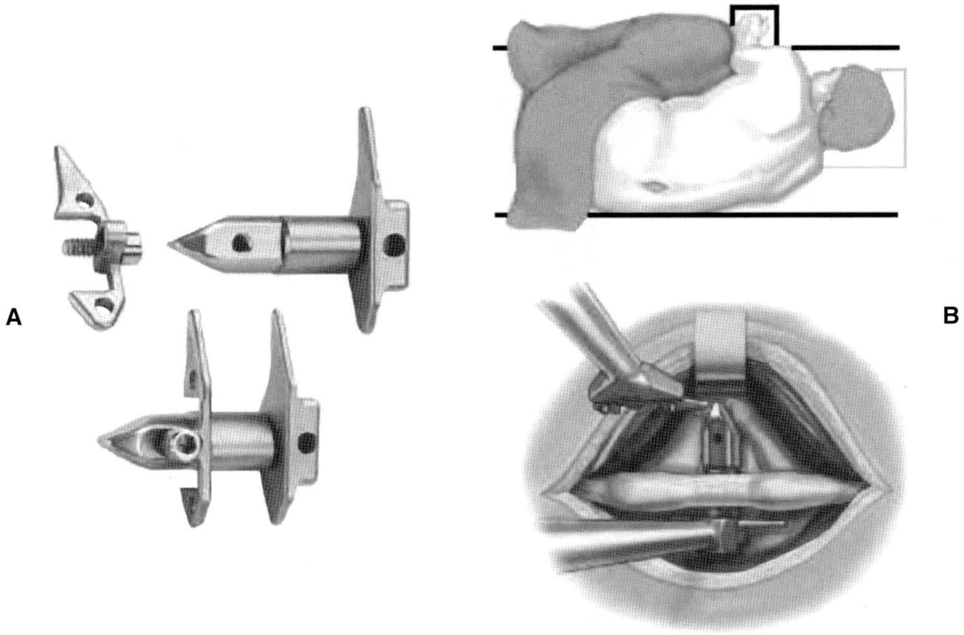

Fig. 10-5 The X STOP (introduced by St. Francis Medical Technologies, Inc.). **A,** The implants. **B,** The schematic representation of surgical implantation. (From St. Francis Medical Technologies, Inc., The X STOP interspinous process decompression system [IPD] for the treatment of lumbar spinal stenosis, 2001. www.sfmt.com/ipd.html.)

spine in flexion, reducing the stenosis. This device may be implanted via a minimally invasive approach with a local anesthetic, and may be useful in elderly patients with degenerative spinal stenosis who would prefer to avoid open surgery because of comorbid conditions (Fig. 10-5).

Interspinous Compression Devices

Elastic Ligament

The interspinous ligament devices may be applied directly around the spinous processes without any metal anchorage. Caserta et al[6] reported their experience of using elastic ligament alone or to supplement the adjacent segment to fusion (Fig. 10-6). The authors have used the system in 82 cases since 1994 and describe encouraging results; unfortunately, their report does not provide any details of the implant material or the clinical results.

Loop System

Garner et al[16a] described the Loop system (Spineology Inc., Stillwater, MN), a new tension-band device for stabilization of the spine across the spinous

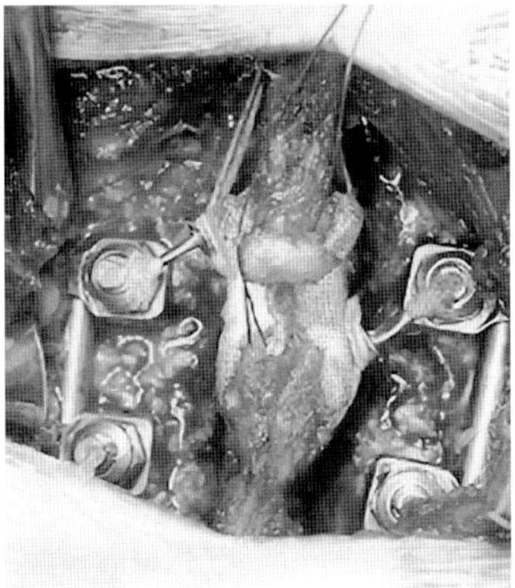

Fig. 10-6 The elastic interspinous ligament as described by Caserta et al. Perioperative picture of L4-5 elastic stabilization following rigid fixation of the L5-S1 segment. (From Caserta S, La Maida GA, Misaggi B, et al. Elastic stabilization alone or combined with rigid fusion in spinal surgery: A biomechanical study and clinical experience based on 82 cases. Eur Spine J 11[Suppl 2]:S192-S197, 2002.)

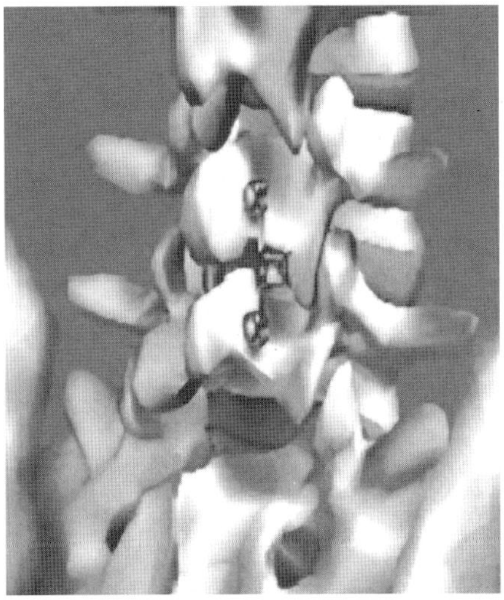

Fig. 10-7 The Loop system. (From Garner MD, Wolfe SJ, Kuslich SD. Development and preclinical testing of a new tension-band device for the spine: The Loop system. Eur Spine J 11[Suppl 2]:S186-S191, 2002.)

processes (Fig. 10-7). It consists of a braided polyethylene cable, a locking clip, and an optional ferrule that can be placed in the spinous process. After tension is applied by use of a tensioning tool, a locking clip secures the construct (Fig. 10-7). Garner et al[16a] compared the static tensile and fatigue strength, stiffness, and creep properties as well as the literature on different spine cables and wire fixation systems; they concluded that the Loop system has strength similar to a titanium cable system and has a no-slip locking clip designed to maintain the construct tension. It combines the advantages of the metallic system (lower creep) with the advantages of the polymer cables (high fatigue strength) without sacrificing strength, stiffness, or ease of use.

Ligaments Across Pedicle Screws

Graf Ligament

Ligaments across the pedicles are the systems that truly address the goal of a dynamic stabilization for degenerative instability of the lumbar spine. The most widely used device in this category is the Graf ligament, invented by Henri Graf.[18] The system consists of a nonelastic braided polyester ligament (Dacrilene) in the form of a loop, which is applied around the pedicle screws (Fig. 10-8). The ligaments are applied to the pedicle screws under tension to lock the motion segment in extension, with the intention that, once the facet joints were locked, rotation would not occur. Graf was of the view that "instability" was related to the development of an abnormal rotary movement, and if this were stopped, the system would still allow limited flexion, but within the range of normal flexion, which would therefore probably not be painful. There was no clinical or experimental basis for this view about the cause of instability or the efficacy of the ligament. Despite this fact, the Graf ligament has been used by several independent surgeons in Europe and the Far East with clinical success comparable to that of fusion.* The Graf ligamentoplasty procedure also produces a significant increase in lateral canal stenosis, especially if there is any preexisting degenerative change in the facet joints or infolding of the ligamentum flavum, owing to the marked lordosis of the segment instrumented; indeed, early clinical failure was often associated with this surgical complication.[19] The Graf ligament transfers the load from the anterior aspect of the disc to the posterior anulus and increases the disc pressure profile towards the posterior anulus, which was further substantiated by an experimental study with disc profilometry.[19] It is not known whether the clinical success was related to the restriction of motion or to the transfer of load to the posterior aspect removing loading from the painful anterior part of the disc. However, this may explain

*References 12, 43, 44, 50, 56, 59.

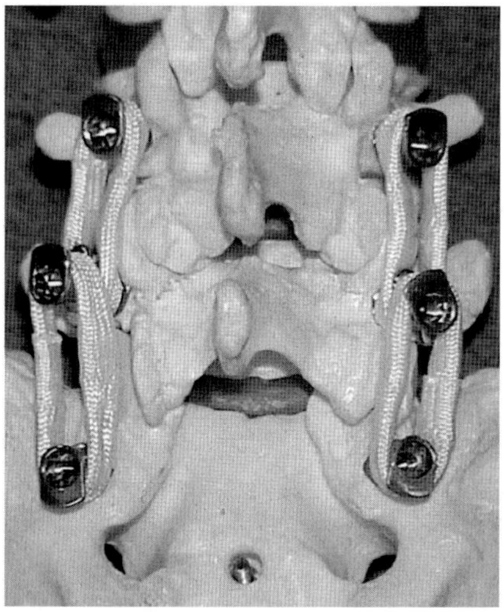

Fig. 10-8 The Graf ligament system, applied between pedicle screws at L4-5 and L5-S1 segment in saw-bone. (From Mulholland RC, Sengupta DK. Rationale, principles and experimental evaluation of the concept of soft stabilization. Eur Spine J 11[Suppl 2]:S198-S205, 2002.)

the late failure of the Graf ligament, which may accelerate the disc degeneration by overloading the posterior part of the disc.[41]

Dynesys Device

The Dynesys (dynamic neutralization system)[57] was developed by Gilles Dubois in 1994. In the present form the system consists of titanium alloy (Protasul 100) pedicle screws, polyester (Sulene-PET) cords, and polycarbonaturethane (Sulene-PCU) spacers (Fig. 10-9). The screws anchor the Dynesys system in the pedicle and in the vertebral body. The modular spacer fits between the pedicle screw heads. The stabilizing cords connect the pedicle screw heads via the hollow core of the spacer in place. According to the authors, its preload provides a uniform system rigidity, the stabilizing cord carries tensile forces, and the spacers resist compressive forces. The system is said to establish a mobile load transfer and controls motion of the segment in all planes.

The biomechanical testing of the system, as published in the literature, is limited to fatigue testing of the whole construct, and biocompatibility of the nonmetallic components. No data are available for the load-sharing characteristics or kinematics of the spinal motion segments after implantation of the Dynesys system.

Stoll, Dubois, and Schwarzenbach[57] presented their initial results on 83 patients. The indications included a mixed bag of degenerative conditions including spinal stenosis, degenerative discopathy, disc herniation, spondylolisthesis, and revision surgery. The clinical results have been described as encouraging and safe. However, unlike the Graf ligament, screw loosening was observed in seven cases treated with the Dynesys device. Early surgical intervention was needed in four cases, and late surgery was needed in five cases in the same segment and in seven cases for adjacent segment disease. The authors concluded that dynamic

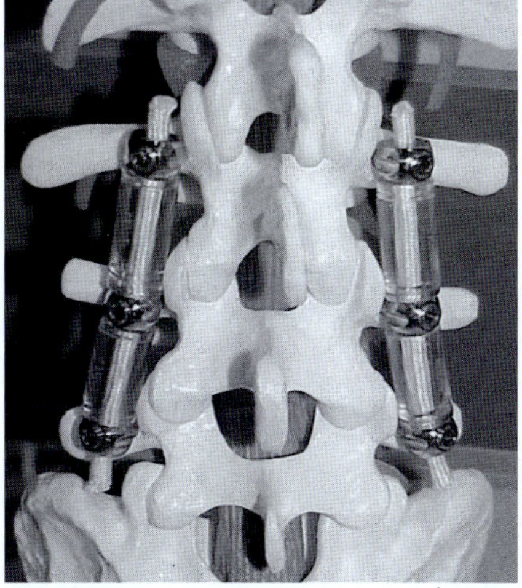

Fig. 10-9 The Dynesys system. (From Mulholland RC, Sengupta DK. Rationale, principles and experimental evaluation of the concept of soft stabilization. Eur Spine J 11[Suppl 2]: S198-S205, 2002.)

neutralization proved to be a safe and effective alternative in the treatment of unstable lumbar conditions.

A closer look into the system clarifies that introduction of the spacers between the pedicle screws leads to loss of lordosis of the segment. If the spinal extensor muscles can restore lordosis of the segment, they will do so by distracting the disc space while the spacer acts as a load-bearing fulcrum. This will unload the disc. Rajaratnam et al recently reviewed a group of 60 patients treated with the Dynesys device, with postoperative standing films with a plumb line; they found that the patients who failed to benefit from the Dynesys system are those who could not achieve lordosis at the stabilized segments.[49] Therefore the lordosis and load sharing by the plastic cylinder depend very critically on the placement of the implant and on the ability of the patient to achieve lordosis with the extensor muscles.[41]

Semirigid Metallic Devices Across the Pedicle Screws

Fulcrum-Assisted Soft Stabilization (FASS) System

I developed the FASS system (Fig. 10-10) to address what were perceived to be disadvantages of the Graf system.[52] There are two problems commonly experienced with the Graf system:

1. The lordosis produced by the Graf ligament system invariably results in narrowing of the lateral recess, leading to root entrapment, especially if there was any preexisting facet arthropathy.
2. The Graf system increases the loading of the posterior anulus, which is a feature of the painful degenerative disc.

A

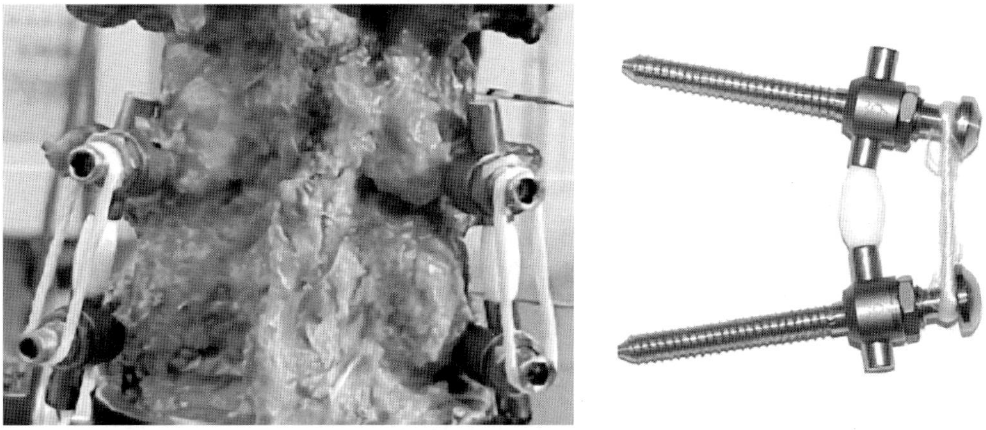

B

Fig. 10-10 A and **B,** The FASS system, as applied to a cadaver spine. In this prototype the fulcrum is made up of flexible polytetrafluoroethylene and the ligament is made up of elastic fabric band containing polyurethane.

The presence of the fulcrum in the FASS system prevents both these problems. The fulcrum is placed between the pedicle screws in front of the ligament, thereby distracting the posterior anulus. The elastic ligament is placed posterior to the fulcrum to compress between the heads of the pedicle screws. The fulcrum transforms this posterior compression force into an anterior distraction force, which distracts and unloads the disc. It is imperative that the FASS device should be inserted with sufficient tension in the ligament to create the required lordosis. The FASS system can unload the disc, unaided by the posture or muscle action; unlike the Dynesys system, it does not allow the segment to be put into kyphosis. The lordosis is created by the implant and is not dependent on the patient's ability to achieve lordosis with his or her own muscles.

The implant experimentally unloads the disc by sharing load. The degree of disc unloading depends on the relative tension and compression produced by the fulcrum and the ligament. For a given distraction by the fulcrum, the higher the compressive force applied by the ligament the greater would be the disc unloading. However, laboratory experiments in spine models and cadaver spines demonstrate that greater disc unloading also imparts higher stiffness of the motion segment.[53] In other words, as greater unloading of the disc is achieved by adjustment of the tension in the ligament and the fulcrum, the system shares higher load and the motion segment loses flexibility. Clearly, if a very stiff system is implanted, screw loosening and implant failure are more likely to occur in the long term. To maintain the normal physiologic environment in the disc, it may be desirable to unload the disc partially and allow the segment mobility as close to normal as possible. The fulcrum should act as a load-sharing device and not as a load-bearing device. The system is still under development (sponsored by AO International, Davos, Switzerland) and a clinically applicable prototype is yet to be made available.

Dynamic Soft Stabilization (DSS) System

The DSS system has been developed by the author (sponsored by Spinal Concepts, Inc., Austin, TX), but it has not been used clinically yet. Two designs of the DSS system have been tested in the laboratory (Fig. 10-11). The DSS-I system consists of a titanium spring, made of spring grade titanium wires 3 mm in cross-sectional diameter. The DSS-II system consists of an elliptical coil spring, made from 4 mm spring-grade titanium rods. Both the springs are applied to the motion segment by pedicle screws. Pre-tension at the spring during its application would unload the disc at rest. The flexibility of the spring will permit limited flexibility of the motion segment. The disc unloading during motion will be dependent on the location of the instant axis of rotation (IAR) of the springs and that of the motion segment. If the location of these IARs remains close to each other, the disc unloading and load sharing would be uniform throughout the range of motion and will only depend on the flexibility of the

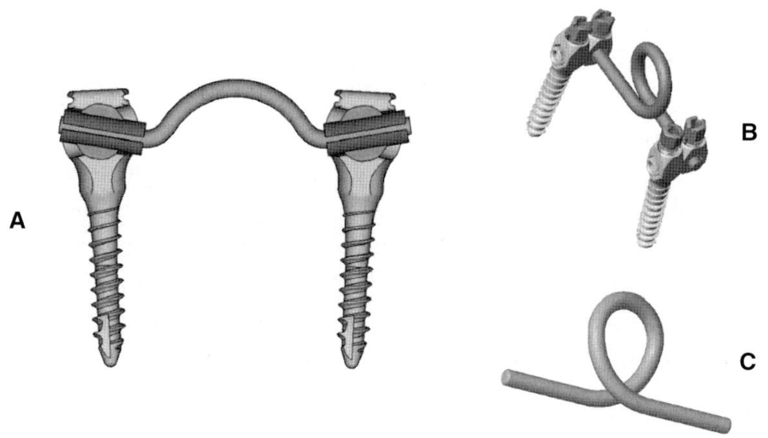

Fig. 10-11 A, The DSS-I system consists of a C-shaped titanium spring. **B** and **C,** The DSS-II system consists of a titanium coil spring, which can be attached to the pedicle screws of different designs.

spring. On the other hand, if there is a discrepancy in the relative location of the IAR, the DSS system may become an increasingly load-bearing structure at certain ranges of motion (see Fig. 10-3), which may lead to early implant failure or loosening. Recent cadaver tests show that the DSS-II system offers a more favorable kinematics and promises to achieve the objectives of soft stabilization with optimum load sharing, disc unloading, and control of motion.

A prospective clinical trial is underway with the DSS-II system for activity-related mechanical back pain patients who do not have leg pain and do not require any decompression. The DSS-II is introduced through a minimally invasive technique. The rationale is to examine whether the system can relieve such back pain clinically when used alone as an isolated treatment method. This evidence is essential before its use can be recommended for other indications, such as stabilization of a segment following decompression or of an adjacent segment following fusion. An example of the DSS-II's clinical application is presented in Fig. 10-12.

Soft Stabilization as an Adjunct to Disc Prosthesis

As stated earlier, disc replacement is only an equivalent to a partial joint replacement. In the presence of significant facet joint arthritis, disc replacement may not relieve pain. When radicular pain warrants decompression involving a partial facetectomy, disc replacement may destabilize the motion segment. A posterior soft stabilization system promises to add stability after decompressive lumbar laminectomy or facetectomy. In effect, adding a posterior soft stabilization to disc replacement may make it equivalent to total joint replacement.

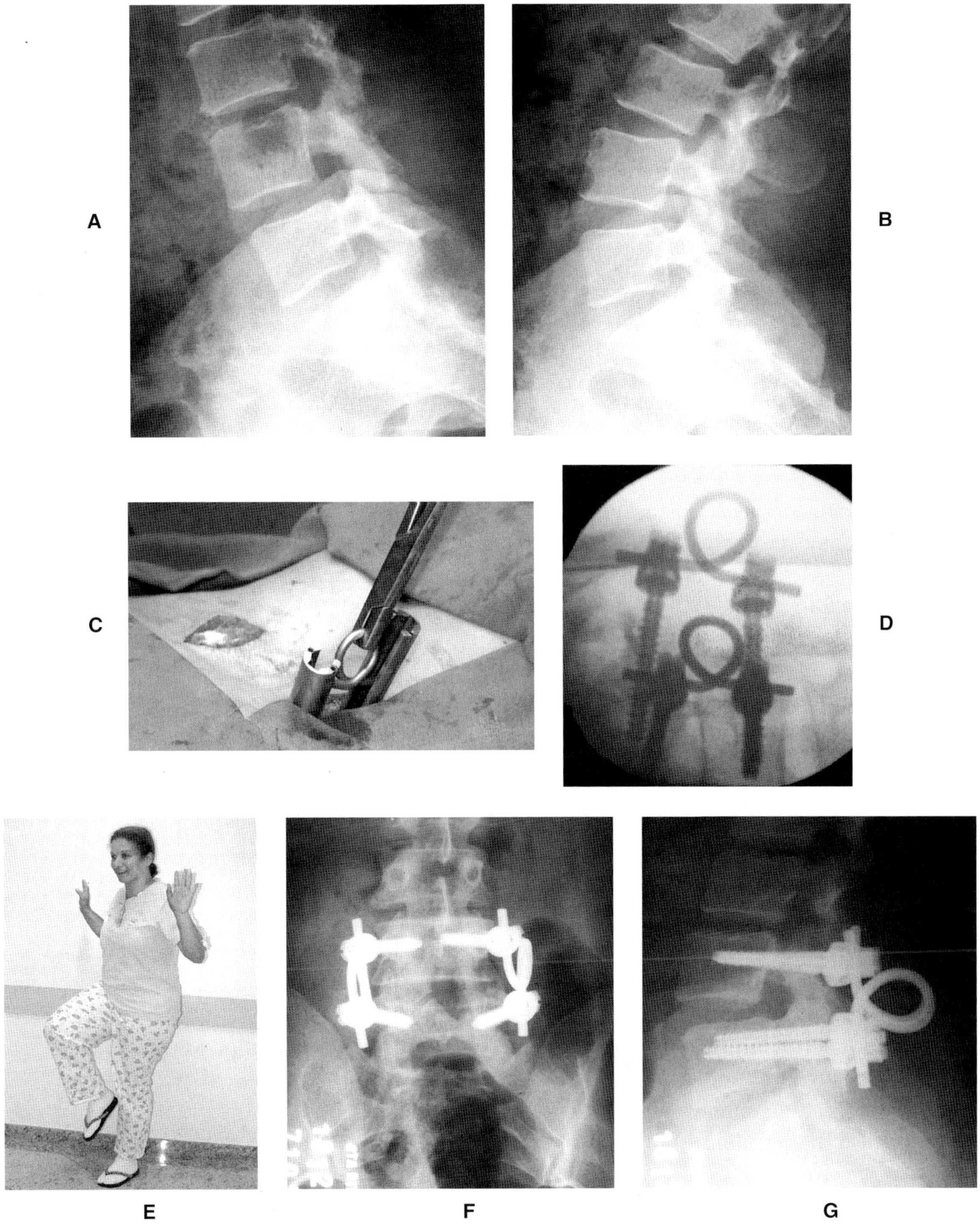

Fig. 10-12 A, Flexion and **B,** extension preoperative radiographs in a 46-year-old woman with a previous L4-5 discectomy and recurrence of mechanical back pain. MRI showed disc degeneration and a discogram reproduced concordant pain at the L4-5 segment. **C,** The DSS spring is pushed downward toward the percutaneously placed pedicle screws to which it will be attached. **D,** Fluoroscopic oblique view shows the devices in place bilaterally. **E,** Since the postoperative morbidity was minimal, the patient could ambulate just a few hours after surgery and experienced significant relief of her mechanical back pain. **F** and **G,** Postoperative AP and lateral views showing the device in place.

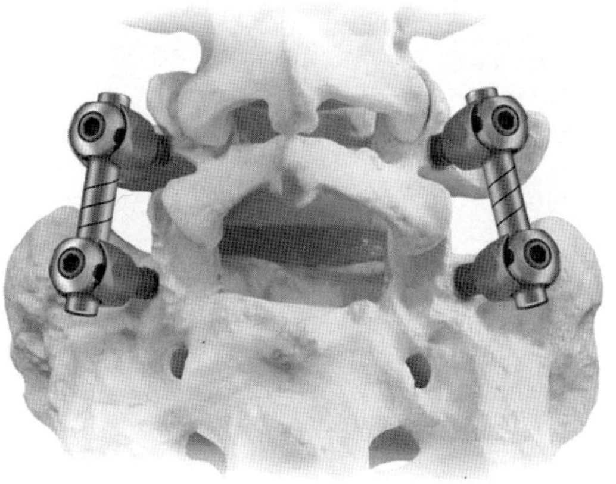

Fig. 10-13 The AccuFlex system (Globus Medical Inc., Phoenoxville, PA).

This system consists of a flexible titanium rod that can be inserted in a minimally invasive technique to the pedicle screws. Cannulated pedicle screws can be inserted percutaneously. Biomechanical tests have shown the fatigue life of this flexible rod system to last more than 10 million cycles. The advantage of this system is that the flexible segment can form pat of a solid fusion rod for application to an adjacent segment. A preliminary clinical trial has been started, but an IDE study for FDA approval is due (Fig. 10-13).

Conclusion

In summary, soft stabilization plays an important role in the treatment of the degenerative lumbar spine. Fusion of one or two motion segments may not make a big difference in the total range of motion of the lumbar spine, but preserving the flexibility of a motion segment may prevent adjacent disease and may permit disc replacement, even when facet joints need to be excised. Additionally, if a favorable environment can be created in the motion segment by unloading the disc and permitting near-normal motion, the disc may be able to repair itself. Gene therapy in degenerative disc diseases, either by promoting enzymes to produce proteoglycans or by preventing the release of enzymes like proteases that damage the disc, is an emerging technology that holds a lot of promise. Soft stabilization may further enhance the reparative process activated by gene therapy.

Although soft stabilization appears to be promising, any new implant system should be viewed with caution. A fusion implant only has to serve as a temporary stabilization device until fusion has taken place; on the other hand, a soft stabilization system has to provide stability throughout its life. In fusion surgery, loosening is common in the presence of pseudarthrosis. After soft stabilization the implant has to stay anchored to the bone while allowing near-normal spinal movement, which sounds like an impossible task. However, the flexibility of the implant system should protect it from loosening where it is anchored into the bone. Finally, the soft stabilization system is intended to load-share with the disc and the facet joint only partially and unloads the motion segment. However, any mismatch between the kinematics of the implant system and the motion segment, in particular, any discrepancy between their IAR would result in the implant bearing an unexpected load at certain ranges of motion. If that happens, it would guarantee early implant failure or loosening. Thus the need for a bench test in the laboratory cannot be overemphasized. To date, the few soft stabilization systems that have had clinical applications produced a clinical outcome comparable to that of fusion. No prospective randomized controlled trials have been reported yet, which is essential for the practice of evidence-based medicine.

REFERENCES

1. Agazzi S, Reverdin A, May D. Posterior lumbar interbody fusion with cages: An independent review of 71 cases. J Neurosurg 91:186-192, 1999.
2. Ariga K, Miyamoto S, Nakase T, et al. The relationship between apoptosis of endplate chondrocytes and aging and degeneration of the intervertebral disc. Spine 26:2414-2420, 2001.
3. Bjarke Christensen F, Stender Hansen E, et al. Long-term functional outcome of pedicle screw instrumentation as a support for posterolateral spinal fusion: Randomized clinical study with a 5-year follow-up. Spine 27:1269-1277, 2002.
4. Boos N, Webb JK. Pedicle screw fixation in spinal disorders: A European view. Eur Spine J 6:2-18, 1997.
5. Brechbuhler D, Markwalder TM, Braun M. Surgical results after soft system stabilization of the lumbar spine in degenerative disc disease—long-term results. Acta Neurochir (Wien) 140:521-525, 1998.
6. Caserta S, La Maida GA, Misaggi B, et al. Elastic stabilization alone or combined with rigid fusion in spinal surgery: A biomechanical study and clinical experience based on 82 cases. Eur Spine J 11(Suppl 2):S192-S197, 2002.
7. Chou WY, Hsu CJ, Chang WN, et al. Adjacent segment degeneration after lumbar spinal posterolateral fusion with instrumentation in elderly patients. Arch Orthop Trauma Surg 122:39-43, 2002.
8. Christensen FB, Thomsen K, Eiskjaer SP, et al. Functional outcome after posterolateral spinal fusion using pedicle screws: Comparison between primary and salvage procedure. Eur Spine J 7:321-327, 1998.
9. Dahl B, Gehrchen P, Blyme P, et al. Clinical outcome after spinal fusion with a rigid versus a semirigid pedicle screw system. Eur Spine J 6:412-416. 1997.
10. Eck JC, Humphreys SC, Hodges SD. Adjacent-segment degeneration after lumbar fusion: A review of clinical, biomechanical, and radiologic studies. Am J Orthop 28:336-340, 1999.
11. Etebar S, Cahill DW. Risk factors for adjacent-segment failure following lumbar fixation with rigid instrumentation for degenerative instability. J Neurosurg 90:163-169, 1999.
12. Friberg O. Lumbar instability: A dynamic approach by traction-compression radiography. Spine 12:119-129, 1987.
13. Fritzell P, Hagg O, Wessberg P, et al. Chronic low back pain and fusion: A comparison of three surgical techniques: A prospective multicenter randomized study from the Swedish lumbar spine study group. Spine 27:1131-1141, 2002.
14. Fujiwara A, Lim TH, An HS, et al. The effect of disc degeneration and facet joint osteoarthritis on the segmental flexibility of the lumbar spine. Spine 25:3036-3044, 2000.

15. Fujiwara A, Tamai K, An HS, et al. The relationship between disc degeneration, facet joint osteoarthritis, and stability of the degenerative lumbar spine. J Spinal Disord 13:444-450, 2000.
16. Gardner A, Pande KC. Graf ligamentoplasty: A 7-year follow-up. Eur Spine J 11(Suppl 2):S157-S163, 2002.
16a. Garner MD, Wolfe SJ, Kuslich SD. Development and preclinical testing of a new tension-band device for the spine: The Loop system. Eur Spine J 11(Suppl 2):S186-S191, 2002.
17. Gibson JN, Grant IC, Waddell G. The Cochrane review of surgery for lumbar disc prolapse and degenerative lumbar spondylosis. Spine 24:1820-1832, 1999.
18. Graf H. Lumbar instability. Surgical treatment without fusion. Rachis 412:123-137, 1992.
19. Grevitt MP, Gardner AD, Spilsbury J, et al. The Graf stabilisation system: Early results in 50 patients. Eur Spine J 4:169-175, 1995.
20. Guigui P, Chopin D. Assessment of the use of the Graf ligamentoplasty in the surgical treatment of lumbar spinal stenosis. Apropos of a series of 26 patients. Rev Chir Orthop Reparatrice Appar Mot 80:681-688, 1994.
21. Hadlow SV, Fagan AB, Hillier TM, et al. The Graf ligamentoplasty procedure. Comparison with posterolateral fusion in the management of low back pain. Spine 23:1172-1179, 1998.
22. Hukins DW. A simple model for the function of proteoglycans and collagen in the response to compression of the intervertebral disc. Proc R Soc Lond B Biol Sci 249:281-285, 1992.
23. Kanayama M, Hashimoto T, Shigenobu K, et al. Adjacent-segment morbidity after Graf ligamentoplasty compared with posterolateral lumbar fusion. J Neurosurg 95:5-10, 2001.
24. Kawakami M, Tamaki T, Ando M, et al. Lumbar sagittal balance influences the clinical outcome after decompression and posterolateral spinal fusion for degenerative lumbar spondylolisthesis. Spine 27:59-64, 2002.
25. Keller TS, Hansson TH, Abram AC, et al. Regional variations in the compressive properties of lumbar vertebral trabeculae. Effects of disc degeneration. Spine 14:1012-1019, 1989.
26. Korsgaard M, Christensen FB, Thomsen K, et al. The influence of lumbar lordosis on spinal fusion and functional outcome after posterolateral spinal fusion with and without pedicle screw instrumentation. J Spinal Disord Tech 15:187-192, 2002.
27. Krag MH, Seroussi RE, Wilder DG, et al. Internal displacement distribution from in vitro loading of human thoracic and lumbar spinal motion segments: Experimental results and theoretical predictions. Spine 12:1001-1007, 1987.
28. Kumar MN, Baklanov A, Chopin D. Correlation between sagittal plane changes and adjacent segment degeneration following lumbar spine fusion. Eur Spine J 10:314-319, 2001.
29. Lazennec JY, Ramare S, Arafati N, et al. Sagittal alignment in lumbosacral fusion: Relations between radiological parameters and pain. Eur Spine J 9:47-55, 2000.
30. Legaye J, De Cloedt P, Emery R. Supple intervertebral stabilization according to Graf. Evaluation of its use and technical approach. Acta Orthop Belg 60:393-401, 1994.
31. Mahvi DM, Zdeblick TA. A prospective study of laparoscopic spinal fusion. Technique and operative complications. Ann Surg 224:85-90, 1996.
32. Markwalder TM, Wenger M. Adjacent-segment morbidity. J Neurosurg 96:139-140, 2002.
33. McAfee PC. Interbody fusion cages in reconstructive operations on the spine. J Bone Joint Surg Am 81:859-880, 1999.
34. McMillan DW, McNally DS, Garbutt G, et al. Stress distributions inside intervertebral discs: The validity of experimental "stress profilometry." Proc Inst Mech Eng 210:81-87, 1996.
35. McNally DS. The objectives for the mechanical evaluation of spinal instrumentation have changed. Eur Spine J 11(Suppl 2):S179-S185, 2002.
36. McNally DS, Adams MA. Internal intervertebral disc mechanics as revealed by stress profilometry. Spine 17:66-73, 1992.

37. McNally DS, Shackleford IM, Goodship AE, et al. In vivo stress measurement can predict pain on discography. Spine 21:2580-2587, 1996.
38. Minns RJ, Walsh WK. Preliminary design and experimental studies of a novel soft implant for correcting sagittal plane instability in the lumbar spine. Spine 22:1819-1825, 1997.
39. Mochida J, Suzuki K, Chiba M. How to stabilize a single level lesion of degenerative lumbar spondylolisthesis. Clin Orthop 126-134, 1999.
40. Moore RJ, Vernon-Roberts B, Fraser RD, et al. The origin and fate of herniated lumbar intervertebral disc tissue. Spine 21:2149-2155, 1996.
41. Mulholland RC, Sengupta DK. Rationale, principles and experimental evaluation of the concept of soft stabilization. Eur Spine J 11(Suppl 2):S198-S205, 2002.
42. Nachemson AL. Disc pressure measurements. Spine 6:93-97, 1981.
43. Ogston NG, King GJ, Gertzbein SD, et al. Centrode patterns in the lumbar spine. Baseline studies in normal subjects. Spine 11:591-595, 1986.
44. Okawa A, Shinomiya K, Komori H, et al. Dynamic motion study of the whole lumbar spine by videofluoroscopy. Spine 23:1743-1749, 1998.
45. Panjabi M, Yamamoto I, Oxland T, et al. How does posture affect coupling in the lumbar spine? Spine 14:1002-1011, 1989.
46. Pearcy M, Portek I, Shepherd J. The effect of low-back pain on lumbar spinal movements measured by three-dimensional x-ray analysis. Spine 10:150-153, 1985.
47. Polikeit A OT, Nolte L-P. Factors affecting the behaviour of interbody cages in the lumbar spine—finite element analysis. Presented at the Annual Meeting of the International Society for the Study of the Lumbar Spine, Adelaide, Scotland, June 2000.
48. Rahm MD, Hall BB. Adjacent-segment degeneration after lumbar fusion with instrumentation: A retrospective study. J Spinal Disord 9:392-400, 1996.
49. Rajaratnam SS SG, Mueller M, Shepperd JAN, et al. Dynesis stabilization of the lumbosacral spine. Presented at Britspine, Birmingham, England, 2002.
50. Seligman JV, Gertzbein SD, Tile M, et al. Computer analysis of spinal segment motion in degenerative disc disease with and without axial loading. Spine 9:566-573, 1984.
51. Senegas J, Etchevers JP, Vital JM, et al. Recalibration of the lumbar canal, an alternative to laminectomy in the treatment of lumbar canal stenosis. Rev Chir Orthop Reparatrice Appar Mot 74:15-22, 1988.
52. Sengupta DK, Ohnmeiss DD, Guyer RD, et al. Fulcrum-assisted soft stabilisation in the treatment of low back pain—a new concept. Presented at the Annual Meeting of the International Society for the Study of the Lumbar Spine, Hawaii, March 1999.
53. Sengupta DK, Ohnmeiss DD, Webb JK, et al. Can soft stabilization in the lumbar spine unload the disc and retain mobility? A biomechanical study with fulcrum-assisted soft stabilization on cadaver spine. Presented at the Annual Meeting of the International Society for the Study of the Lumbar Spine, Edinburgh, Scotland, June 2001.
54. Simpson EK, Parkinson IH, Manthey B, et al. Intervertebral disc disorganization is related to trabecular bone architecture in the lumbar spine. J Bone Miner Res 16:681-687, 2001.
55. St. Francis Medical Technologies, Inc. The X STOP interspinous process distraction system (IPD) for the treatment of lumbar spinal stenosis, 2001. www.sfmt.com/ipd.html.
56. Stokes IA, Frymoyer JW. Segmental motion and instability. Spine 12:688-691, 1987.
57. Stoll TM, Dubois G, Schwarzenbach O. The dynamic neutralization system for the spine: A multi-center study of a novel non-fusion system. Eur Spine J 11(Suppl 2):S170-S178, 2002.
58. Thomsen K, Christensen FB, Eiskjaer SP, et al. 1997 Volvo Award winner in clinical studies. The effect of pedicle screw instrumentation on functional outcome and fusion rates in posterolateral lumbar spinal fusion: A prospective, randomized clinical study. Spine 22:2813-2822, 1997.
59. Weiler PJ, King GJ, Gertzbein SD. Analysis of sagittal plane instability of the lumbar spine in vivo. Spine 15:1300-1306, 1990.

60. Whitecloud TS III, Castro FP Jr, Brinker MR, et al. Degenerative conditions of the lumbar spine treated with intervertebral titanium cages and posterior instrumentation for circumferential fusion. J Spinal Disord 11:479-486, 1998.
61. Wilke H, Neef P, Hinz B, et al. Intradiscal pressure together with anthropometric data—a data set for the validation of models. Clin Biomech 16(Suppl 1):S111-S126, 2001.
62. Zuckerman JF, Hsu KY, Hartjen CA, et al. A prospective randomized multi-center study for the treatment of lumbar spinal stenosis with the X STOP interspinous implant: 1-year results. Eur Spin J 13:22-31, 2004.

CHAPTER

11

Microsurgical Anular Reconstruction (Anuloplasty) Following Lumbar Microdiscectomy

Joseph C. Cauthen

Anular repair is a technique that is still evolving to meet current and future requirements. In this chapter preliminary results from an ongoing anuloplasty series will be presented. A selected review of published work on lumbar disc reherniation is summarized to highlight definitional issues in the belief that standardized definitions will strengthen the case for anular repair techniques. The future role of anular repair in the treatment of disc herniation and disc replacement will also be discussed.

RATIONALE

Surgical repair of the defective lumbar disc anulus (anuloplasty) immediately raises the question: "Why?" The starting point of the standard technique involves removal of a disc fragment extruding through an opening in the disc anulus. The traditional end result is a gaping anulotomy incision or an anular tear created by the centrifugal path of the disc nucleus (Fig. 11-1). Traditionally, the anular defect has not been addressed as a *portal for reherniation.* We will present several possible advantages of closing this anular opening to aid postoperative anular healing.

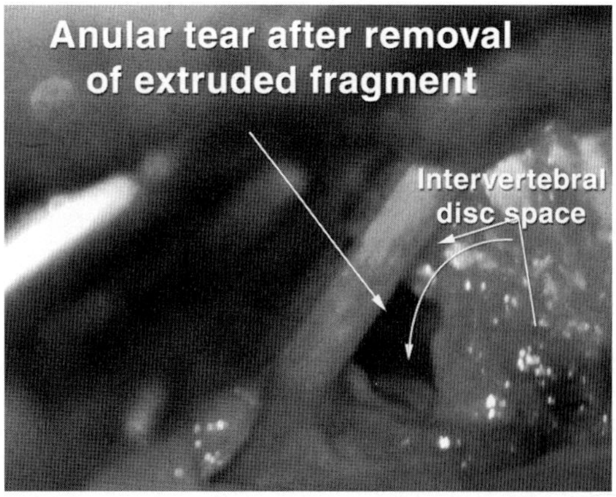

Fig. 11-1 Traditional end result (gaping anulotomy).

Preoperative Treatment and Evaluation

Before patients with lumbar disc herniation are considered for a procedure including anuloplasty, they are required to undergo nonoperative therapy for 1 to 3 months if the pain level and neurologic status permit. Nonoperative treatment includes physical therapy as tolerated, nonnarcotic analgesics, nonsteroidal antiinflammatory drugs (NSAIDs) as tolerated, epidural steroid therapy, and 3 to 5 days of bed rest at the onset of acute symptoms. Herniations are confirmed with magnetic resonance imaging (MRI) and/or lumbar myelography with computed tomography (CT).

Surgical Technique

Approach to the Anulus and Subanular Space

After surgical extradural fragment removal, all subsequent considerations are subanular. Current surgical techniques indicate that subanular access can be gained by cutting a rectangular opening in the anulus *(box anulotomy)*. This procedure provides excellent access to the interdiscal space and improves the chances of identifying and removing residual subanular fragments, a source of nuclear reherniation. Box anulotomy is less physiologic and more likely to allow recurrent herniation because of the open pathway from the disc center through the anulus to the epidural space.

Dilation and spreading of anular fibers by blunt perforation is an alternative that has been advocated by Williams[63-66]; however, subanular access is limited, reducing the opportunity for retrieval of additional subanular fragments.

An improved technique has been developed using *slit anulotomy* and anular repair. In contained nuclear herniation, subanular access is gained via a linear incision with greater potential for early healing (slit anulotomy). In an extruded nuclear herniation, gaining subanular access by traversing the existing anular defect is desirable. Either pathway allows anular repair if sufficient exposure and sufficient anular tissue is present.

Microsurgical Discectomy

The present technique includes a 5 to 8 mm sharp incision at the anular midpoint, equidistant from the endplates, allowing subanular disc fragment removal and nerve decompression using microoperative technique. Following experimentation with one suture, closure now requires two or three 4-0 absorbable sutures on half-circle needles placed equidistant along the slit anulotomy incision. Additionally, in a variation of suture anular reapproximation, a subanular fascial autograft can be used to augment the strength of the anuloplasty.

Microsurgical knot-tying technique secures the fascial autograft in the subanular loop of the sutures and closes the anulotomy incision. An autologous fat graft is placed in the epidural space to reduce the incursion of fibroblastic epidural scar and its associated inflammatory response.

Microsurgical anular reconstruction was used after removal of a subanular fragment indicated in the axial view of an L4-5 discal herniation (Fig. 11-2). The approach involved the minimal adequate skin incision of 4 cm over the target interspace, confirmed by intraoperative x-ray. A limited laminotomy and removal of sufficient ligamentum flavum allowed entry into the epidural space. The anulus was palpated at the midpoint between the endplates with the lumbar dura retracted medially and the medial aspect of the exiting nerve root clearly demonstrated (Fig. 11-3). A 5 to 8 mm anular incision was made equidistant from the endplates. With the dura protected with a nerve retractor and the exiting nerve root well visualized, incision with a Beaver 6400 ophthalmic blade has been useful (Fig. 11-4). After withdrawal of the subanular fragment with resulting nerve decompression, the interspace was thoroughly explored with straight and angled pituitary rongeurs and by application of irrigation and suction to the subanular space with the intent of dislodging additional fragments.

Initiation of the first needle pass with a 4-0 Vicryl suture (Ethicon 504) on a P-2 needle allowed retrieval of the needle point medial to the nerve, as indicated in the intraoperative photograph (Fig. 11-5), completing the suture path.

Regardless of which method of anuloplasty is used (one, multiple sutures alone, or multiple sutures with fascial autograft), 4-0 Vicryl sutures on half-circle needles are used to reapproximate the sides of the anular incision. Each suture is

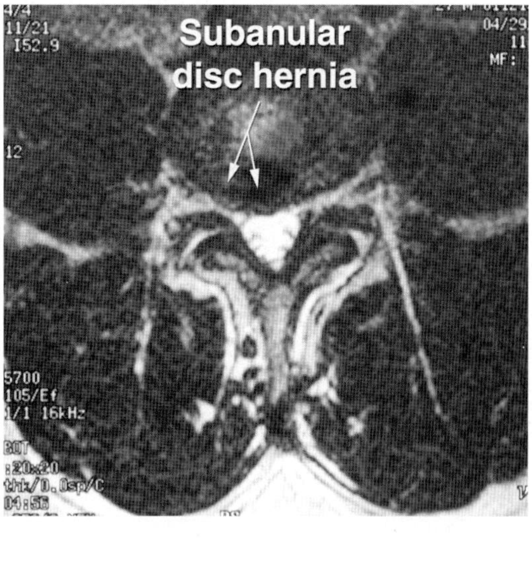

Fig. 11-2 Axial view: subanular disc hernia.

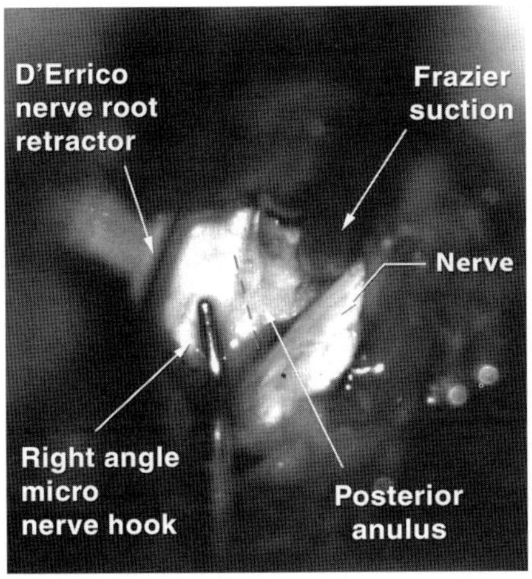

Fig. 11-3 Palpation of anulus at midpoint between endplates.

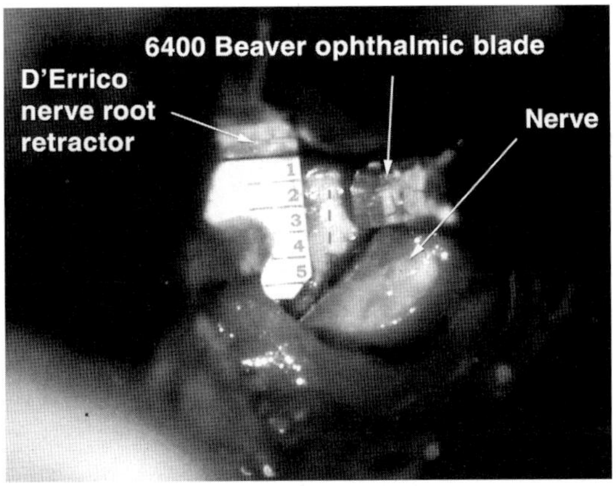

Fig. 11-4 Initiation of 6 mm incision of anulus at midpoint between endplates.

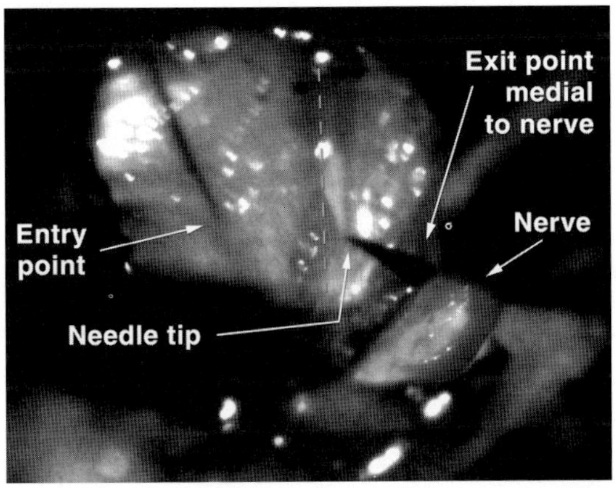

Fig. 11-5 Initiation of first needle pass.

placed through the inferior and superior sides of the anulotomy, which is then closed using microsurgical knot-tying technique.

When subanular fascial autograft is used, a 10 by 4 mm fascial autograft is harvested from the lumbodorsal fascia and placed in a subanular position suspended in the subanular loops of two or more sutures. Each suture is then tied in succession, securing the autograft in place.

The completed needle pass with the entry point approximately 3 mm lateral to the anular opening and exit point medial to the nerve at the same distance from the anular opening completes the first suture placement. At least two approximating sutures on each side of the anulotomy are separated, in preparation of placing the subanular fascial autograft. Occasionally, there is sufficient room to place three approximating sutures on each side of the anular opening. These sutures are microsurgically tied over the subanular fascial autograft, which was harvested from the lumbodorsal fascia through the initial incision used for the laminotomy.

The fascial autograft is positioned for subanular placement in the subanular loops of either two or three reapproximating sutures (Fig. 11-6). The anulus is then reapproximated and the strength of the anular repair is augmented by the subanular fascial autograft (Fig. 11-7). After anular closure, the incision is irrigated thoroughly with normal saline solution containing bacitracin. Topical 0.25% local anesthetic and epidural steroid preparations are placed on the exposed dural surfaces beneath an autologous fat graft.

The incision is closed in typical fashion. The patient is encouraged to ambulate within hours after completion of the procedure. Discharge is anticipated on the same day as surgery and, in many cases, within 24 hours of admission.

Postoperative Follow-up

Follow-up office visits are scheduled at 1 and 3 weeks after surgery. Patients are encouraged to perform gentle stretching and strengthening exercises for leg, abdominal, and lumbar musculature for 12 weeks to avoid compression loading and torque to the lumbar spine, allowing healing of the anular repair. Thereafter, supervised physical therapy is initiated, emphasizing muscle strengthening and avoidance of compression and torque stresses for 4 weeks.

Outcome Evaluation: Chart Review and Patient Survey

Research Methods

The charts of all patients who underwent microsurgical discectomy with anuloplasty between April 1994 and February 1999 were reviewed for demographic

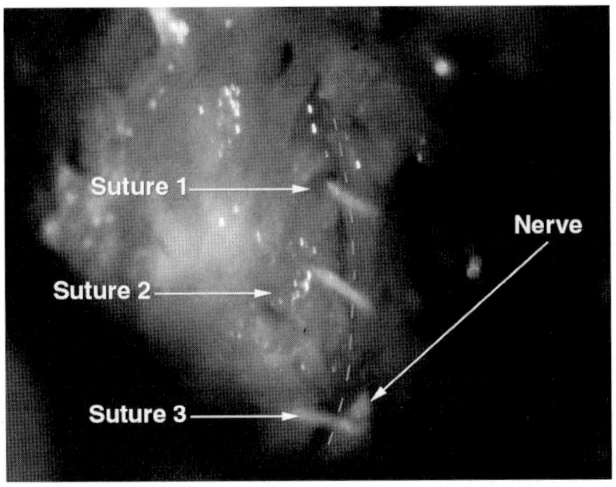

Fig. 11-6 Three approximating sutures on each side of anulotomy ready for microsurgical tying over subanular fascial autograft.

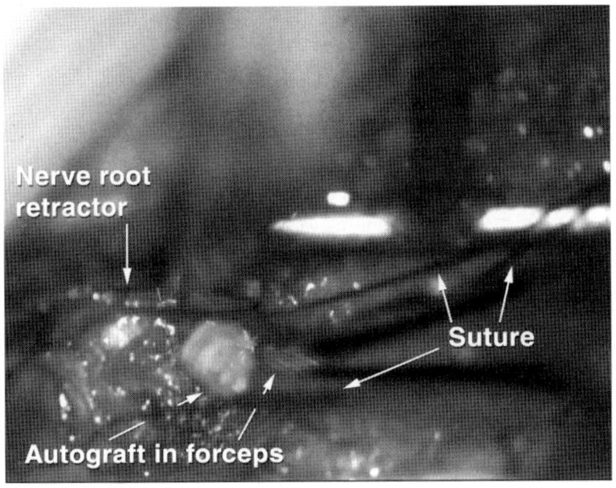

Fig. 11-7 Fascial autograft positioned for subanular placement.

data, diagnoses, procedures, complications, and recurrences (as established by radiology reports and reoperations). Charts were also reviewed for a control group of patients who underwent microsurgical discectomy for herniated lumbar disc without anuloplasty during the 4 years preceding the anuloplasty group (January 1991 to December 1994).

A two-page questionnaire was mailed to patients in both groups at least 1 year after the anuloplasty procedure. Patients who did not return the questionnaire were contacted by phone. (Of 197 responses obtained for the control group, 140 were mailed in and 57 were obtained through telephone interview. Of 117 responses obtained for the anuloplasty group, 81 were mailed in and 36 were obtained by phone.) All patients were given space on the questionnaire to encourage comments, confirm answers, and address issues not explicitly covered elsewhere in the questionnaire.

Inclusion criteria for patients in this study were: (1) a diagnosis of symptomatic herniated nucleus pulposus (HNP); (2) a microdiscectomy procedure with or without anuloplasty with at least 1-year follow-up; (3) a questionnaire response.

Patients who underwent fusion operations concurrent with microdiscectomy were excluded from the control group. However, previous lumbar surgery at another level did not exclude a patient from this study.

Patient Population

Demographic information is presented for patients in all groups in Table 11-1: sex, age at time of surgery, smoking, employment, workers' compensation, disability status, incidence of accident-related litigation, and previous surgeries.

In all cases, nerve compression was noted as a consequence of HNP. In some patients, cauda equina compression, extruded fragment, disc protrusion, and

TABLE 11-1 PATIENT DEMOGRAPHICS: CONTROL AND THREE TYPES OF ANULOPLASTY

	Control (N = 197)	One Suture (N = 35)	Two+ Sutures (N = 42)	Fascial Autograft (N = 40)
Male (N = 178; 57%)	117 (59%)	21 (60%)	22 (52%)	18 (45%)
Female (N = 136; 43%)	80 (41%)	14 (40%)	20 (48%)	22 (55%)
Age (17.2-82.1 years; mean = 46.9)	46.9 (17.2-75.9)	45.3 (20.4-81.1)	46.6 (18.9-82.1)	48.2 (19.3-74.8)
Smokers, before operation (N = 105; 33.4%)	66 (33.5%)	13 (37.1%)	15 (35.7%)	11 (27.5%)
Working at time of surgery (N = 249; 79.3%)	157 (79.7%)	27 (77.1%)	35 (83.3%)	30 (75.0%)
Receiving workers' compensation (N = 97; 30.9%)	66 (33.5%)	14 (40.0%)	14 (33.3%)	3 (7.5%)
Receiving other disability claims (N = 40; 12.7%)	25 (12.7%)	10 (28.6%)	1 (2.4%)	4 (10.0%)
Injury-related litigation (N = 44; 14.0%)	28 (14.2%)	4 (11.4%)	9 (21.4%)	3 (7.5%)
Previous Surgeries				
Any lumbar	12	3	4	6
Discectomy, same level/side as index	22	1	2	1
None	163	31	36	33

radiculopathy were present. Five patients had far lateral disc herniation, and 12 had recurrent disc herniation. Table 11-2 presents the population by number and distribution of levels on which surgery was performed. Table 11-3 presents additional diagnoses found within both study groups, in order of frequency. No concurrent diagnoses were believed to pose any problems or require any modifications for the microdiscectomy or anuloplasty procedures.

TABLE 11-2 OPERATIVE VARIABLES

	Control (N = 197)	One Suture (N = 35)	Two+ Sutures (N = 42)	Fascial Autograft (N = 40)
Single-level (N = 276; 87.9%)	166 (84.3%)	32 (91.4%)	39 (92.9%)	39 (97.5%)
L1-2	1 (0.5%)	0	0	0
L2-3	4 (2.0%)	1 (2.9%)	0	1 (2.5%)
L3-4	20 (10.2%)	4 (11.4%)	2 (4.8%)	8 (20.0%)
L4-5	63 (32.0%)	9 (25.7%)	15 (35.7%)	18 (45.0%)
L5-S1	78 (39.6%)	18 (51.4%)	22 (52.4%)	12 (30.0%)
Two-level	28 (14.2%)	3 (8.6%)	3 (7.1%)	1 (2.5%)
L1-3	1 (0.5%)	0	0	0
L2-4	1 (0.5%)	0	0	0
L3-5	8 (4.1%)	0	0	0
L4-S1	18 (9.4%)	3 (8.6%)	3 (7.1%)	1 (2.5%)
Three-level	3 (1.5%)	0	0	0
L3-S1	3 (1.5%)	0	0	0

TABLE 11-3 CONCURRENT DIAGNOSES

Additional Diagnosis	Number of Patients	Group(s)
Lumbar degenerative disc disease	91	Both
Spinal stenosis	20	Both
Lateral recess stenosis	13	Both
Foot drop	4	Both
Nerve root entrapment	4	Control
Cauda equina syndrome	3	Control
Spondylolysis	3	Control
Spondylosis	3	Control
Other diagnoses*	19	Anuloplasty

*Anular fissure, chronic obstructive pulmonary disease, coronary artery disease, degenerative osteophyte, diabetes mellitus, epidural scar, ischemic cardiomyopathy, junctional nevi, lumbar degenerative joint disease, lumbar scoliosis, morbid obesity, multiple myeloma, neurogenic bladder, spondylolisthesis, and vertebral osteophyte formation.

Data Analysis

Patient data were evaluated for all patients with 1-year follow-up who had responded to the questionnaire (anuloplasty N = 117; control N = 197). An objective evaluation of recurrences was important for this study, and questionnaire follow-up (by mail or phone) was the only method of confirming whether a patient had undergone additional surgery elsewhere for recurrent disc herniation.

A patient was considered to have a recurrent disc herniation if the herniation occurred at the same level and side as the original operation (control or anuloplasty). Confirmation of recurrences by subsequent operations and/or radiologic findings (MRI, lumbar myelography with CT) was considered adequate, making this study's results more inclusive than results of other discectomy-effectiveness studies that define recurrences by reoperation only. For six patients, recurrences were confirmed by MRI, but not by reoperation. Three of these patients were candidates for additional surgery but cancelled their scheduled reoperations and discontinued office visits for personal reasons. One patient, whose reherniation was confirmed by MRI, experienced noted improvement after epidural steroid treatment and required no further visits. A fifth patient had additional surgery in another city following MRI evaluation. For the sixth patient, the appropriate information could not be gathered. Nonetheless, all six patients were included. All data management and statistical analysis were performed using JMP software (SAS Institute, Inc., Cary, NC).

Results

Lumbar *reoperations* were performed on 84 patients (27% of 314) and are grouped by their relation to index surgery (Table 11-4). The term *residual* disc herniation was applied to two control patients who did not experience pain-free intervals following index surgery, indicated by residual disc fragments found at reoperation. Discectomies for *recurrent* disc herniations were revisions at the same level and side as index surgery; *contralateral* disc herniations refer to subsequent discectomies at the same level, opposite side; *new* disc herniations were treated by discectomies at other vertebral levels. Concurrent arthrodesis (posterior lumbar interbody fusion [PLIF]) procedures involving the discectomy level (or levels) were performed for 35% (24/69) of these reoperations (control 25% [11/44]; anuloplasty 59% [13/22]). Subsequent anuloplasty procedures were performed on three patients who underwent reoperation for contralateral or new disc herniation. Reoperations in the *other* category refer to laminotomies, laminectomies, fusions (with and without instrumentation), and osteophytectomies that did not also involve discectomy. Sixteen patients (5.1% of 314) underwent a second reoperation (control 12; anuloplasty 4), six of which were for a second recurrence of herniation.

TABLE 11-4 LUMBAR REOPERATIONS IN RELATION TO INDEX SURGERY

	Control (N = 197)	One Suture (N = 35)	Two+ Sutures (N = 42)	Fascial Autograft (N = 40)
Time to reoperation (average years)	2.1	1.6	1.6	0.8
Discectomies				
Residual disc herniation	2 (1.0%)	0	0	0
Recurrent disc herniation	37 (18.8%)	6 (17.1%)	2 (4.8%)	3 (7.5%)
Contralateral disc herniation	1 (0.5%)	3 (8.6%)	4 (9.5%)	2 (5.0%)
New disc herniation	4 (2.0%)	2 (5.7%)	0	2 (5.0%)
Other lower back	13 (6.6%)	1 (2.9%)	2 (4.8%)	0
TOTAL	57 (28.9%)	12 (34.3%)	8 (19.0%)	7 (17.5%)

Recurrences were evaluated at both 1-year and 2-year follow-ups. Results at 1-year follow-up (Table 11-5) were established using this study's more inclusive criteria: patients who returned questionnaires, with reherniation confirmed by reoperation and/or radiologic evaluation. These criteria explain the difference in recurrence figures in Table 11-4, which deals only with recurrences determined by reoperation. Of 56 total recurrences, 7 (12.5%) were identified by MRI alone (control 2; anuloplasty 5). Results are presented at the 2-year follow-up (Table 11-6) for comparison with results of other discectomy-effectiveness studies, using more standard criteria. Two-year results include only patients who underwent one-level procedures and who returned questionnaires, with reherniation confirmed by surgery only. Table 11-7 outlines complications noted in this patient sample.

HISTOLOGIC OBSERVATIONS

In six postoperative anuloplasty patients who experienced *contralateral* same-level nuclear herniation, ipsilateral anulus resection at the original anular repair site was possible as part of a bilateral discectomy required for PLIF. The macroscopic appearance viewed through an operating microscope was that of a continuous, smooth, anular surface with no extradural fibrotic reactive or discernible suture line. In several patients with ipsilateral reherniation, the recurrent fragment presented in the subarticular recess lateral to a healed anulus, accompanied by robust extradural adhesions in the immediate area of the reherniation.

Table 11-5 Recurrences at One-Year Follow-up

Group	Total Patients (N = 314)	Recurrences (N = 58)	Recurrence Rate (%)	Average Follow-up (years)	Average Time to Recurrence (years)
Control	197 (63%)	42	21.3	7.3 (5.1-9.1)	1.4 (0.10-5.9)
One suture	35 (11%)	7	20.0	4.8 (3.3-5.8)	1.4 (0.25-2.9)
Two+ sutures	42 (13%)	4	9.5	4.1 (1.4-5.5)	1.1 (0.08-2.0)
Fascial autograft	40 (13%)	5	12.5	2.0 (1.1-2.7)	0.8 (0.16-1.2)

Table 11-6 Recurrences at Two-Year Follow-up

Group	Total Patients (N = 254)	Recurrences (N)	Recurrence Rate (%)
Control	166 (65%)	35	21.1
One suture	32 (13%)	3	9.4
Two+ sutures	37 (15%)	2	5.4
Fascial autograft	19 (7%)	1	5.3

Table 11-7 Complications

Complication	Control (N = 197)	One Suture (N = 35)	Two+ Sutures (N = 42)	Fascial Autograft (N = 40)
Incisional pain	0	0	0	1 (3%)
Prolonged back pain (>3 mo)	0	2 (6%)	2 (5%)	0
Prolonged leg pain (>3 mo)	22 (11%)	2 (6%)	4 (10%)	0
Subcutaneous fluid collection	7 (4%)	1 (3%)	4 (10%)	5 (13%)
Subcutaneous fluid loss	3 (2%)	2 (6%)	1 (2%)	1 (3%)
Staphylococcal wound infection	2 (1%)	0	0	1 (3%)
Urinary retention	0	0	2 (5%)	0
Unhealed incision	1 (1%)	0	0	0

By contrast, the macroscopic appearance of the anulus repair of patient PM showed a smooth surface with no obvious suture remnants or significant epidural scar. Postoperative histologic examination of the site indicated a healed appearance at the anuloplasty site 35 months following repair (Fig. 11-8).

Following excision of a healed anulotomy site contralateral to a new same-level herniation that required discectomy and interbody fusion, the patient shown in Fig. 11-9 appeared to be a healed at the microscopic level with a refractile suture artifact 38 months after repair. Collagen realignment with a Gelfoam vacuole formation at 38 months is demonstrated with no evidence of inflammatory change or reaction to the polylactic acid (Vicryl) sutures that were used to stabilize the anulus repair (Fig. 11-10).

Discussion

Anular Healing

In a study of canine intervertebral discs, Key[37] demonstrated that surgical defects in the anulus primarily heal in the superficial outer laminae, with persistent surgical defects in more central layers. Similarly, Smith and Walmsley[60] found the deeper layers of anulus in rabbits to be inert, attributing the persistent defects to the avascularity of more central anular fibers.

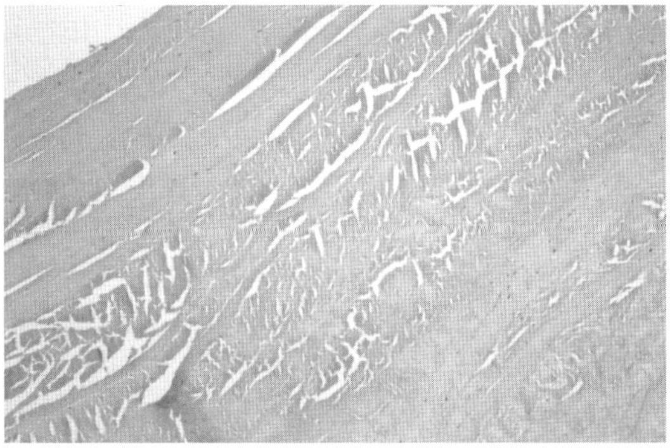

Fig. 11-8 Histology of anuloplasty site showing no elastic fibers or inflammatory changes 35 months following anular repair.

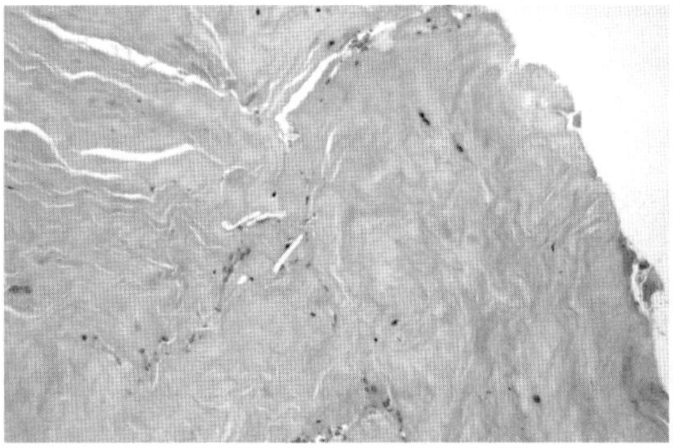

Fig. 11-9 A refractile suture artifact is evident 38 months after repair.

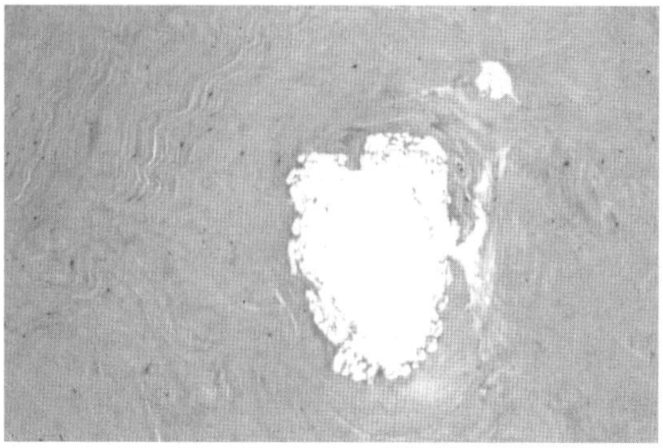

Fig. 11-10 A Gelfoam vacuole is shown 38 months after repair.

More recent studies confirm these early findings.[1,19,26] In canines, Hampton et al[26] compared the healing potential of 3 by 5 mm rectangular (box) anulotomies with 5 mm anular linear incisions. In the linear anulotomy tracts, there was no evidence of healing aside from small caps of fibrous tissue at the periphery. In rectangular excisions of anulus, solid healing was observed in the form of fibrous *plugs*, which the authors concluded would prevent further leakage of nuclear fluid. Ethier et al[19] verified these findings with a similar comparison of various anulotomies in a goat model. However, their evaluation of the anular window technique was more critical, given that rapid and severe disc degeneration and untoward histologic features were demonstrated in this group. Using a sheep model, Ahlgren et al[2] also found that box anulotomies withstood significantly less saline injection pressure and exhibited greater range of motion than slit anulotomies (in comparison with unincised control discs), concluding that slit anulotomy leads to stronger anular closure. In another study by Ahlgren et al[1] designed to evaluate the effect of anular repair techniques in a sheep model, competency of the repair at 6 weeks in a *slit with repair* group demonstrated leakage of injected saline at 1590 kPa injection pressure. Because 1 kPa unit equals 0.14504 pound per square inch, Ahlgren's injection pressure of 230.6 pounds per square inch is probably an unrealistic challenge for an epianular patch with six weeks of healing. It appears reasonable then to take issue with the Ahlgren's conclusion that the experimental attempts to repair the anulus were unsuccessful, in view of the nonphysiologic endpoint of resistance to injected saline solution at high pressure. To prevent reherniation, a competent anulus need only withstand the intradiscal pressure sufficient to propel a nuclear fragment through the anulus repair site, not noncompressible saline indicated in the Ahlgren work.

Numerous authors have suggested that such unhealed anular incisions may be a factor in lumbar disc reherniation.[1,11,45,50,63] In an outcome study of discectomy operations, Pappas et al[50] speculated that recurrences less than 6 months after the original discectomy tended to occur through the original anular defect. In further support, Matsui et al[45] reported a case of lateral disc reherniation 2 months after percutaneous discectomy, observing that the extrusion occurred through the first anulotomy site. To my knowledge, a technique of anular reconstruction to prevent such recurrences in a clinical setting has not been previously addressed.

Other surgeons have emphasized the need to minimize the anular incision. Williams[65] advocated blunt perforation of the anulus in his minimally invasive microlumbar discectomy. Other surgeons applied the technique, usually with their own modifications.[22,36,69] However, Williams's technique is intended for removal of only the offending disc fragment. In an analysis of existing microdiscectomy studies, Apostolides[4] showed that recurrence rates were invariably higher for those surgeons who completed only partial removal of disc fragments as opposed to more generous disc excision. Dilation and spreading of anular fibers by blunt perforation gives only limited subanular access, thus preventing the adequate identification and removal of all disc fragments. Incidentally, Williams[65] noted in reoperation of recurrent herniations that even his blunt anular perforations left gaping circular openings.

In defense of conservative minimal discectomy, the more radical procedure needs review because it has been shown that extensive discectomy can create lumbar instability. Mochida et al[46] compared the postoperative disc space height of patients who underwent either open discectomy or percutaneous nucleotomy. They found a significantly higher risk of disc space collapse when large amounts of nuclear material were removed. Similarly, in an in vitro biomechanical study, Brinckmann and Grootenboer[7] found that disc height decreases approximately in proportion with the mass of tissue excised, which leads to increased disc bulge and the possibility of nerve compression. Hanley and Shapiro[27] reported 98% of patients undergoing lumbar disc excision showed disc space narrowing as well, although this finding showed no correlation with postoperative pain. Hypermobility of lumbar segments may also be a factor following lumbar discectomy. Goel et al[23,24] found that subtotal discectomy allowed significantly less motion at the test site than total discectomy in cadaver studies. Panjabi et al[49] demonstrated that increased motion after nucleus removal is greater than after anular injury alone. They proposed a cascade of events that takes place after posterolateral injury of the lumbar disc, which disturbs the kinematics of levels adjacent to the surgical level, leading to cartilage degeneration, osteoarthritis, and facet atrophy.

The Ideal Procedure

In light of these findings, the ideal nerve decompression procedure requires excision of sufficient nuclear mass to prevent acute recurrence (which requires an adequate anulotomy), without compromising lumbar stability. How to prevent recurrent nuclear extrusion through a partially healed anular incision is an unanswered challenge. We have proposed that anuloplasty is a good first step toward achieving this goal. We define anuloplasty as repair of the surgically incised anulus to reestablish anular competence and prevent reherniation.

Although few authors have addressed the possibility of repairing the anulus, techniques such as intradiscal thermal anuloplasty (IDTA) and intradiscal electrothermal anuloplasty (IDET) have been developed for patients with symptoms of internal disc disruption (IDD), which is a condition characterized by a degraded nucleus pulposus with radial fissures extending into the peripheral anulus.[34] Thermal anuloplasty techniques developed by Saal and Saal[56,57] use an intradiscal catheter to destroy anular nociceptors and shorten subanular collagen fibers. In 2000 Karasek and Bogduk[34] published their controlled, clinical study of IDTA, reporting improvements in pain ratings for 89% of patients 3 months after the procedure. In contradistinction, my anuloplasty technique is indicated for lumbar disc herniation, as opposed to IDD, and incorporates anular sutures, a subanular fascial autograft, microsurgical knot-tying technique, and nerve decompression during microdiscetomy.

Historical Context

Suture anuloplasty has been attempted previously. During a series of microdiscectomies that began as early as 1967, Professor MG Yasargil[68] adopted the practice of suturing the anulus with one 7.0 suture. His stated rationale was not anular repair to prevent recurrence, but to reduce adhesions.

The biomechanical study by Ahlgren et al[1] in 2000 more closely approximates the technique and rationale of this chapter. Using a sheep model, they conducted pressure-volume evaluations of three types of anulotomy incisions (box, slit, and cruciate). Half of the anulotomies were left to heal secondarily, and the other half was repaired with Vicryl suture. Repaired box anulotomies were closed by suturing a fascial graft over the defect. The study found minimal increases in resistance to increasing levels of injection pressure in repaired discs, with all groups except the *slit repair group* proving significantly weaker than the control level discs. Although results indicated no significant differences between repaired and nonrepaired discs, maximum follow-up was only 6 weeks.

To my knowledge, the technique of anuloplasty for the purpose of reducing reherniation has not been used in a clinical setting, and deserves an objective evaluation.

Reduction of Reherniation Rates

Anular repair can be considered as a technique with the possibility of reducing the risk of disc nucleus reherniation. There are two obvious reasons to repair the anulus and several other, less obvious reasons. Regarding reduced reherniation rates, in my experience, a 21% range for disc reherniation rate was demonstrated based on 166 patients followed for 7 years. The average time to recurrence was 1.4 years. Based on literature review that includes the clinical outcomes of Asch et al[5] and the MRI study of Van Goethem et al,[62] the true reherniation rate probably ranges from 1.3% to 20% or even 30%.

In a prospective multiple outcomes study, Asch et al[5] concluded that although success rates for lumbar microdiscectomy have been reported as high as 95%, overall success rates of 75% to 80% are more realistic. Moderately successful outcomes for leg pain (80%), back pain (77%), Oswestry disability index (78%), and satisfaction with surgery (76%) were contrasted with poorer outcomes for return-to-normal-activity and return-to-work measures (65% versus 61%, respectively). This study and my experience indicate a significant tendency to underreport negative outcomes for this most common operative spine procedure. In a study evaluating standard lumbar discectomy solely through MRI, Van Goethem et al[62] found 20% of patients to have recurrent disc herniation. However, all 34 patients were considered to have had excellent clinical outcome and no symptoms.

Intuitively, we expect a progressive reherniation rate as a result of the aging process in the anular wall *(anular incompetence)*. Recognizing the cascade of disc degeneration described by Kirkaldy-Willis[38] and Selby,[58] anular incompetence progresses to disc space narrowing, facet degeneration, spinal stenosis, and, frequently, disc nuclear herniation through an anular defect.

If laminotomy and disc fragment excision is followed by recurrent disc herniation in 10% to 30% of patients, typically through the same anular defect, restoring anular competence through anular repair (anuloplasty) deserves the attention of spine surgeons.

Recurrence rates for lumbar disc herniation cited in the literature range from 0% to 20%, although these numbers vary by operative technique.*

Among surgeons who use microsurgical techniques, such as microsurgical discectomy (MSD) introduced by Yasargil and Caspar[68] in 1977 and microlumbar discectomy (MLD) introduced by Williams[65] in 1978, published recurrence rates do not exceed 9.5%.†

This level is less than half of the highest rates published for standard lumbar discectomy (SLD), which is 19% to 20%.[44,62] However, Barrios et al[6] reported recurrences in 6.6% of patients who underwent MSD and in 1.3% of patients who underwent SLD. Three reoperations were reported in their microsurgical

*References 3, 6, 9-13, 15-18, 20-22, 25, 27, 29-32, 35, 39-44, 48, 50, 51, 53, 54, 59, 61-68.
†References 3, 6, 10, 11, 17, 21, 22, 25, 30, 35, 39, 40, 43, 48, 50, 51, 53, 59, 61, 63-68.

group that were necessitated by incomplete disc removal. These reoperations were performed within 1 month of the first operation (although they used generous disc excision rather than Williams's minimal technique). According to Postacchini and Cinotti[52] (1998), these procedures are better classified as failed surgeries than recurrences, because newly formed tissue is unlikely to be the source of disc prolapse within 3 months after surgery. In 1991 Caspar et al[10] conducted a similar comparison that produced more favorable results for microsurgical technique. Their 3.3% recurrence rate for MSD was compared with 7.6% for standard operations. The authors credited this improvement to the effectiveness of the operating microscope in helping to identify disc fragments. Thomas and Afshar[61] also acknowledged the benefits of microscopic discectomy in preventing recurrence after establishing a 1.6% recurrence rate for their MSD series.

Among those surgeons using variations in microsurgical technique, there have been claims of superiority in preventing recurrences. Williams[65] proposed that blunt perforation of the anulus, as used in MLD operations, minimizes the occurrence of reherniation. In support of MSD, Wilson and Harbaugh[67] attributed improved results to subtotal disc excision. However, among published studies of MLD, the average recurrence rate was 4.2% (range 1.5% to 9.4%). In published studies of MSD, the average rate was 3.9% (range 0% to 9.5%).*

Hudgins[31] reported a comparable recurrence rate (5.5%) for a series of patients undergoing a modified microdiscetomy procedure, incorporating the blunt anular perforation of MLD with laminotomy and disc curetting. While each technique may propose valid mechanisms for recurrence prevention, if recurrence rates are assumed to be directly comparable, neither seems to have an advantage over the other.

However, recurrence rates in the literature are rarely directly comparable because of the wide variation in the way authors define and evaluate recurrences. Among studies of discectomy effectiveness in which the authors clearly indicate their reherniation criteria, 11 studies consider all subsequent herniations, regardless of level or side, to be recurrences.†

These occurrences may be more appropriately labeled *pseudorecurrences*.[55] In comparison, 12 studies restrict the definition of recurrences to be herniations at the same level and side as the initial operation.‡

The fact that the former group has a higher average recurrence rate than the latter (10% versus 4.7%) is not surprising in light of its more inclusive criteria for defining reherniation. Because the objective of the present study is to eval-

*References 3, 6, 10, 11, 17, 21, 22, 25, 30, 35, 39, 40, 43, 48, 50, 51, 53, 59, 61, 63-68.
†References 12, 13, 15, 18, 21, 29, 31, 32, 41, 44, 54.
‡References 11, 22, 25, 39, 43, 48, 51, 53, 61-66.

uate the effectiveness of anuloplasty in preventing reherniation at a particular level and side, recurrences in this report are defined as subsequent symptomatic herniations at the same site as the initial procedure. In short, these are symptomatic recurrences on the same side and at the same level.

Most authors include recurrences in study results only when reherniations have been confirmed by reoperation.*

Studies that evaluate recurrences based on radiological findings alone are rare, primarily in response to reports that MRI exams frequently disclose disc herniation in asymptomatic patients.[14,33,62] In a study evaluating postoperative standard lumbar discectomy procedures through MRI, Van Goethem et al[62] found 20% of patients to have recurrent disc herniation. However, all 34 patients, were considered to have had excellent clinical outcome and no symptoms.

As Postacchini et al[52] have argued, in limiting recurrence evaluations to revision patients alone, investigators cannot determine the exact incidence of recurrent and new herniations. Regardless of this argument, studies that evaluate recurrences based on both reoperation and radiological/clinical findings are rare. In an effectiveness study of microlumbar discectomy, Maroon and Abla[43] reported four "true recurrences" out of 120 operations (3.3%). Of these, three patients had recurring disc fragments retrieved in reoperation, and one was diagnosed with recurrence by computed tomography scan, refusing to have additional surgery. The tendency for authors to evaluate recurrences of revision patients only was explicitly challenged by Martin[44] in a study of laminectomy and discectomy procedures. Martin established a 19% recurrence rate, with 9% of these patients having their recurrences confirmed at reoperation, and 10% determined by clinical evaluation only. Myelography was not considered a useful diagnostic tool in Martin's study because of its inability to distinguish between recurring disc lesion and scar tissue. The wide discrepancy between the recurrence rates of these two studies can be explained by their differing operative techniques and by the criteria each author used to define recurrences. Martin defined recurrence as any subsequent herniation, regardless of level or side. Maroon and Abla limited recurrences to subsequent herniations at the same level and side as the initial operation, as in the present study.

Length of Follow-up Period

Another variable is the length of the follow-up period. It has been suggested that rates will typically rise with longer periods of follow-up, given that patients in longer-term studies have had more time for recurrent symptoms to develop.[29] However, among articles that clearly indicated follow-up periods, there

*References 3, 6, 9-13, 15-18, 20-22, 25, 27, 29, 30-32, 35, 39-44, 48, 50, 51, 53, 54, 59, 61, 63-67.

was little difference among the average recurrence rates published in short-term (less than 5 years follow-up), mid-term (5 to 10 years follow-up), and long-term (greater than 10 years follow-up) studies. In reports that followed patients up to five years after surgery, the average recurrence rate was 6.2%.*

In studies following patients from 5 to 10 years after surgery, the average rate was 5.8%.†

In studies that followed patients into the long-term, the average rate was 7.1%.‡ A variable that may provide more value than follow-up range is the average time to recurrence, which is one variable considered in the present study. By reviewing the average time to recurrence, additional predictive information is available.

Concluding Observations

Anular repair is a reality, reducing the reherniation rate in a human clinical trial by 50% in my experience. It can be predicted that as the technology and efficacy of anular repair evolve, the indicated surgical response after nerve decompression has occurred will be restoration of anular competence. Additionally, it is important to recognize transanular migration of inflammatory chemicals that are produced in the degenerated disc center, which has been well demonstrated.[8,28,47] Preliminary observations of healed anulotomy sites suggest that further clinical research is needed to determine if anulus repair is sufficient to block the emergence of proinflammatory substances and inflammatory cells at the site of the herniation, reducing epidural scar formation. Finally, anular reconstruction is important for at least three reasons: (1) strengthening the barrier to reherniation of secondary nuclear fragments, (2) eliminating displacement of prosthetic nucleus components, and (3) reducing the transport of intradiscal inflammatory substances, which are injurious to the overlying nerve and may perpetuate the cascade of disc degeneration.

*References 3, 6, 9, 10, 22, 25, 29, 39, 40, 43, 50, 51, 61-67.
†References 10-12, 17, 21, 27, 30, 35, 44, 48, 53, 59, 67, 68.
‡References 13, 15, 32, 40, 41, 54, 59, 63, 64, 66.

REFERENCES

1. Ahlgren B, Lui W, Herkowitz H, et al. Effect of anular repair on the healing strength of the intervertebral disc. Spine 25:2165-2170, 2000.
2. Ahlgren B, Vasavada A, Brower R, et al. Anular incision technique on the strength and multidirectional flexibility of the healing intervertebral disc. Spine 19:948-954, 1994.
3. Andrews D, Lavyne M. Retrospective analysis of microsurgical and standard lumbar discectomy. Spine 15:329-335, 1990.
4. Apostolides P. Lumbar discectomy microdiscectomy: The "gold standard." Clin Neurosurg 43:228-238, 1996.
5. Asch H, Lewis P, Moreland D, et al. Prospective multiple outcomes study of outpatient lumbar microdiscectomy: Should 75 to 80% success rates be the norm? J Neurosurg Spine 96:34-44, 2002.
6. Barrios C, Ahmed M, Arrotegui J, et al. Microsurgery versus standard removal of the herniated lumbar disc. Acta Orthop Scand 61:399-403, 1990.
7. Brinckmann P, Grootenboer H. Change of disc height, radial disc bulge, and intradiscal pressure from discectomy. Spine 16:641-646, 1991.
8. Burke JG, Watson RW, McCormack D, et al. Intervertebral discs which cause low back pain secrete high levels of proinflammatory mediators. J Bone Joint Surg Br 84:196-201, 2002.
9. Carragee E, Han M, Kim D, et al. Fragment type and anular competence as predictive factors in lumbar discectomy. Presented at the Annual Meeting of the American Association of Neurological Surgeons, San Francisco, April, 2000.
10. Caspar W, Campbell B, Barbier D, et al. The Caspar microsurgical discectomy and comparison with a conventional standard lumbar disc procedure. Neurosurgery 28:78-87, 1991.
11. Cinotti G, Roysam G, Eisenstein S, et al. Ipsilateral recurrent lumbar disc herniation. J Bone Joint Surg 80:825-832, 1998.
12. Connolly E. Surgery for recurrent lumbar disc herniation. Clin Neurosurg 39:211-216, 1992.
13. Davis R. A long-term outcome analysis of 984 surgically treated herniated lumbar discs. J Neurosurg 80:415-421, 1994.
14. Deyo R. Magnetic resonance imaging of the lumbar spine: Terrific test or tar baby? New Engl J Med 331:115-116, 1994.
15. Dvorak J, Gauchat M, Valach L. The outcome of surgery for lumbar disc herniation: A 4-17 years' follow-up with emphasis on somatic aspects. Spine 13:1418-1422, 1988.
16. Ebeling U, Kalbarcyk H, Reulen H. Microsurgical operation following lumbar disc surgery. J Neurosurg 70:397-404, 1989.
17. Ebeling U, Reichenberg W, Reulen H. Results of microsurgical lumbar discectomy. Acta Neurochir Wien 81:45-52, 1986.
18. Epstein J, Lavine L, Epstein B. Recurrent herniation of the lumbar intervertebral disk. Clin Orthop 52:169-178, 1967.
19. Ethier D, Cain JE, Yaszemski MJ, et al. The influence of anulotomy selection on disc competence. Spine 19:2071-2076, 1994.
20. Fandino J, Botana C, Viladrich A, et al. Reoperation after lumbar disc surgery: Results in 130 cases. Acta Neurochir Wien 122:102-104, 1993.
21. Findlay G, Hall B, Musa B, et al. A 10-year follow-up of the outcome of lumbar microdiscectomy. Spine 23:1168-1171, 1968.
22. Goald H. Microlumbar discectomy: Follow-up of 477 patients. J Microsurg 2:95-100, 1980.
23. Goel VK, Goyal S, Clark C, et al. The kinematics of the whole lumbar spine: Effect of discectomy. Spine 10:543-554, 1985.
24. Goel VK, Nishiyama K, Weinstein JN, et al. Mechanical properties of lumbar spinal motion segments as affected by partial disc removal. Spine 11:1008-1012, 1986.

25. Haglund M, Moore A, Marsh H, et al. Outcome after repeat lumbar microdiscectomy. Br J Neurosurg 9:487-495, 1995.
26. Hampton D, Laros D, McCarron R, et al. Healing potential of the anulus fibrosis. Spine 14:398-401, 1989.
27. Hanley E, Shapiro D. The development of low-back pain after excision of a lumbar disc. J Bone Joint Surg 71:719-721, 1989.
28. Harrington JF, Messier AA, Bereiter D, et al. Herniated lumbar disc material as a source of free glutamate available to affect pain signals through the dorsal root ganglion. Spine 25:929-936, 2000.
29. Herron L. Recurrent lumbar disc herniation: results of repeat laminectomy and discectomy. J Spinal Disord 7:161-166, 1994.
30. Hirabayashi S, Kumano K, Ogawa Y, et al. Microdiscectomy and second operation for lumbar disc herniation. Spine 18:2206-2211, 1993.
31. Hudgins WR. The role of microdiscectomy. Orthop Clin North Am 14:589-603, 1983.
32. Jackson RK. The long-term effects of wide laminectomy for lumbar disc excision. J Bone Joint Surg Br 53:609-616, 1971.
33. Jensen M, Brant-Zawadzki M, Obuchowski N, et al. Magnetic resonance imaging of the lumbar spine in people without back pain. N Engl J Med 331:69-73, 1994.
34. Karasek M, Bogduk N. Twelve-month follow-up of a controlled trial of intradiscal thermal anuloplasty for back pain due to internal disc disruption. Spine 25:2601-2607, 2000.
35. Kelly A, Griffith H, Jamjoom A. Results of day-case surgery for lumbar disc prolapse. Br J Neurosurg 8:47-49, 1994.
36. Kelly R, Dinner M, Lavyne M, et al. The effect of lumbar disc surgery on postoperative pulmonary function and temperature. Spine 18:287-290, 1993.
37. Key J. Experimental intervertebral disc lesions. J Bone Joint Surg 30:621-630, 1948.
38. Kirkaldy-Willis WH. Managing Low Back Pain. New York: Churchill Livingstone, 1983.
39. Kotilainen E, Valtonen S, Carlson C. Microsurgical treatment of lumbar disc herniation: Follow-up of 237 patients. Acta Neurochir Wien 120:143-149, 1993.
40. Kulali A, Wild KV. Microsurgical management of the lumbar intervertebral disc-disease. Neurosurg Rev 18:183-188, 1995.
41. Lewis P, Weir B, Broad R, et al. Long-term prospective study of lumbosacral discectomy. J Neurosurg 67:49-53, 1987.
42. Loupasis G, Stamos K, Katonis P, et al. Seven- to 20-year outcome of lumbar discectomy. Spine 24:2313-2317, 1999.
43. Maroon J, Abla A. Microlumbar discectomy. Clin Neurosurg 33:407-417, 1986.
44. Martin G. Recurrent disc prolapse as a cause of recurrent pain after laminectomy for lumbar disc lesions. N Z Med J 91:206-208, 1980.
45. Matsui H, Aoki M, Kanamori M. Lateral disc herniation following percutaneous lumbar discectomy. Int Orthop 21:169-171, 1997.
46. Mochida J, Nishimura K, Nomura T, et al. The importance of preserving disc structure in surgical approaches to lumbar disc herniation. Spine 21:1556-1564, 1996.
47. Nygaard OP, Mellgren SI, Osterud B. The inflammatory properties of contained and noncontained lumbar disc herniation. Spine 22:2484-2488, 1997.
48. Nystrom B. Experience of microsurgical compared with conventional technique in lumbar disc operations. Acta Neurol Scand 76:129-141, 1987.
49. Panjabi M, Krag M, Chung T. Effects of disc injury on mechanical behavior of the human spine. Spine 9:707-713, 1984.
50. Pappas C, Harrington T, Sonntag V. Outcome analysis in 654 surgically treated lumbar disc herniations. Neurosurgery 30:862-866, 1992.
51. Patel N, Pople I, Cummins B. Revisional lumbar microdiscectomy and analysis of operative findings and clinical outcome. Br J Neurosurg 9:733-737, 1995.

52. Postacchini F, Cinotti G, Gumina S. Microsurgical excision of lateral lumbar disc herniation through an interlaminar approach. J Bone Joint Surg Br 80:201-207, 1998.
53. Postacchini F, Cinotti G. Recurrent and new herniations. In Postacchini F, ed. Lumbar Disc Herniation. New York: Springer-Verlag, 1999.
54. Raaf J. Some observations regarding 905 patients operated upon for protruded lumbar intervertebral disc. Am J Surg 97:388-399, 1959.
55. Reith C, Lausberg G. Risk factors of recurrent disc herniation. Neurosurg Rev 12:147-150, 1989.
56. Saal JA, Saal JS. Intradiscal electrothermal anuloplasty (IDET) for chronic disc disease: Outcome assessment with minimum 1 year follow-up. Presented at the Fourteenth Annual Meeting of the North American Spine Society, Chicago, Oct 1999.
57. Saal JA, Saal JS. Intradiscal electrothermal anuloplasty (IDET) treatment for chronic multi-level discogenic pain: Prospective 1-year follow-up outcome study. Presented at the Fourteenth Annual Meeting of the North American Spine Society, Chicago, Oct 1999.
58. Selby DK. The structural degenerative cascade. In White AH, ed. Spine Care, vol 1. St Louis: Mosby, 1995, pp 8-26.
59. Silvers HR. Microsurgical versus standard lumbar discectomy. Neurosurgery 22:837-841, 1988.
60. Smith J, Walmsley R. Experimental incision of the intervertebral disc. J Bone Joint Surg Br 33:612-625, 1951.
61. Thomas A, Afshar F. The microsurgical treatment of lumbar disc protrusion. Follow-up of 60 cases. J Bone Joint Surg Br 69:696-698, 1987.
62. Van Goethem J, Van de Kelft E, Biltjes I, et al. MRI after successful lumbar discectomy. Neuroradiology 38(Suppl 1):S90-S96, 1996.
63. Williams R. Microdiskectomy—myth, mania, or milestone? An 18-year surgical adventure. Mt Sinai J Med 158:139-145, 1991.
64. Williams R. Microlumbar discectomy: A 12-year statistical review. Spine 11:851-852, 1986.
65. Williams R. Microlumbar discectomy: A conservative surgical approach to the virgin herniated lumbar disc. Spine 3:175-182, 1978.
66. Williams R. Microlumbar discectomy: A surgical alternative for initial disc herniation. In Cauthen J, ed. Lumbar Spine Surgery. Baltimore: Williams & Wilkins, 1988, pp 171-183.
67. Wilson D, Harbaugh R. Microsurgical and standard removal of the protruded lumbar disc: A comparative study. Neurosurgery 8:422-427, 1981.
68. Yasargil MG, Caspar W. Microsurgical operation of herniated lumbar disc. Adv Neurosurg 4:81, 1977.
69. Zahrawi F. Microlumbar discectomy (MLD). Spine 13:358-359, 1988.

CHAPTER

12

Total Disc Replacement: Implants and Clinical Results

Richard D. Guyer ▪ Timothy A. Burd
Steven H. Hochschuler ▪ Paul C. McAfee

The twenty-first century has ushered in many novel and exciting alternatives to the traditional treatment of chronic low back pain secondary to internal disc derangement. Historically, spine surgeons have addressed symptomatic disc disease with a variety of procedures, most commonly spondylodesis of the diseased dysfunctional spinal unit. Fusion has shown satisfactory long-term results; however, this procedure is fraught with complications, including symptomatic pseudarthrosis, hardware failure in instrumented cases, graft collapse, autograft harvest site pain, loss of normal sagittal balance, transitional syndrome secondary to increased stress at adjacent levels, and lost motion across the fused segments.

Lehmann et al[32] reported on the long-term success of lumbar fusion with 21- to 52-year follow-up (average 33 years). The authors determined that 50% of patients suffered low back pain requiring medication and 15% required additional surgical procedures during the study period. More striking, 42% of patients experienced lumbar spinal stenosis and 45% of patients had adjacent-level segmental lumbar instability. Hilibrand et al[25,26] also demonstrated the rates of symptomatic adjacent segment degeneration, defined as new radiculopathy or myelopathy in levels adjacent to cervical fusion, to be approximately 3% per year over a 10-year period. Using Kaplan-Meier survivorship analysis, the authors predicted that approximately 25% of patients would develop new adjacent-level disease over the next 10 years following index surgery. The authors also concluded that achieving an adjacent fusion in patients who have had previous cervical arthrodesis is more difficult using interbody grafting compared with corpectomy and strut grafting.

No other large joint in the musculoskeletal system has arthrodesis as its primary method of treatment for degenerative osteoarthrosis. Therefore, why should the motion segments within the lumbar spine be treated otherwise? In harmony with the Arbeitsgemeinschaft fur Osteosynthesfragen (AO) principle—"movement is life and life is movement"—this axiom would intuitively apply to the lumbar spine by saving motion segments and replicating normal spinal physiology.[49]

The primary goals of spinal arthroplasty are:

- To restore normal anatomy (that is, disc height and posterior foraminal patency)
- To preserve mobility at the affected disc level
- To relieve low back and discogenic pain

Various design proposals have focused on two main principles: (1) to create an implant that reproduces the viscoelastic properties of the intervertebral disc via polymers, silicon spacers or injectable monomers that undergo in situ polymerization, and (2) to reproduce the characteristic motion of the functional spinal unit. In this chapter, we focus on motion-preserving implants and provide a framework to enhance understanding of the conceptual and practical basis for total disc arthroplasty. Operative indications, contraindications, rationale, and an in-depth discussion of biomechanical considerations are addressed in separate chapters.

History

Nachemson[50,51] first attempted to restore the viscoelastic properties of the intervertebral disc by injecting liquid silicon rubber into cadaveric discs and testing them biomechanically. He discovered that the implants catastrophically disintegrated after 20 to 30 million cycles under simulated walking conditions. Most early implants consisted of rubber silicon composites or polyurethane and were manufactured in a variety of different shapes and sizes including helicoids,[2] hydrogel beads encased in semipermeable membranes,[1] and a host of expandable prostheses.[4,7,36,53] Although these early promising devices, along with many other implants, have been patented or reported in the literature, they have not been clinically used for various reasons.[56]

Many devices that were designed to restore physiologic motion were never used clinically. The first of these prostheses was the lumbar prosthesis designed by Weber[59] in 1978, which consisted of two polyethylene structures embedded into the superior and inferior endplates of adjacent vertebrae and a ceramic ovoid core interposed between them. Other promising prostheses that did not gain clinical acceptance were the Kostuik chromium-molybdenum hinged device[22-24,31] and the Keller biconvex metallic core implant.[30] More recently designed implants that are under investigation include various ball-and-socket devices[17,44,54] and articulating implants that mimic total knee arthroplasty.[55,62]

In addition to lumbar spine arthroplasty, cervical disc prostheses[29,48,52,60] and facet arthroplasty[15,40] techniques have been studied in the laboratory and animal models; however, few have been implanted into humans for clinical examination. In Chapter 2, Dr. Garcia described the early results of Fernström[14] and intervertebral stainless steel spheres implanted following posterior discectomy; he presented the early successes and failures of various small clinical and laboratory studies, ultimately concluding with the current recensions, the total disc arthroplasty.

There are currently four lumbar disc arthroplasty devices actively implanted in patients in the United States. All of these devices are implanted anteriorly. Although there are various anterior approaches to the spine, Chapter 9 presented one technique in detail. IDE studies on the CHARITÉ Artificial Disc (Johnson & Johnson/DePuy Spine, formerly Waldemar Link GmbH & Co of Hamburg, Germany) and the ProDisc II (Spine Solutions/Synthes, New York, NY) began in March 2000 and October 2001, respectively. These devices will be discussed later in this chapter. The third lumbar implant, the MAVERICK prosthesis (Medtronic Sofamor Danek, Memphis, TN) (see Chapter 13), is a metal-on-metal device with its axis of rotation centered posteriorly.[41] This device has a hydroxyapatite crystalline coating for improved osteointegration; however, because the implant is a chrome cobalt, metal-on-metal device, further testing is necessary. Matthews et al[42] recently presented their results evaluating CoCrMo wear debris in the rabbit spine. The authors used dosage levels of the metal alloy debris equivalent to 10, 30, and 60 years of exposure, and injected the particles within the epidural space. Multiple visceral tissues and lymph nodes were sampled following exposure to determine pathologic changes. Local response to the particles was minimal to nil. No foreign body giant cells were identified. The authors concluded that no significant histologic changes were present after comparing particle-injected animals and control subjects. These findings have been corroborated by Cunningham et al.[10] Hence a prospective randomized study was launched in 2003 to compare the MAVERICK prosthesis with stand-alone lumbar tapered titanium cages. The fourth disc, described by Errico,[13] is the FlexiCore disc. This device has a ball-and-socket design with chrome- cobalt bearing surfaces. Similar to the MAVERICK prosthesis from Medtronic Sofamor Danek, the FlexiCore disc (Stryker Spine, Allendale, NJ) is metal-on-metal. This design allows for a 34-degree flexion-extension arc without translation and titanium–plasma sprayed endplates. Their IDE study is currently ongoing.

Another novel articulated lumbar disc prosthesis was recently presented. South African scientists have implanted the new disc into 15 patients.[21] The prosthesis consists of two titanium endplates and a radiation cross-linked mobile polyethylene core—recently redesigned with a mobile metal core, Kineflex™ (SpinalMotion, Mountain View, CA). The center of rotation is located posteriorly. All three components are implanted simultaneously using a unique insertion jig that allows for reproducible centralization of the prosthesis. Clinical results are pending; a U.S. IDE study is to begin in the second quarter of 2005.

Two cervical disc arthroplasty devices are also currently being studied in human trials: the Bryan Total Cervical Disc® (Medtronic Sofamor Danek, Memphis, TN) (see Chapter 13), and the Bristol/Gill cervical implant (also known as the Prestige I disc also by Medtronic Sofamor Danek), which consists of a ball-and-socket stainless steel device that is mounted and screwed into the adjacent endplates.[16] The early results of the Bryan cervical disc, reported by Bryan,[5] demonstrate an 87% clinical success rate in 46 patients, with success graded as excellent, good, or fair at one-year follow-up. Eight of nine patients had clinical success using the same grading scale at 2 years. The preliminary results appear to be approximately as good as results for one-level anterior discectomy and fusion; therefore further data is needed to address whether or not the device is efficacious in obviating adjacent disc disease and preserving segmental motion. In a recent review, Traynelis[57] reported unpublished data from Robertson's experience with the Bristol disc after 1 year. The study compared the cervical disc with a standard one-level arthrodesis and demonstrated improved scores on the Neck Disability Index, visual analog scale (VAS), and SF-36 in the arthroplasty cohort. Moreover, segmental motion was maintained in the nonfusion group. The latest recension of the Bristol/Cummins disc is the Prestige SS, which has been implanted as part of an FDA approved IDE study as of 2002.[58] (For a more extensive discussion of the cervical artificial disc describing the clinical and biomechanical results, see related chapters.)

Biomechanics

The three basic biomechanical roles of the spine are:

- To act as a load-bearing support for bipedal ambulation
- To transfer stresses throughout the spine in concert for movement in space
- To protect the spinal cord and thecal sac

Because the spine functions primarily through coordinated, coupled movements, it absorbs and recognizes the multiple stresses applied simultaneously to maintain stability. Under normal conditions, the spine experiences compressive, shear, tensile, bending, and torsional stresses, and, when functioning correctly, handles these forces without compromise. However, when normal physiologic stresses are unable to be resisted by the inherent anatomic restraints, the anulus fibrosis, nucleus pulposus, facet joints, and surrounding ligaments, symptomatic multidirectional instability may occur. As defined by White and Panjabi,[61] "Clinical instability is the loss of the ability of the spine under physiologic loads to maintain relationships between vertebrae in such a way that there is neither damage nor subsequent irritation to the spinal cord or nerve roots, and, in addition, there is no development of incapacitating deformity or pain due to structural changes." Traditionally, clinical instability has been measured radiographically using the criteria espoused by White and Panjabi. According to these criteria, clinical instability is defined as (1) greater than 3.5 mm of translational motion on dynamic flexion and extension radiographs and (2) greater than 11 degrees of segmental rotational difference from the adjacent segment on flexion and extension views.

There are two fundamental design strategies in total disc technology that are related to spinal movement: unconstrained and constrained prosthesis. The unconstrained prosthesis has a mobile bearing core allowing the ultrahigh molecular weight polyethylene (UHMWPE)–bearing surface to translate with 6 degrees of segmental motion, as seen in a normal spine. In theory, it follows that by allowing for both translation and rotation about all three planes, the stress concentrations at the polyethylene core surface would be minimized, thereby reducing the incidence of cold flow.[6] The Charité total disc replacement is unconstrained; the ProDisc is a semiconstrained model with the UHMWPE core inserted within the superior endplate of the caudal vertebral body. Therefore motion occurs along one interface—between the inferior endplate of the cephalad vertebra and the polyethylene core. Debate continues regarding which model, semiconstrained or unconstrained, is better. Long-term studies and further in vitro and in vivo mechanical analysis is needed.

IMPLANTS

CHARITÉ Artificial Disc

The original version of the Charité artificial disc prosthesis was developed in 1982 by Karin Büttner-Janz and Kurt Schellnack in East Germany at the Charité Hospital. The development was described by Dr. Büttner-Janz in Chapter 6. The design was based on the low friction principle, which had been deemed biomechanically sound in the peripheral joint literature using UHMWPE as a bearing surface that articulates with adjacent 1.0 mm-thick steel endplates.

The original design, the SB Charité I artificial disc prosthesis, was first implanted in September 1984 in Berlin. This model caused axial plane migration, leading to the development of a second version (SB Charité II) in 1985. This version had a larger endplate contact area and wings bilaterally in the coronal plane to mitigate subsidence. Both of these models, the Mark I and Mark II, were manufactured solely in the German Democratic Republic and were never available commercially. Because of endplate fractures and poor instrumentation for implantation, the designers enlisted the help of the Link Company to develop another implant similar to the first two versions, without the inherent complications. The Link SB CHARITÉ III was designed in 1987 and remains the currently used design (the CHARITÉ Artificial Disc, Johnson & Johnson/DePuy Spine). This disc has improved metallurgic qualities using casted CoCrMo alloy (ISO 5832/IV, ASTM F75-82) endplates and six teeth per endplate to integrate with the adjacent vertebral bodies. Multiple sizes have been developed to allow for modularity and patients' unique anatomy. The endplates are available in four sizes, with lordosis fixed into the prostheses at 0, 5, 7.5, and 10 degrees. Endplate lordosis can be mixed to provide optimal lordotic angulation and to reproduce normal lumbar anatomy. Additionally, five sizes of UHMWPE sliding cores (ISO 5834/II, ASTM 648-83) are available, ranging from 7.5 to 11.5 mm in 1.0 mm increments.

To improve osteointegration at the implant-bone interface, a bioactive coating consisting of three layers was developed. Two layers of commercially pure titanium were sintered and sprayed onto the endplates. The second layer allows for optimal porous ingrowth with a pore size of 75 to 300 μm. The final layer is composed of a ceramic, calcium phosphate with a 10 to 25 mm thickness that accelerates osteoblastic endplate attachment. This open-cell, porous structure provides for optimal biologic ingrowth and implant stabilization. Recently, McAfee et al[46] demonstrated a 47.9% porous ingrowth using electrochemically bonded hydroxyapatite coating in a nonhuman primate model. Link has developed a trade name of TiCaP to refer to this unique new coating. More than 99% of this ceramic coating is resorbed by 6 weeks after surgery. Compared with appendicular skeletal implants, the degree of osteointegration in the spine is much greater with the former, ranging from 0% to 43% ingrowth, depending on the type of surface material and coating techniques.

Operative Technique

The operative technique for the CHARITÉ Artifical Disc is included in this discussion because this disc has been approved by the FDA. As other discs are approved, operative techniques specific to those devices will be reported. The general principles, however, apply to all disc replacements.

Patient Preparation and Positioning

Anterior exposure of the spine is an important part of the artificial disc implantation procedure. Proper execution of discectomy is critical to the success of this operation, and good exposure is key to ensuring that the rest of the technique proceeds smoothly.

Few measures need to be taken to prepare patients for implantation of the artificial disc. Bowel preparation is not necessary. A Foley catheter is not usually needed, unless the procedure will be lengthy. However, the surgeon may consider using a Foley catheter if the L5-S1 approach is used.

The patient should be placed in a supine position with the arms across the chest on a radiolucent operating table. Care is taken to align the break in the table directly under the affected disc; many surgeons adjust the table during the procedure to open up the disc space during discectomy. Alternatively, many surgeons use a Jackson table, which does not break or hinge in the middle. An inflatable lumbar pillow can be placed under the patient's lumbar spine during positioning before antibacterial skin preparation. In this manner, the operative disc space can be extended open like a book during discectomy and at the initial insertion of the CHARITÉ Artificial Disc prosthetic endplates. The lumbar spine needs to be flatter, in more physiologic standing orientation, when the CHARITÉ Artificial Disc endplates are being advanced in the posterior half of the vertebral bodies. They will otherwise impinge, and excessive force can be avoided if intraoperative adjustment of lumbar lordosis/kyphosis can be accommodated. Patients are positioned with their arms across the chest, leaving space for circumferential C-arm movement over and around the operative level. After the patient is in proper position, deep venous thrombosis prophylaxis should be administered; however, a central venous line and/or arterial line are generally not needed.

Approach

Anterior approaches to the spine may be either transperitoneal or retroperitoneal. The left retroperitoneal approach is preferred because it avoids several complications and allows better visualization (see Chapter 9).

The skin incision may be midline or paramedian. A midline incision is preferred because it allows better midline visualization of the disc space for more accurate midline placement of the prosthesis. The skin incision may also be either transverse or vertical; however, exact placement of a transverse incision is critical, whereas a vertical incision may be extended if placement is not exact. The surgeon should determine incision placement by locating the iliac crest on lateral radiographs. Preoperative C-arm visualization may be used as well. A vertical incision allows easier exposure for more than one level. A vertical incision should be used in any case that may be difficult, for example, exposure of an adjacent level to a previously fused space, previously operated retroperitoneum, or in patients with a history of discitis. If vascular injury occurs, this incision can be extended for better control of the major vessels.

After the appropriate type of incision is chosen, the midline fascia is cut with a Bovie cautery unit. After the incision is made, the arcuate line or semilunar line of the posterior rectus sheath will be visible (Fig. 12-1). The retroperitoneal space is located at L5-S1, directly below the arcuate line. The surgeon

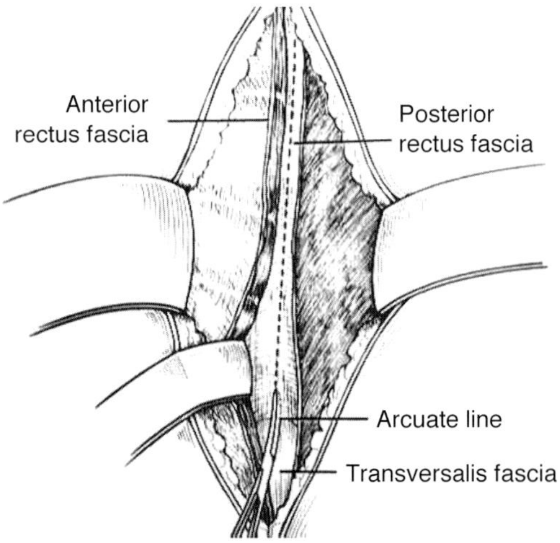

Fig. 12-1 Exposure of the rectus sheath, showing the arcuate line beneath the anterior rectus fascia. (From Wilder JR. Atlas of General Surgery, 2nd ed. St Louis: Mosby, 1964.)

may have to cut the posterior rectus sheath to expose L4-5 or above to enter the retroperitoneal space.

To enter the retroperitoneal space, the arcuate line may be bluntly dissected off the peritoneum before it is cut by pushing the peritoneum medially by hand. The fascia is then cut laterally. The retroperitoneal space is an avascular plane, allowing for bloodless blunt dissection. The peritoneum is pushed off the anterior abdominal wall laterally to the crest, and then posteriorly back to the psoas muscle. Once the psoas muscle is encountered, the peritoneum can be lifted, which also lifts the ureter along with it. There should be no bleeding.

Below the L5-S1 area, one may encounter the vas deferens or round ligament in the retroperitoneal space. The dissection should be lateral and superior to the vas deferens or round ligament. Sometimes the peritoneum on the psoas muscle will resist elevation, and it may help to use a peanut to get under it. Care must be taken to position the peanut directly on the psoas muscle to lift the ureter with the posterior peritoneum.

After the retroperitoneal space has been entered, the surgeon can begin inserting the retractors. Handheld retractors are recommended. A Wiley retractor, which has a smooth curved lip that gently retracts the vena cava or common iliac vein, can be used to retract the vessels to the right. It has a concave surface, unlike the Deaver retractor, and vessels gently drape around it. This retractor is handheld by the assistant. A vein retractor is then used on the left side.

There are several differences between disc exposure of L5-S1 and L4-5. The exposure of L5-S1 is between the bifurcation of the iliac veins, whereas the exposure of L4-5 is above or right at the bifurcation. At L4-5, the vessels should be retracted to the right, and the sympathetic chain should be retracted to the left.

At L5-S1, extreme care should be taken to protect the left and right common iliac vessels. The ureter and everything else should be pushed away from the iliac vein (Fig. 12-2). The dissection is made directly on top of the left iliac vein and

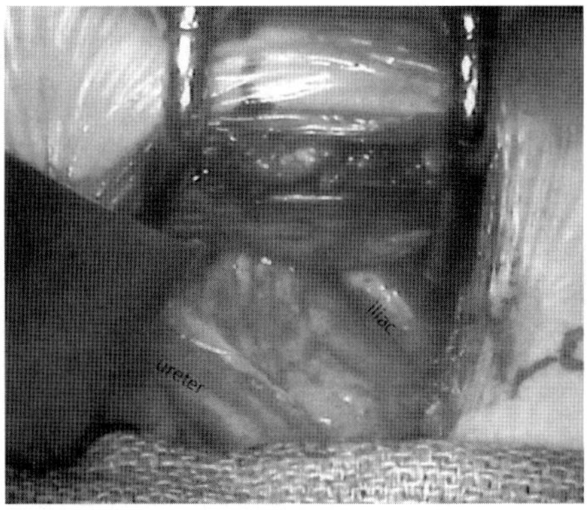

Fig. 12-2 The surgeon should take extreme care to protect the ureter and iliac vessels.

A

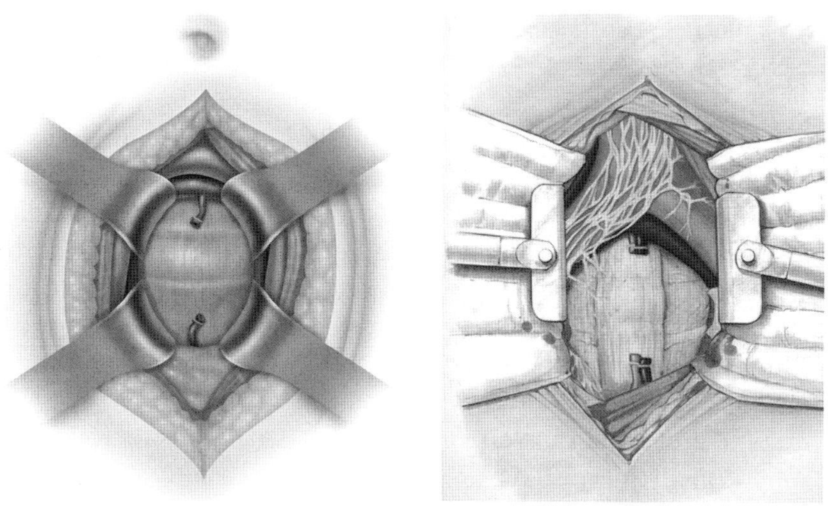

B

Fig. 12-3 A and **B,** Final exposure of the disc. Note that the median sacral vessels must be ligated and then retracted. (**B** courtesy John J. Regan, MD.)

directly over the edge of the vein. The surgeon should lift the layer with the ureter and posterior peritoneum because the hypogastric plexus is located here. This retroperitoneal approach creates fewer instances of retrograde ejaculation when compared with a transperitoneal approach, because the hypogastric plexus is lifted and retracted to the right. Incising the posterior peritoneum via the transperitoneal approach is more likely to cause injury to the hypogastric plexus and cause retrograde ejaculation. However, there are also precautions that need to be taken with the retroperitoneal dissection. For example, it is important to stay directly on the iliac veins at L5-S1 to lift the posterior peritoneum and areolar tissue that contains the hypogastric plexus off of the disc space.

Next the median sacral vessels are ligated or hemoclipped and transected. Further dissection of the tissue anterior to the intervertebral disc is performed mainly by blunt dissection with a Kittner dissector. Often there is an aberrant branch from the left iliac vein over the space. This should be hemoclipped and transected as well to avoid avulsion or tearing of the iliac vein.

Sometimes it may help to use a 4 × 4 sponge to clean off the areolar tissue on the disc space. This is done by placing this sponge over the L5-S1 disc and pushing it down into the space in front of the sacrum.

The final exposure is shown in Fig. 12-3 with the vessels ligated and the disc exposed. All of the vessels are retracted laterally and occasionally superiorly.

Exposure of the L4-5 disc space is obtained with blunt dissection, pushing the aorta and vena cava to the right. The genitofemoral and sympathetic nerves remain laterally to the left with the psoas muscle. An ascending lumbar branch courses from the left iliac vein posteriorly along the body of L5 and is often un-

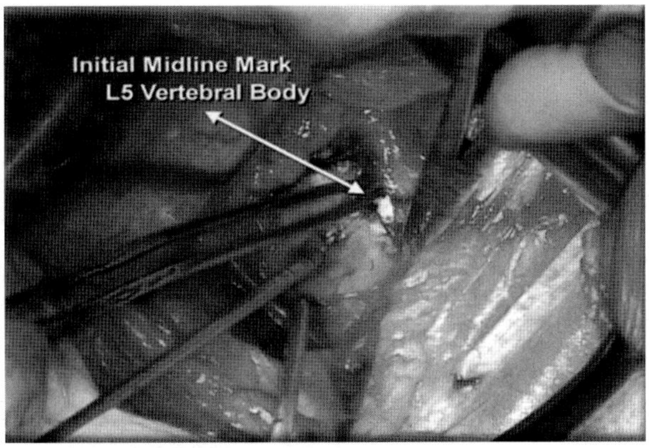

Fig. 12-4 Identification of the midline is an essential part of the surgery, allowing correct placement of the CHARITÉ Artificial Disc.

der tension, with retraction of the vessels to the right. If this branch is under tension, it should be clipped or ligated and transected. Avulsion of this vessel can cause significant bleeding, and tension can rip a large hole in the vena cava at its origin. A Wiley retractor is then placed under the vena cava and aorta and rests over the right curve of the vertebral body and disc space.

Discectomy: Preparation of the Disc Space

Discectomy is a crucial component of artificial disc implantation. With disc replacement, the disc space must be completely cleaned out down to the endplates, leaving two flat surfaces. Without an extensive discectomy, the surgeon will not be able to proceed to the next step of the artificial disc implantation.

It is crucial to use C-arm fluoroscopy for every single patient and for every single step, especially if the surgeon is becoming accustomed to the technique. The C-arm and anteroposterior images will help the surgeon identify the midline.

The initial midline should be determined using a 25 mm screw in the disc space (Fig. 12-4). The use of the screw allows differentiation of the head and shaft of the screw. Using Bovie cautery, the midline can be marked on the inferior portion of the L5 vertebral body, approximately 5 mm superior to the endplate.

The initial discectomy can be performed in one of two ways. The anulus can be removed anteriorly or it can be cut down the middle to create two flaps, which are retracted laterally. The discectomy begins with a disc elevator, an important tool for elevating and removing the disc. The endplate is cut and a sharp Cobb elevator is used to elevate and remove as much of the disc as possible during the initial discectomy.

Most surgeons use a headlamp to adequately view the posterior disc. Some choose to use magnifying loupes.

A

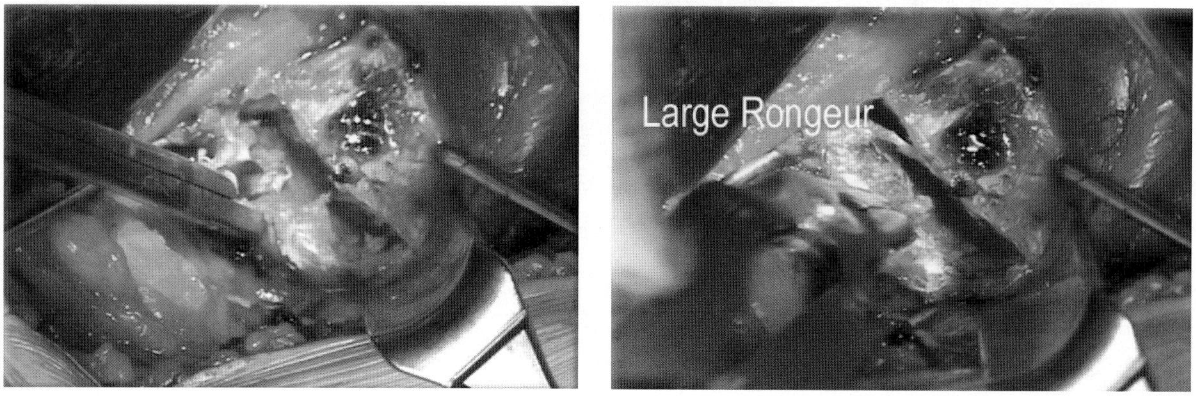

B

Fig. 12-5 **A,** Preparation of the anterior lip. **B,** The long rongeur should be used to resect the osteophyte.

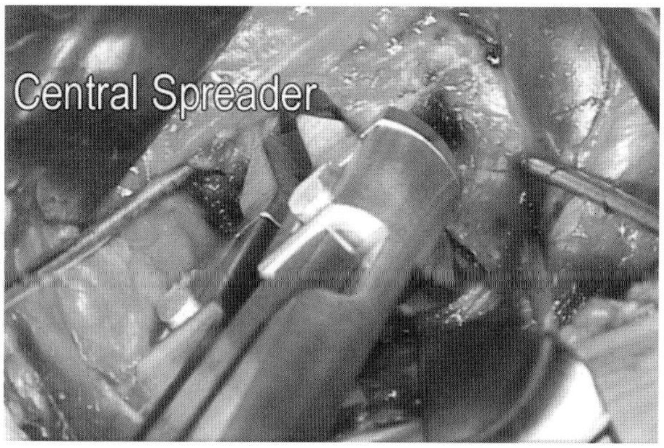

Fig. 12-6 The central spreader (spreading and insertion forceps) is inserted into the disc space to allow for controlled distraction.

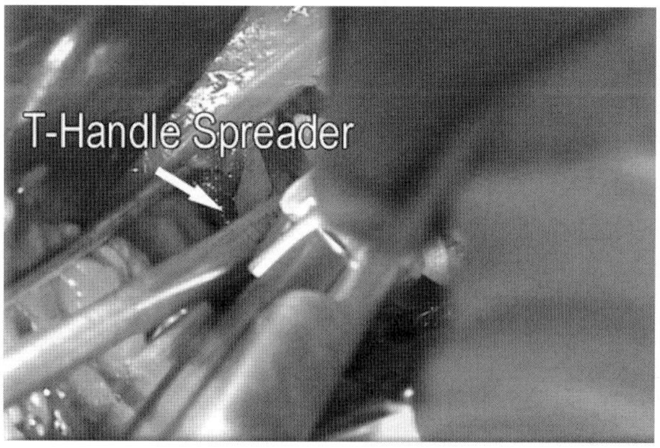

Fig. 12-7 The T-handles (distraction spacers) are inserted into the central spreader. They permit parallel distraction and prevent a fishmouth.

Ring curettes are used to prepare the endplate initially. These instruments are effective for removing the cartilage without removing the bone. The surgeon must be careful not to damage the bony endplate.

Next the anterior lip is prepared (Fig. 12-5, *A*). If an anterior osteophyte is present, it should be resected because it will disturb the placements. Almost all degenerative discs show some ossification. If there is a significant anterior lip that might interfere with the surgeon's ability to judge how to position the prosthesis and how far back it should be placed, it is easier to resect the osteophyte using a rongeur (Fig. 12-5, *B*).

Preparation with the ring curette should be thorough. Adequate time must be spent preparing the disc space. It will take 5 or 10 minutes longer to adequately prepare the disc space for implantation of the CHARITÉ Artificial Disc than it would for an anterior lumbar interbody fusion.

Some surgeons use self-retainers that attach to the table. At our institution, handheld retainers are used because we have enough fellows and assistants.

Next the tension in the anulus must be addressed. The amount of release of the posterior anulus depends on the amount of disc space collapse. For controlled distraction, the David spreader or the central spreader (spreading and insertion forceps) is inserted into the disc space (Fig. 12-6). The T-handles (distraction spacers) are inserted through the spreading and insertion forceps (Fig. 12-7); they are inserted parallel and then turned 90 degrees. The T-handles *must be* positioned to the back of the spreader. They provide parallel distraction and prevent a *fishmouth*. When there is a collapsed disc space, the surgeon may hear a popping sound when the disc space is distracted to the proper tension. This noise is caused by the release of the posterior longitudinal ligament complex in the posterior disc. If the disc is tall, the pop will not be heard, because the surgeon is placing the proper amount of tension in the disc space.

When a sufficient amount of distraction has been obtained, the posterolateral corners can be accessed. With the spreading and insertion forceps, access to the posterolateral corners can be gained with relative ease. The lamina spreader can then be inserted into the disc space. The surgeon can gain better access to the disc if the patient is positioned over a break in the table and the table is hyperextended.

The discectomy is not complete at this point; the surgeon still needs to remove the remaining disc material from the posterolateral corner. Any of the following situations will prevent inserting the prosthesis back far enough:

- Failure to remove enough of the disc from the disc space
- Failure to remove enough of the disc from the posterolateral corner
- Failure to remove a posterior lip from the L5-S1 vertebrae

It is often easier to hyperextend the table after the spreading and insertion forceps have been placed. When this is done, the spreading and insertion forceps are not in the way, and the entire expanse of the disc space can be viewed. Between the curettes and the pituitary rongeurs, the surgeons can gain access as far back as needed.

It is important to double-check the posterolateral corner to ensure that the entire disc has been removed. Very rarely, the epidural veins will bleed like an iliac vein with use of the spreading and insertion forceps or with the removal of the posterior disc, the posterior anulus, or the epidural veins. If that occurs, the distraction should be taken down, and the break should be taken out of the table. The surgeon should then pack the area and wait. The bleeding stops in 90% of patients. If it does not, Gelfoam or Surgicel or even one of the more advanced hemostatic agents can be used. The surgeon needs to be prepared—to know what to do when bleeding occurs. If the bleeding is stopped quickly enough, the patient may lose only 25 ml instead of 1500 ml of blood.

Most of the time the disc space will need to be stretched but occasionally, after the spreading and insertion forceps are inserted, the surgeon will hear a popping noise and encounter diastasis of the fibers. At that time the surgeon will be looking at the epidural space. The temptation is to clean the rear of this area with a Kerrison punch; however, caution is advised because this response sometimes causes epidural bleeding.

The lamina spreader can also be used to gain access to the disc (Fig. 12-8, *A*). Using the lamina spreader and a radiograph, the surgeon can achieve great distraction (Fig. 12-8, *B*). This distraction also allows access to the posterolateral corners, allowing the surgeon to ensure that enough of the disc has been removed in that area.

We frequently use a curette to remove the posterior lip at L5 and the L5-S1 disc. This removal is important because the posterior lip can sometimes prevent the prosthesis from being placed as far posteriorly as desired. To gain a better view and avoid placing the prosthesis too far back into the canal, the C-arm fluoroscope can be used. It is important to avoid the dural sac and to smooth the posterolateral corner to place the disc as far posteriorly as possible.

Next the posterior endplate is prepared. If additional help is needed at this point, the surgeon can use a Kerrison punch. However, using a curette usually works well enough to remove the posterior lip, similar to the removal of an anterior cervical disc. Endplate preparation is extremely important. Even after the entire disc is removed, it is likely that the surgeon will be able to remove still more disc from the posterolateral corners. The completed discectomy is shown in Fig. 12-9.

A 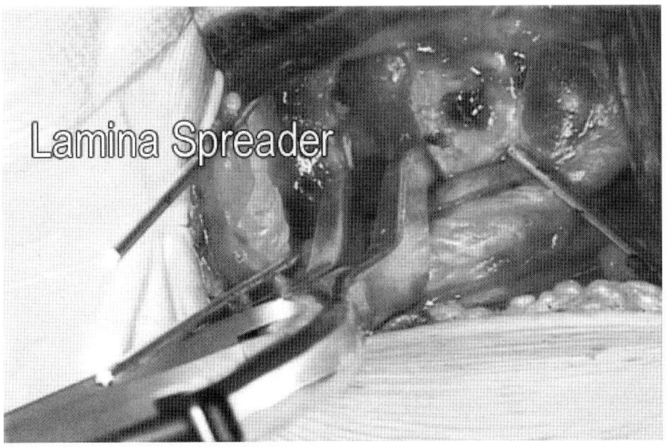 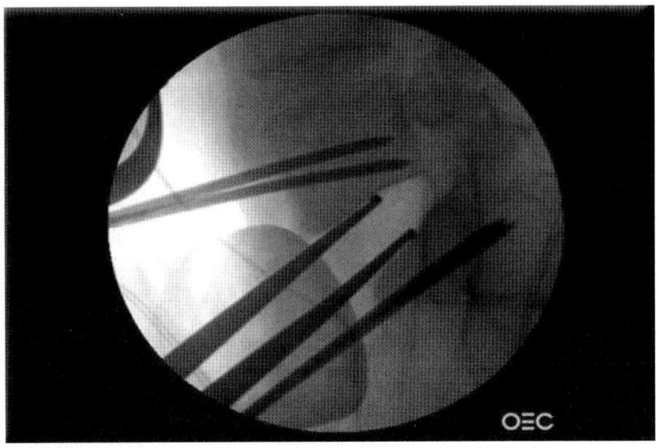 B

Fig. 12-8 A, The lamina spreader is used to gain more exposure, allowing more disc to be removed. **B,** A lateral image can help the surgeon to determine whether all of the disc material has been removed.

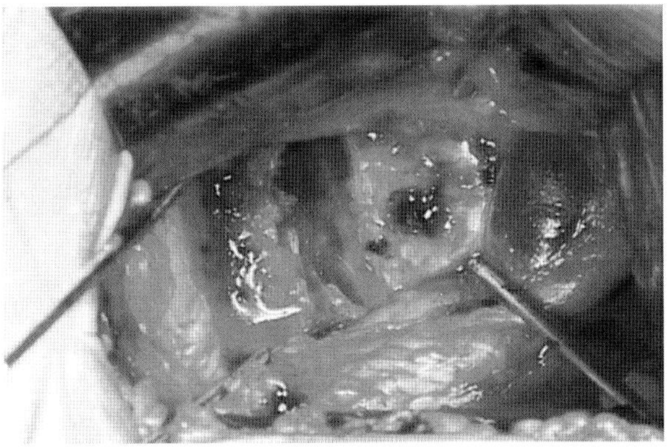

Fig. 12-9 A completed discectomy.

Implant Insertion

FOOTPLATE TEMPLATING. Following adequate disc space preparation, the CHARITÉ Artificial Disc can be inserted. The first step of implant insertion is determining the correct footprint size. The two prosthetic endplates are available in footprint sizes 2, 3, 4, and 5. The correct footprint size is determined using the sizing gauges, which correspond to the four available endplate footprint sizes. The correct size is verified by lateral fluoroscopy.

The prosthetic endplates are relatively flat on their metal-bone surface; therefore in addition to determining the ultimate size that will be used, it is critically important to ensure that there is a flat surface for insertion. To do this, the in-

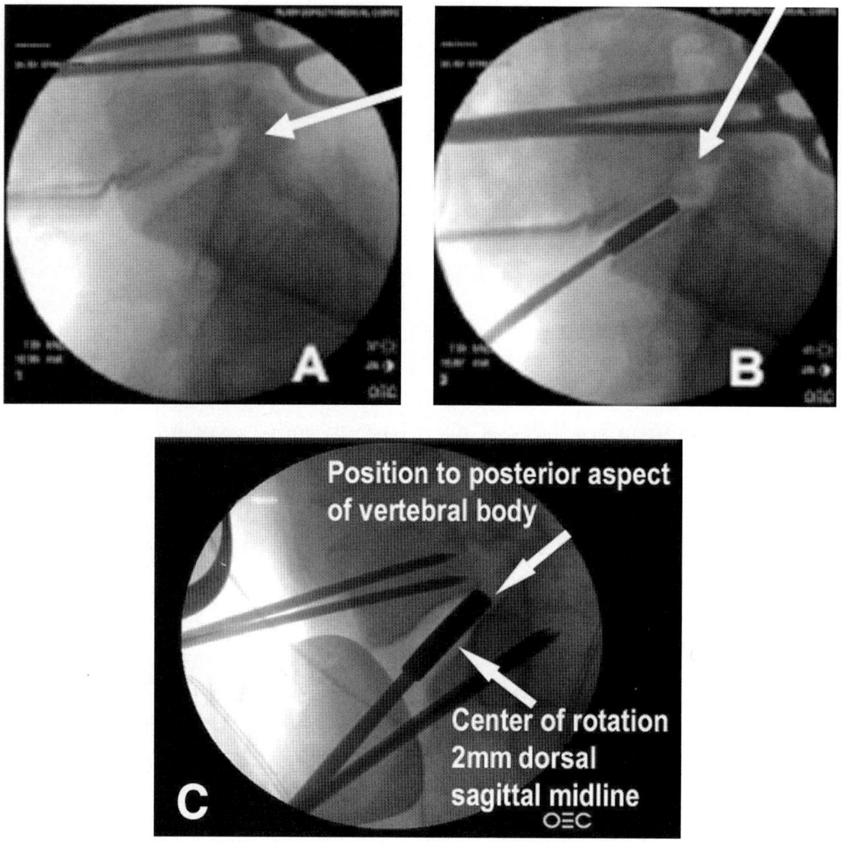

Fig. 12-10 **A** and **B,** A lateral radiograph is obtained to ensure that the posterior lip has been adequately removed, which will allow proper posterior positioning of the implant. **C,** Following removal of the posterior lip, a lateral radiograph confirms that the position of the template extends to the posterior aspect of the vertebral body. Note that the center of rotation should be 2 mm of the dorsal sagittal midline.

strument (usually a curette or osteotome) can be scraped against the surface until the cartilaginous endplate and osteophytes are removed. We used a burr for this purpose in the past; however, over the past 2 years we have switched to strictly using handheld equipment—mainly long, straight curettes—to make the surface as flat as possible. This change has helped to preserve the subchondral bone, which prevents postoperative prosthesis subsidence. The sizing gauges have a flat surface and thus can be used to assess the flatness of the vertebral endplates. If there are sclerotic ridges or irregularities in the bony surface, they must be flattened with curettes or osteotomes, because the prosthesis needs to sit flush with the bony surface and be *press-fit*. When determining the appropriate implant size, the insertion instrument is larger than the trial template.

The posterior lip needs to be removed to allow proper posterior positioning (Fig. 12-10). This procedure has proved controversial among some of the IDE study investigators. Frequently the back of the vertebrae curve at L5-S1, and European investigators have shown that if the surgeon goes straight in with a pilot driver or implant, it is possible to fracture the back endplate, which is very difficult to see on fluoroscopy. The patient then wakes up with leg pain from the fracture, which can be observed on computed tomography (CT) scan. The posterior teeth on the implant or the posterior teeth on a pilot driver can act as a stress riser, causing a posterior vertebral fracture fragment to displace into the spinal canal. The best technique to use to avoid any bony fracturing is to never use force after the sliding core has been inserted and the teeth have been distracted into the bone. It is important to adjust the position of the prosthesis into its final resting location in both anteroposterior and lateral planes. The sliding core is inserted only after the surgeon is assured of the correct prosthetic endplate position. After this point, no force or hammering is ever applied to try to shift or tweak the prosthesis position. When inserting the device, the surgeon will not be able to discern whether the vertebra curves in a fishmouth shape or whether the inferior L5 vertebral endplate has a downward-sloping posterior lip. Previously, we used a Kerrison rongeur to remove the back lip; now we use only curettes as well as the ring curette. These instruments allow safe removal of bone without entering the spinal canal and irritating the epidural veins. The surgeon starts posteriorly and drags the curette forward to effectively create two flat surfaces.

Another possible stumbling block that can be encountered when inserting the template is an extremely fishmouth-shaped L5 vertebra. With the CHARITÉ Artificial Disc it is impossible to compensate for a large hump in the middle of the vertebra, because there is no type of space or wedge that can be placed exactly in the middle of the prosthesis. If a large central hump is encountered, the top part should be made straight.

INSERTION OF THE RADIOLUCENT TRIAL WITH INSERTION GUIDE. A total discectomy should have been completed before insertion of the radiolucent trial with insertion guide. Two flat surfaces must first be created on the endplates before the radiolucent trial is inserted; it will have the correct vertebral footprint and the correct lordotic angulation, but not necessarily the correct final prosthesis thickness (UHMWPE core height). The trials all have a metal radiopaque alignment guide that contains a radiolucent circle to help the surgeon align the radiolucent circle with the theoretical *floating center of rotation* (FCOR). The radiolucent circle represents the centroidal (elliptical) shape of the motion pattern; it can only be recreated with a mobile bearing prosthesis like the CHARITÉ Artificial Disc, which has been biomechanically shown to restore mobility.

The radiolucent trials mimic the footprint, angulation, and height of the endplates and sliding core. Correct sizing, placement, and lordotic angle are critical to ensure optimal performance. Obtaining a good anteroposterior film to define

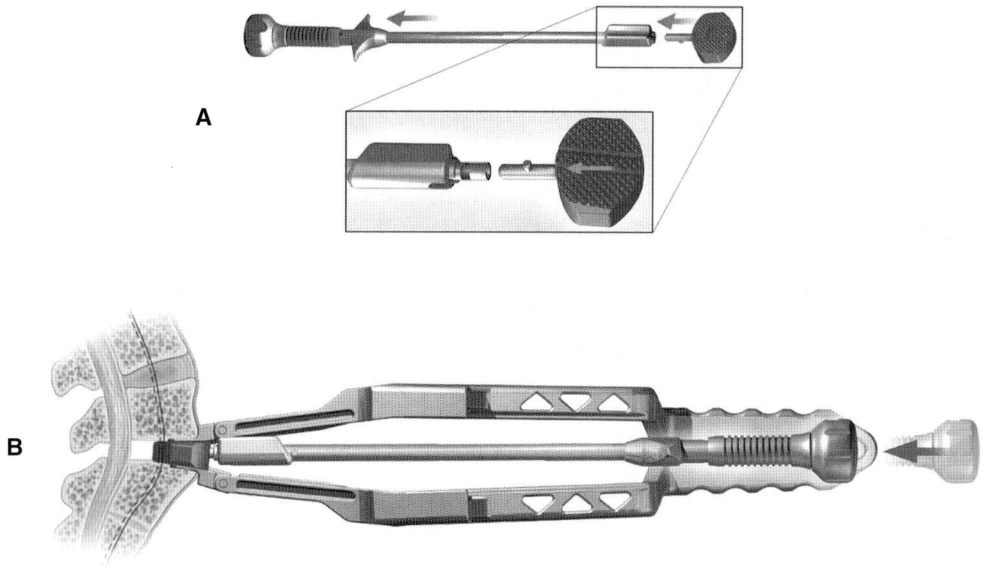

Fig. 12-11 A, Insertion of the trial insertion guide and trial. **B,** The radiolucent trial is placed with the marker side oriented superiorly. Note the retraction of all vascular structures.

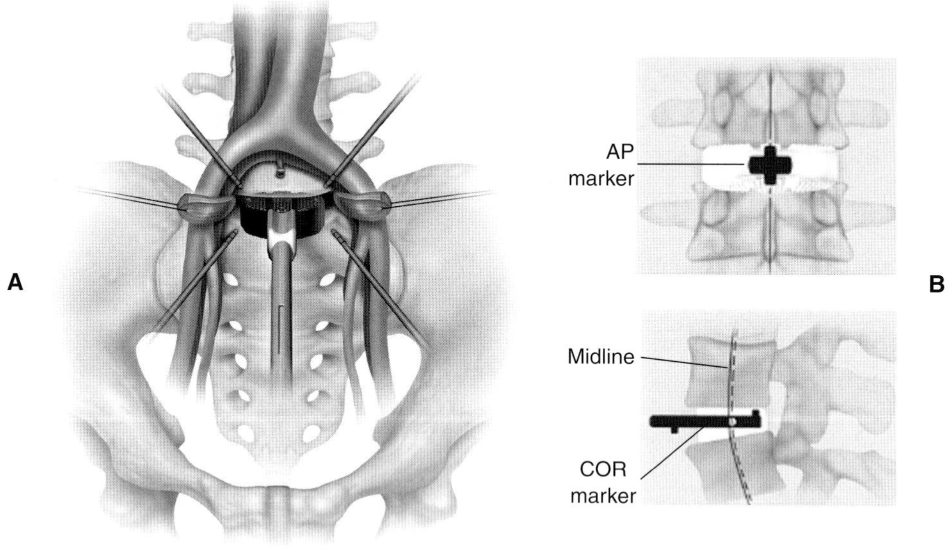

Fig. 12-12 A and **B,** Anteroposterior and lateral radiographs confirm the trial is perpendicular to the coronal plane and is in the midline (+). The radiographs also confirm proper lordosis.

the midline of the vertebral body is critical to proper placement of the device. Positioning the fluoroscopic x-ray machine at the correct angle and position to get a good anteroposterior film can be challenging but is worth the effort in time to obtain an optimal patient outcome. The fluoroscopic equipment should be positioned so that the pedicles are of equal size in magnification and equidistant from the spinous process.

Next the trial insertion guide is inserted into the disc space, placing the marker side superiorly (Fig. 12-11). Based on the footprint size, as determined by the sizing gauge in the previous step, the surgeon can then select the appropriate lordotic trial and load it onto the trial insertion guide to assist in placing the trial guide. The larger lordotic angle is placed inferiorly to reduce shear forces and to help protect the prosthesis and posterior elements. The trial insertion guide is then removed from the disc space, leaving only the trial. Proper size, placement, and lordotic angulation are imperative.

After the trial insertion guide is in the perfect position, the midline marker is placed in the midline of the superior vertebral body. It is important to insert a midline marker to indicate the correct midline position, and to help the surgeon gain orientation during the subsequent insertion of the instruments and implant. After the trial guide has been inserted, an anteroposterior radiograph is taken to verify the following (Fig. 12-12):

- The trial insertion guide is perpendicular to the coronal plane, indicated by +.
- The trial insertion guide is placed on the midline, indicated by +.
- There is no lucency between the trial insertion guide and the vertebral endplate, which indicates proper restoration of lordosis.

It is absolutely mandatory that the C-arm image be positioned directly parallel (colinear) with the endplates. To obtain this C-arm image, the radiography technician is instructed that the surgeon needs a perfect circle to continue the procedure. To ensure that the technician gets the C-arm endplate alignment perfectly parallel—and this is very important—it should be briefly viewed on continuous fluoroscopy.

Another helpful method is to use the shaft on the trial as a guide. The technician is told that the surgeon needs to have a circle; therefore the best approach would be for the technician to shoot the x-ray beam "straight down the pipe" on the trial. Even a beginning technician will be able to provide direct AP and lateral views. The radiograph must be set up properly to obtain a perfect circle and ultimately ensure optimal positioning of the prosthesis.

A 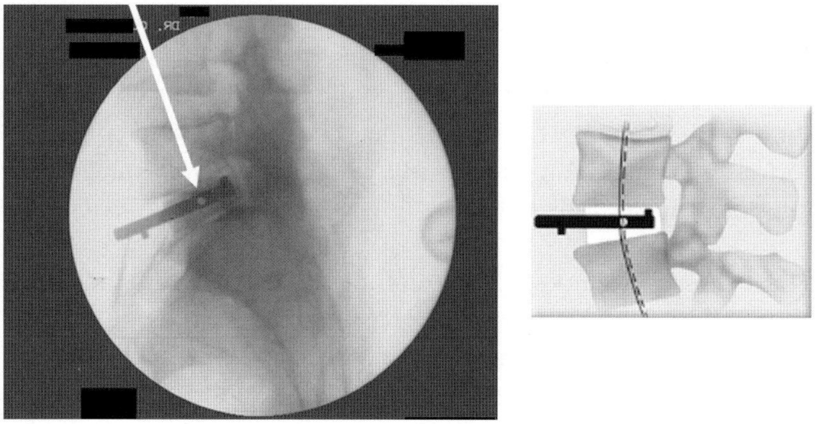 B

Fig. 12-13 A, To obtain a proper lateral image, the eyelet position on the inserter shaft should be aligned bilaterally to obtain a circular opening. **B,** The eyelet position is confirmed 2 mm posterior to the vertebral body sagittal midline.

A 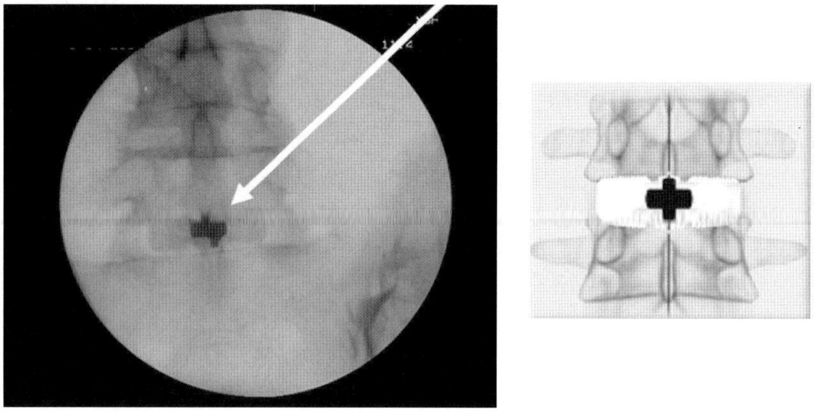 B

Fig. 12-14 A, Improper positioning is indicated by misaligned crosshairs. **B,** Proper positioning is confirmed by superior and inferior crosshair alignment. Center of CHARITÉ Artificial Disc = center of intervertebral disc space.

To obtain a lateral view, the radiography technician should align the bilateral eyelets on the inserter shaft to form a circular opening (Fig. 12-13, *A*). The eyelet position can be confirmed at 2 mm posterior to the vertebral body sagittal midline (Fig. 12-13, *B*). The superior and inferior crosshairs should align with the midsagittal axis on the anteroposterior radiograph. Notice on the anteroposterior radiograph shown in Fig. 12-14, *A*, that the crosshairs are out of alignment. This misalignment can be confirmed by keeping the C-arm where it is and moving it back and forth. In this situation, the radiology technician should readjust the x-ray position to make the image colinear with the marker (Fig. 12-14, *B*). This readjustment ensures that the prosthesis is as ideally positioned as possible.

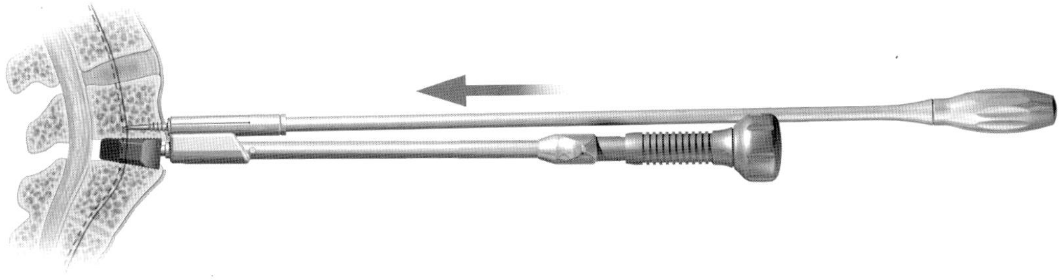

Fig. 12-15 Insertion of the midline marker.

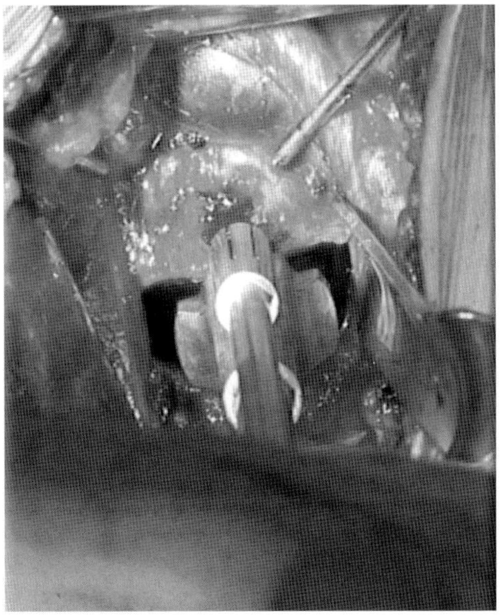

Fig. 12-16 Insertion of the radiolucent trial.

INSERTION OF THE MIDLINE MARKER. A second important consideration when viewing the radiolucent trial is to ensure that the trial is countersunk to the correct depth. The anteroposterior view can indicate whether the prosthesis has the correct width, which is required for a good footprint fit. If there are no gaps above or below, the angulation is good. Fig. 12-15 shows a midline marker inserter that is used to place the midline marker. After correct placement of the trial is verified, the midline marker is inserted into the anteroposterior midline of the superior vertebral body by placing the loaded marker inserter into the grooves on the trial insertion instrument.

The radiolucent trial is shown in Fig. 12-16. This trial has a metal attachment that locks in place. The midline marker is placed in the vertebra above. Occasionally, because of exposure, the surgeon will need to take a different approach at L4-5, placing the marker inferior to the endplate and placing the screw into the L5 vertebral body. The midline marker is needed to ensure correct placement of the instruments and the CHARITÉ Artificial Disc.

On the midline marker anteroposterior radiograph, it is essential to look for landmarks. One is the actual trajectory of the pin. The position of the midline helps to establish alignment, which can also be done using the trajectory of the marker to guide the alignment. Because the marker has a long stick attached to it, the surgeon can ensure that the trajectory is lined up evenly from front to back by looking at the radiographic image.

INSERTION OF THE PILOT DRIVER. It is critical to have shaped any curved vertebral surfaces before pilot driver impaction to reduce the potential for vertebral body or endplate fracture during this procedure.

The pilot driver is used to confirm positioning by matching the footprint geometry and approximating the height of the implanted endplates. The middle tooth of the pilot driver and handle must be in line with the midline marker and spinous processes to ensure maintenance of the midline (Fig. 12-17, *A*). The center of the pilot driver should be 2 mm posterior to the lateral midline. The pilot driver must be inserted parallel to the endplates to prevent endplate violation (Fig. 12-17, *B*). If resistance is encountered when inserting the pilot driver, a lateral C-arm image should be obtained to confirm that the pilot driver is absolutely parallel to the endplates to avoid breaking off part of the bone or gouging part of the endplate.

As the pilot driver is inserted, it is important to make certain that the center tooth is aligned with the midline marker. The next step is to impact the pilot

A

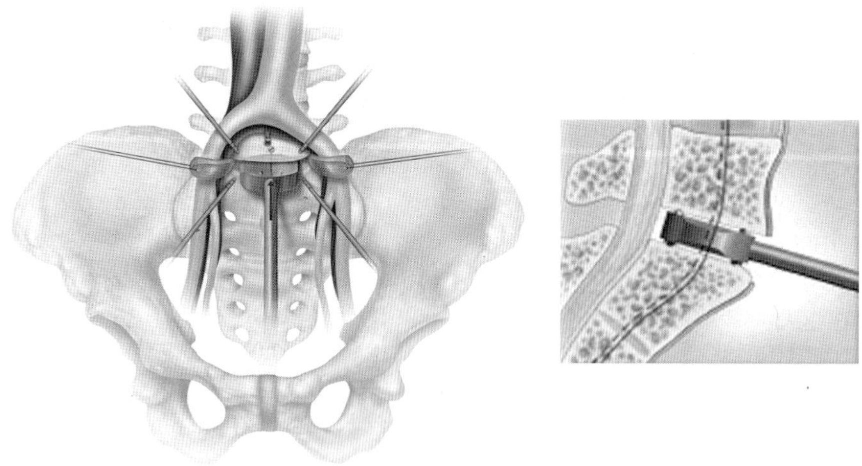

B

Fig. 12-17 Insertion of the pilot driver. **A,** The middle tooth and handle of the pilot driver must be in alignment with the midline marker and spinous process to ensure maintenance of the midline. **B,** The pilot driver must be inserted parallel to the endplates to prevent endplate violation.

driver to make three grooves for the endplates. Each of the surfaces should be flat at 0 degrees and 0 degrees.

A lateral C-arm image is taken of the pilot driver. If the driver is not exactly coplanar or parallel with the vertebral endplates, the hand is moved caudal or cephalad to stay within the endplate margins. The table must be in the neutral supine position when the pilot driver is halfway into position for final posterior advancement of the pilot driver. If there are problems identifying the midline, there is no need to use anteroposterior fluoroscopy at any point, because the surgeon can work off of the midline marker, and every instrument has a central etch on it. The endplate holding forceps, sizing templates, and pilot drivers all have a midline etch on them, and the arrows should always point directly to the midline marker during their insertion.

The pilot driver is more useful for more sclerotic bone. When finished, the surgeon will be impacting the endplates when inserting the prosthesis. The slap hammer is used to safely remove the pilot driver from the disc space.

INSERTION OF THE ENDPLATES. The next step in the implantation process is endplate insertion. CentreLine total disc replacement instruments, such as the endplate insertion tips, the spreading and insertion forceps, and the guided impactor, have been developed for implant insertion. Compared with instruments that we used previously, these instruments are greatly improved. Initially, we used 30-degree offset angles for implant insertion because it was thought that the surgeon needed to come in from the side to work around the peritoneum. Then several investigators used a 15-degree offset angle for insertion and achieved better results. Now there are lines on all of the instruments so that everything can be lined up directly down the middle.

The endplate insertion tips that correspond to the chosen endplate size are attached to the spreading and insertion forceps. The selected endplates are loaded into the endplate insertion tips, placing the more angled of the two endplates inferiorly (Fig. 12-18). When an oblique endplate is used, the sur-

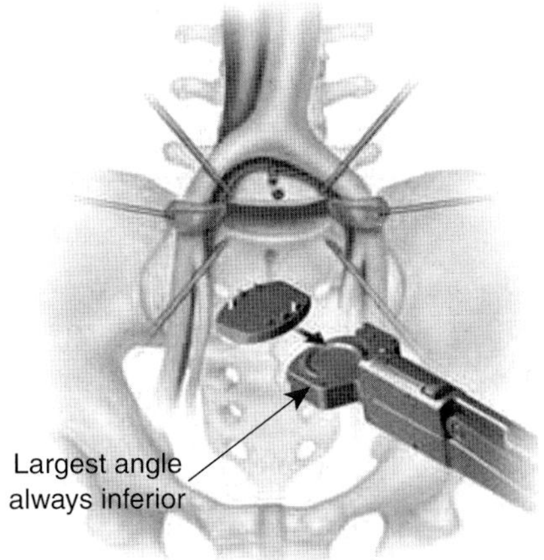

Fig. 12-18 The selected endplates are loaded into the endplate insertion tips. The thicker margin should be loaded into the endplate insertion tip first.

geon should load the thicker margin into the endplate insertion tip first. The thick margin should be placed anteriorly within the vertebral disc space.

The spreading and insertion forceps should be carefully positioned, paying particular attention to the anteroposterior midline. The endplates are carefully inserted into the disc space with the assistance of the guided impactor. Endplate insertion is carefully monitored with fluoroscopy to accurately control the posterior depth and to verify the appropriate lordotic angle.

When inserting a prosthesis, the surgeon must remember to remove the break from the table or deflate the lumbar pillow. Alternatively, lordosis can be increased to initiate impaction of the implant; however, the table should be brought to a neutral supine position when the implant is halfway in the disc space. The angle of the surgeon's hands must be correct to avoid gouging the endplates. On the lateral fluoroscopic view, L5 does not always line up directly over S1, and it may appear that there is a little retrolisthesis. The surgeon should always use the lower corner of the prosthesis as a guide. If the prosthesis is inserted so that the upper part is flush with L5, the surgeon could be back in the spinal canal. Therefore the prosthesis should be set with the lower endplate to maintain the proper orientation with the posterosuperior aspect of the sacrum. While impacting the prosthesis at L5-S1, the surgeon should reference the depth of penetration off of the S1 vertebral body rather than the back of L5, or the prosthesis will end up too deep in the spinal canal.

The ideal disc position is shown in Fig. 12-19. To avoid endplate fracture, the posterior lip is removed. Continuous C-arm monitoring is done during final im-

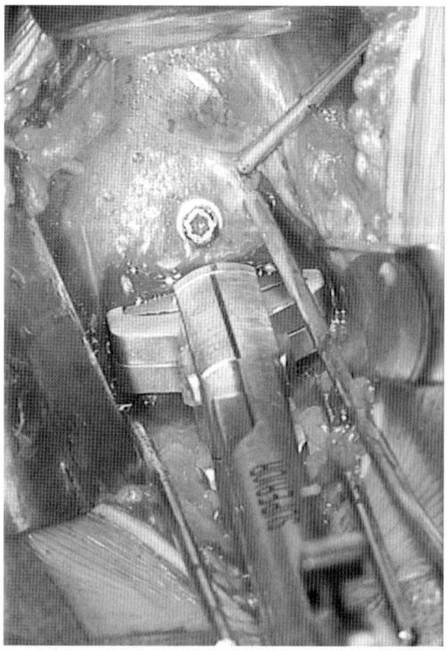

Fig. 12-19 Proper positioning.

plant positioning, and the implant is positioned to ensure that the final position of the center of the endplates is 2 mm posterior to the lateral midline of the vertebral body and centered on the medial-lateral midline. Excessive jacking open or excessive lordosis should be avoided. All the implants should have lines that can be lined up with the midline marker to ensure the most accurate positioning.

THE CORE TRIAL. With the endplates now in place, the next step is to open the disc space using the spreading and insertion forceps. The distraction spacers and modular T-handle are used to achieve proper distraction and core height selection. For controlled distraction, the disc space should first be sequentially distracted. Care must be taken to avoid contact between the distraction spacer and the polished articulating surface of the endplates; therefore a parallel orientation should be maintained between the shaft of the spacer and the spreading and insertion forceps. Once the appropriate distraction is attained, the size indicated on the spacer can be used to select the appropriate core trial. The upper limits of distraction are shown in Fig. 12-20.

The sliding core height can be confirmed by placing the core trial between the distracted endplates. Slight resistance may be felt as the core trial is passed through the rims of the articulating surfaces of the endplates. Once the core trial is in position, it moves within the articulating surface of the endplates. *The core trial should never be impacted.* To enhance visualization, the surgeon may want to release the distraction force of the spreading and insertion forces so that the endplates close around the core trial, demonstrating final position and height. When the surgeon is comfortable with the core trial placement, a lateral radiograph is taken to show the disc height and lordotic angle.

CORE INSERTION AND INSTRUMENT REMOVAL. Next the core trial should be removed and the actual sliding core inserted. Excellent suction is critical to facilitate visualization of the endplates and core placement. To do this, the appro-

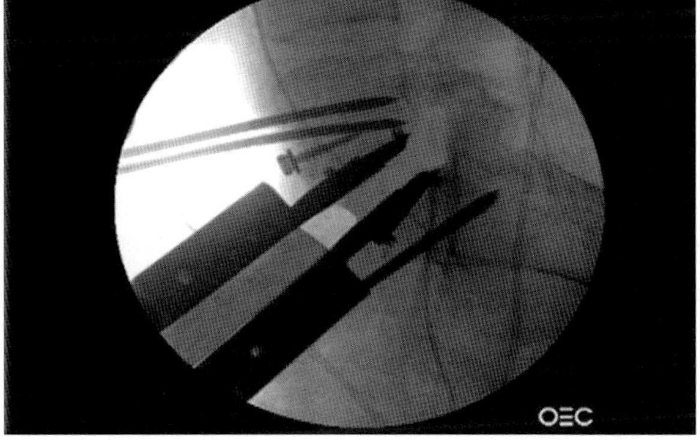

Fig. 12-20 Upper limits of distraction.

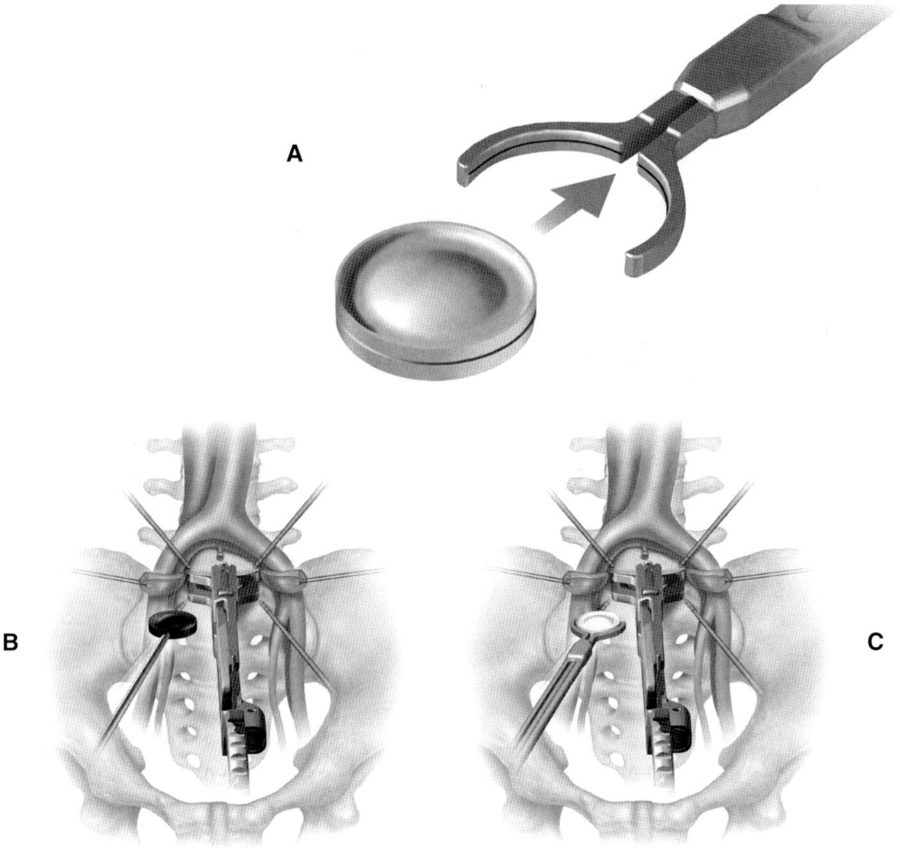

Fig. 12-21 Insertion of the trial core. **A,** The appropriate core insertion tip is loaded into the core insertion instrument. **B,** The core is placed between the endplates in the disc space and the distraction is released. **C,** The core is released by squeezing the core insertion instrument handle.

priate core insertion tip is loaded into the core insertion instrument (Fig. 12-21, *A*). Then the sliding core is placed into the core insertion tip by squeezing the handle. The sliding core is positioned between the endplates in the disc space. If resistance is felt, the distraction is slowly increased. Then the distraction is released on the spreading and insertion forceps, allowing the endplates to close around and engage the sliding core (Fig. 12-21, *B*). Finally, the core is released by squeezing the handle of the core insertion instrument (Fig. 12-21, *C*).

The core insertion instrument can now be removed. To remove the instrument, the surgeon must remove the endplate insertion tips from the vertebral endplates without changing the position of the prosthesis. The slap hammer is then attached to the guided impactor and the combined instrument is used to safely remove the spreading and insertion forceps. The instrument should be pulled directly out, avoiding pivoting and rotating. The intraoperative image and lateral radiograph in Fig. 12-22 demonstrate good implant positioning.

FINAL POSITIONING. The final position of the artificial disc should be verified using fluoroscopy. Proper posterior teeth placement can only be verified by ra-

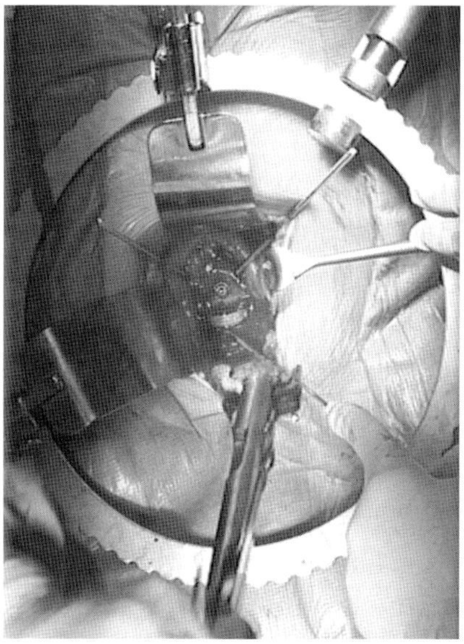

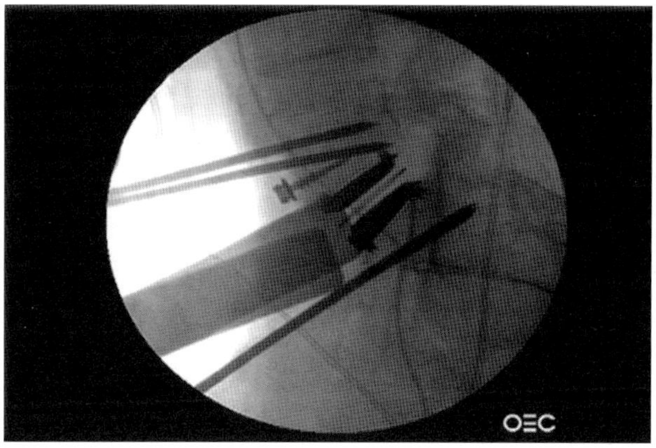

Fig. 12-22 Intraoperative and lateral radiographic views confirm good implant positioning.

A

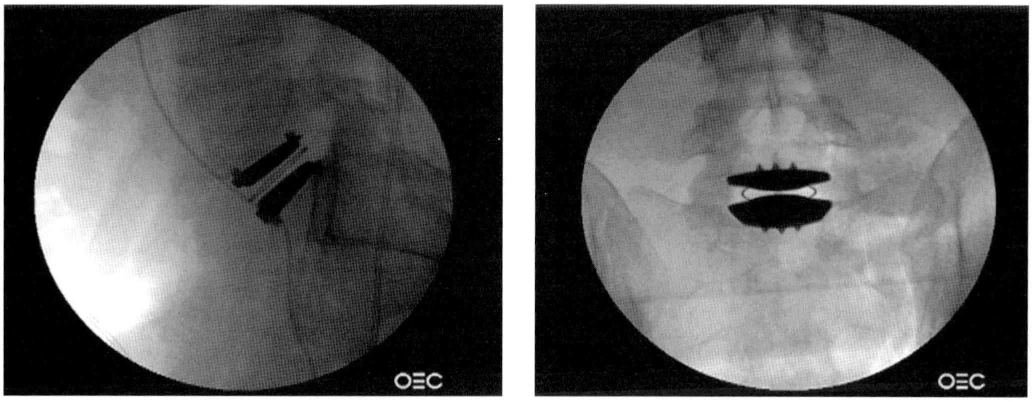

B

Fig. 12-23 A, A lateral radiograph is obtained to ensure that the implant is positioned at proper lordotic angles with maximum footprint coverage. The center of rotation should be 2 mm posterior to the vertebral body sagittal midline. **B,** An anteroposterior radiograph is obtained to confirm that the center spike is positioned at the midline. Although helpful, this radiograph is less than ideal. A Ferguson view offers the best view and should be used to confirm impaction of all six teeth.

diographic imaging. The anterior teeth can be seen by direct vision. The final implant position must not allow the anterior teeth to protrude past the vertebral endplates. It is imperative that the prosthesis be in the correct position in the anteroposterior (AP) and lateral planes. If necessary, final positioning can be altered slightly with the appropriately sized single endplate impactor.

The radiograph of the final positioning should show proper lordotic angles, maximum footprint coverage, and the center of the prosthesis 2 mm posterior to the sagittal midline (Fig. 12-23, *A*). Fig. 12-23, *B*, shows the center tooth positioned on the anteroposterior midline. However, this radiograph is not optimal. A Ferguson view should be achieved to properly assess implant placement. Ideally, all six teeth should be superimposed.

INTRAOPERATIVE REPOSITIONING. If repositioning and adjustment of the prosthesis are needed, they should be done before the sliding core is inserted if possible. If the surgeon waits until after the sliding core has been inserted to reposition the prosthesis with force using a mallet, this may result in breaking off bone or other problems. The inserted core serves as a spacer; if it is moved around, the surgeon may encounter bone fracture. However, the disc can be removed and repositioned or replaced once the sliding core is in place.

If the surgeon notes via radiography or changes in spinal cord monitoring that the disc is positioned back too far or does not appear large enough, the CHARITÉ Artificial Disc may be repositioned intraoperatively. The entire prosthesis can be removed and reimplanted by carefully distracting the interbody space, removing the sliding core, and then removing each endplate, one at a time. This procedure takes several minutes, and an extra core should always be available. The goal is to create a working space to remove the prosthesis without damaging the bone and the surrounding soft tissues.

Care must be taken not to damage the sliding core and the polished surfaces of the endplates. Once the final position has been confirmed, the single endplate impactor may be used to manually engage the anterior fixation teeth of the endplates into the vertebral body, thus providing additional initial fixation.

Closure

The midline marker must be removed before closure. If desired, the anulus can be sutured around the disc space.

The peritoneum is examined to see whether any holes have inadvertently been made in it. We always visualize the ureter and the iliac vein and artery. We double-check anything that we have repaired to ensure hemostasis. The access surgeon and spine surgeon must both examine the important visceral structures at the end of the procedure to ensure that there are no problems.

A better idea of the range of motion can be gained by inflating and deflating the pillow. Sometimes, after wound closure, the patient's legs are flexed and extended to assess the range of motion after impacting the teeth. This can be done while the patient is under general anesthesia. Flexing and extending the patient's hips provides an exact feel for the range of motion of the prosthesis.

POSTOPERATIVE CARE

It is possible with artificial disc replacement to provide early motion to the patient undergoing spinal stabilization with the artificial disc replacement. Unlike spinal fusion, this procedure usually results in rapid resolution of back pain and a more accelerated postoperative rehabilitation as a result of early motion. It is important to encourage core strengthening exercises and avoid overrotation or significant impact loading or hyperextension. Aside from this, most patients in our experience have returned to very active lifestyles within a short time compared with patients undergoing spine fusion.

Immediate Postoperative Care

Rehabilitation is an important part of the patient's recovery after surgery. The surgeon can begin rehabilitation the day of the surgery, if possible, by getting the patient into a sitting position and telling him or her to do a little gentle abdominal flexion. This activity will help to seat the posterior spikes of the implant into the posterior part of the vertebral body. In surgery, the surgeon can knock in the spikes located in the anterior part of the disc; however, the posterior spikes can only be seated after the implant has been loaded. Studies have not demonstrated problems of heterotrophic ossification and stiffness of the implant; this gentle rocking motion simply helps to ensure that the spikes of the implant are impacted into the endplate.

Although the use of a lumbar corset is optional, it may help to avoid *peak loading* of the implant, which occurs with extremes of range of motion (extension, rotation, or lateral bending). Lumbar corsets and lumbar braces were used in the IDE study as standards for comparison because fusion requires the use of a lumbar corset or brace. Some surgeons like to use a corset because it protects patients who plan to be active right after surgery. The lumbar corset slows them down a bit and provides further protection. The surgeon must advise the patient to avoid peak loading of the implant for approximately 3 months. The therapist should be informed of this restriction. Patients should start to ambulate as soon as possible, on the day of surgery or the next day. They should wear TED antiembolic hose and intermittent compression devices to avoid deep venous thrombosis until they are ambulatory.

Early in-hospital physical therapy should include early assisted transferring of patients to a chair, where they can sit as long as tolerable, usually about 20 to 30 minutes. Patients should also do gentle active and passive hip and knee flexion. Ice should be applied to the abdominal incision.

Two to Six Weeks Postoperatively

Patients should be weaned off oral narcotics and nonsteroidal antiinflammatory drugs (NSAIDs), depending on the preoperative pain medication regimen. The pain management team or physician can help to aggressively wean the patient from medication 4 to 6 weeks after surgery, when incisional pain should be nearly resolved. Surgeons can be instrumental in this process by informing patients of this regimen and helping them to develop a mindset that encourages a quicker recovery. Studies show that within 6 weeks most of the recovery has occurred; in 3 months the recovery should be complete.

During the first 2 to 6 weeks after surgery, the patient should avoid hyperextension. The rehabilitation program is then tailored to the patient's preoperative physical conditioning. Progress depends on each patient's unique physical condition. For example, patients who are very fit will progress smoothly through physical therapy. These patients fare much better than patients who are obese and out of shape. Physicians must have realistic expectations of each patient's recovery. For example, overweight patients 55 years of age or older cannot be told they will be playing tennis in 8 weeks. All patients should initiate rehabilitation with a flexibility program, called *flexibility core strengthening,* which is the current method of strengthening their abdominal muscles and teaching balance for trunk stabilization. The program also includes aerobic conditioning that avoids pounding activities such as running or jogging, which could jar the prosthesis. Other activities that should be avoided for at least 3 months include hyperextension exercises, heavy lifting, impact-loading activities such as jumping, contact sports, and sports that involve twisting, such as golf and tennis. The pace of the aerobic and core exercise programs depends on the patient's level of preoperative strength, conditioning, and flexibility.

Two to 6 weeks after surgery, the following exercises are appropriate for patients recovering from disc replacement surgery: stretching, isometric trunk exercises, isometric strengthening, and back strengthening.

Six Weeks to Three Months Postoperatively

Patients should be scheduled for a follow-up visit 6 weeks to 3 months after surgery. Flexion-extension and lateral bending radiographs are obtained approximately 3 months after surgery. Patients should have stopped taking all narcotics unless they have a preoperative history of high-dose narcotic use. Any patient with a new onset of back or leg pain at any time after surgery should be examined with a high-resolution CT scan or CT myelogram, because the implant will create an artifact with magnetic resonance imaging (MRI). Patients with a new onset of leg pain should have an aggressive workup, because there could be a piece of bone or a piece of disc in the canal. It is better to be aware of this complication earlier rather than later. A thin-section, high-resolution CT scan is the most effective way to look at disc material and bone in the canal. Magnetic resonance imaging or CT myelography can be used to look for adjacent-level disc herniations.

The VAS can be used to monitor each patient's pain. According to this scale, a large drop-off is expected at 6 weeks, followed by gradual improvement. Therefore the biggest improvement occurs during the first 6 postoperative weeks.

The same trend, although a bit more gradual, is shown along the disability index. A plateau is evident 3 to 6 months after surgery, with slight degrees of noticeable improvement thereafter. Physicians can expect their patients to follow the same trend. If the patient has a spike in pain, the physician should perform a workup to determine the cause.

Six weeks to 3 months after surgery, physical therapy becomes more aggressive. At 4 weeks, the physical therapy program of flexibility, core training, and aerobic conditioning begins. If possible, this program includes water exercises, especially for overweight, unconditioned patients. At 6 weeks, the abdominal incision should be healed. At this point, patients can perform lumbar spine rotation, side bending, and abdominal strengthening exercises. At 3 months, the patient can begin to play sports that require twisting, such as golf and tennis.

Return to Work

Return to work depends on the patient's occupation. Some patients who are normally sedentary at work can return in 2 to 4 weeks. The average patient returns to work in 3 months. Patients who perform medium and even heavy work activities, such as firefighters and police, may wait 6 months before returning to work. However, every patient is different. One patient, who worked as a driver for a delivery company, returned to work in only 3 months. Studies have shown that patients who have had a CHARITÉ Artificial Disc implanted tend to return to work sooner than patients who have undergone spine fusion, depending on their general conditioning.

Avoiding Complications

Complications can be categorized into those associated with the surgical approach, implantation, and device performance. Strategies to minimize the occurrence of complications and to effectively manage complications will be discussed in depth. There are three major areas in which surgeons encounter the most problems: (1) patient selection, (2) endplate preparation, and (3) positioning of the implant. Surgeons must be aware of those critical areas as they plan and perform artificial disc implantation.

Surgeon Education

It is essential for the surgeon to undergo proper training for implantation of the artificial disc to avoid complications before anterior spine surgery. There is a learning curve for becoming proficient in this procedure of anterior retroperitoneal exposure for disc preparation and implant insertion; therefore a base level of experience is requisite. Surgeons should maintain proficiency and ask, "Is this procedure right for my practice?" They should also follow indications and protocols, and ensure that a qualified access expert (a general surgeon with vascular training who is familiar with the anterior retroperitoneal approach) is available as a resource.

Patient Selection

Patient selection is key to avoiding complications. Patient risk factors include chronic obstructive pulmonary disease, diabetes mellitus, atherosclerotic cardiovascular disease, coagulopathy, massive obesity, and previous abdominal or pelvic surgery. Patients who have any of these risk factors are the most likely to have complications from anterior exposures and are not good candidates for this procedure.

Care must be taken to determine whether the patient has disc-related back pain. Possible spondylolysis should be ruled out. There have been instances in which patients underwent arthroplasty where spondylolysis was not recognized before the surgery. This problem may catch the surgeon unaware because it is possible to miss spondylolysis on CT scans, MRI scans, and even on straight AP and lateral radiographs. Therefore the surgeon must watch extremely carefully for occult spondylolysis.

Patients who have an ankylosed joint or a cartilage space that is barely visible and very irregular cannot be expected to do very well with a CHARITÉ Artificial Disc. The surgeon should rule out advanced degenerative facet disease and make certain the patient has passed a psychological evaluation.

Avoiding Intraoperative Complications

The surgeon can avoid intraoperative complications with careful exposure, adequate retraction, and accurate midline identification. Complications are also avoided with proper disc removal, endplate preparation, accurate sizing, and proper selection and positioning of the implant.

In general, complications of anterior lumbar spine surgery are related primarily to retrograde ejaculation, deep venous thrombosis, ileus, thrombophlebitis, warm leg, abdominal wound incisional hernia, urinary retention, pulmonary infarct, wound infection, vascular injury/hemorrhage, and nerve palsy. These are primarily exposure-related complications, which will be similar in number whether the patient is undergoing artificial disc implantation or fusion.

Approach

Surgeons who have not performed many anterior exposures must be especially careful to avoid complications. The most common complications encountered are vascular in nature. Venous injury or a clot will be the most significant; arterial injury and clots are rare. Occasionally the iliac artery will clot, especially with L4-5 exposure. Some patients may have a transient sympathetic effect or dystrophy. Ureteral injuries are rare; however, if a patient has had previous retroperitoneal surgery, the surgeon should consider putting stents in the ureters. To avoid retrograde ejaculation, the surgeon should be careful to dissect the hypogastric plexus up and off of the vessels. This problem is most easily avoided with a retroperitoneal approach and use of bipolar cautery. Other complications include injuries to the nerve root and/or ileus and injury to the abdominal contents.

It is important to note that from a medicolegal point of view, certain issues will arise if a vascular injury occurs and the surgeon does not have a great deal of experience with the anterior approach. Many feel it is preferable to have a vascular surgeon present during the surgery, even though a venous injury that is difficult to repair occurs in less than 1% of these procedures. It is helpful to coordinate with the vascular surgeon and to have the patient see the vascular surgeon before the operation. This communication sends a message to the patient that this is a team approach. The vascular surgeon should also be involved in the decision-making and informed consent processes. In the patient's preoperative preparations, autologous blood donation should be considered.

Midline Identification

The midline marker helps with the correct placement of the instruments and the artificial disc. Errors during surgery can be identified radiographically. Errors caused by the parallax effect can lead to asymmetry in implant positioning. This new technique allows the surgeon to see the midpoint not only anteriorly but also posteriorly, avoiding the issue of parallax.

Endplate Preparation

Proper endplate preparation can also help the surgeon avoid complications by minimizing the risk of subsidence and vertebral fracture during insertion, thereby optimizing insertion and final positioning. Forceful endplate impaction can result in endplate violation and subsidence. Proper trajectory, bisecting the disc space, is critical.

Accurate Implant Sizing

An undersized prosthesis can lead to subsidence. Either undersizing or angulation of the endplates into the concave part of the vertebral body adjacent to the hard posterior ring apophysis can lead to subsidence. To avoid this complication, patient selection is critical. Preoperative screening for osteoporosis is necessary, even in some male patients; men in their fifties with low testosterone levels might be at risk for osteoporosis. Major complications may occur if the patient has osteoporosis and the surgeon is not aware of this until after the CHARITÉ Artificial Disc has been implanted.

Implant Placement

It is critical that the implant be placed in the dense part of this bone and not into the body where it can end up in a kyphotic position, which will be detrimental to the patient. Inadequate endplate preparation and sizing lead to subsidence.

Accurate placement of the implant is also critical to avoid complications. Ideally the implant is positioned ± 3 mm from the midline. This placement allows a 6 mm leeway and provides a good result. However, an implant positioned 3 to 5 mm from the midline yields a suboptimal result. An implant positioned more than 5 mm from the midline yields a poor result, and the patient is likely to have more pain. Our studies have shown that placement of the implant is statistically significant to clinical results. Complications decreased as surgeons gained more experience.

Implant Migration and Repositioning

An implant is susceptible to migration or retropulsion if the anterior and posterior teeth are not engaged. If the anterior teeth are exposed at the end of the procedure, it means that the device is not back far enough. With the final impactor, the teeth need to be recessed under the vertebral endplate. Ideally they should be engaged under the anterior lip, where they are not going to come out, thereby avoiding implant dislocation. An implant that is too large, or one that is not placed back far enough, can result in dislocation. There are no other causes for dislocation. If implant repositioning is necessary, the UHMWPE core should be removed, allowing the endplates to easily fall out. Keeled implants present greater difficulties in revision or removal.

Postoperative Revision Strategies

Revision in the postoperative period can be done via the anterior approach. If repositioning is done later and the device is in good position, the surgeon can perform posterior fusion, leaving the disc in place. If the device position poses a risk, careful dissection is required to reposition or replace the device. The surgeon can remove the device and perform anterior or 360-degree fusion, or reposition the device and perform a fusion with the disc in place.

Clinical Results

At the time of this writing, more than 9000 Charité Artificial Disc prostheses have been implanted worldwide. In general, although outcomes measures vary among studies, the rates of good to excellent outcomes range from 63% to 75%.[27] The first prosthesis was implanted in the United States in March 2000 at the Texas Back Institute by Dr. Scott Blumenthal. Multiple abstracts have been presented worldwide on clinical results; however, to date, there is a relative paucity of published reports with clinical follow-up available in the English language.*

In 1988 Büttner-Janz et al[8] reported their early results with 76 Charité prostheses implanted in their first 62 patients. The authors did not describe the exact number of each version (SB I, II, or III) implanted. Mean follow-up was 15 months (up to 3 years), with 54% of patients "highly satisfied" with their results and 29% "better than before the operation." Two percent were "worse than before the operation" and 15% of patients had no change from their presurgical condition. Flexion and extension views were obtained and demonstrated 5 degrees of motion preservation at 2 years, compared with 9 degrees preoperatively. Pronounced intraoperative migration was noted in three of 67 (4.5%) endoprostheses. However, the authors demonstrated more significant complications inherent to the SB I and II versions, including postoperative intracorporeal migration, ventral dislocation, and cover plate fissuring and breakage in 26 of 67 prostheses, resulting in a 39% complication rate directly related to the components. In this study, patients' average inpatient stay was 16 days, and patients returned to work by 5 to 6 months (average). Despite these early questionable results, the data provided the foundation for further prosthesis design improvements and clinical testing.[8]

The second report was a multicenter retrospective study investigating the initial European experience in which Griffith et al[18] examined the data from 93 patients who had received the CHARITÉ Artificial Disc with an average follow-up of almost 12 months. The authors also examined the previously implanted SB I and SB II prostheses retrospectively in 49 patients (58 implants). The data were pooled from three different European centers (France, Germany, and the Netherlands) over a 5-year period. One hundred thirty-nine CHARITÉ Artificial Discs were placed in the 93 subjects with the majority (87%) placed at the L4-5 and L5-S1 levels. The preoperative work status revealed that 43.5% of patients were unable to work. Postoperatively, 42% were still not employed ($p = 0.83$). One surgeon noted that all patients had returned to work or were seeking employment at the 1.5 year follow-up, suggesting that both temporal and socioeconomic factors may play a role in patients' motivation and ability to obtain gainful employment. Visual analog scores were significantly improved regarding leg pain bilaterally and low back pain at latest follow-up ($p < 0.001$). The study also reported a 5.7% to 9.4% incidence of increased pain intensity when comparing preoperative to postoperative scores for the right and left legs, respectively. Although back pain increased in 9.7%

*References 8, 9, 18-20, 27, 34, 63.

of patients, it was diminished in nearly two thirds of patients. Neurologic weakness, present in 21% of patients preoperatively, was no longer present in 81% of patients postoperatively. Lumbar flexion improved in 82% of patients, decreased in 7.6%, and remained the same in approximately 10% of patients. Walking distance also increased postoperatively implying improved functional outcomes. Only one of 139 (0.7%) CHARITÉ Artificial Disc implants incurred a complication with the unconstrained UHMWPE sliding core, compared with 40 of 58 (69%) component-related failures in the SB I and SB II groups. The most common reasons for failure were plate fissures and breakage. The authors cautioned that spinal arthroplasty technology should be used judiciously, and stringent adherence to indications must occur to mitigate suboptimal outcomes.

Cinotti et al[9] reported their results with a minimum 2-year follow-up using the CHARITÉ Artificial Disc. This was a retrospective study analyzing 46 patients who were treated with spinal arthroplasty for either degenerative disc disease or failed disc excision. The average follow-up was 3.2 years and 56 prostheses were implanted. Clinical outcomes were rated as excellent in 11 (24%) patients, good in 18 (39%), fair in 14 (30%), and poor in three (7%) patients. Patient-perceived satisfaction postoperatively was described as either a "great benefit" or "great benefit but not complete benefit" in approximately two thirds (31 of 46) of patients. Similarly, 31 patients returned to their normal daily life activities or work; nine patients (20%) were less active. Four patients reported pain that was too severe and prevented them from working, and two patients were unemployed. Twenty-five of 36 patients (69%) with single-level implants were satisfied with their clinical outcomes, and only four of 10 (40%) were satisfied after having two-level arthroplasty. Seventeen of 22 (77%) patients without prior spine surgery had satisfactory results, whereas only 12 of 24 (50%) patients who had undergone previous spine surgery experienced satisfactory outcomes ($p = 0.004$). Segmental motion measured 12 degrees in patients with the prosthesis placed either centrally or posteriorly (approximately 50% of normal sagittal plane motion), and 5 degrees in patients with implants placed anteriorly ($p = 0.01$). These findings are in concert with previous biomechanics studies demonstrating the center of the dynamic disc spacer (nucleus) to be 2 mm dorsal to the center of the vertebral body in the sagittal plane.[45] Patients who began exercises one week after surgery had better mobility than those who wore corsets for three months ($p < 0.05$). In addition, no loss of UHMWPE disc height was identified at the latest follow-up, suggesting little if any third body wear between bearing surfaces. In this series, seven of 17 (41%) patients with unsatisfactory outcomes underwent posterior spinal fusion without removing the artificial disc; only three patients reported satisfactory outcomes at the latest follow-up. The authors concluded that up to 60% of patients with discogenic pain may be treated successfully using total disc arthroplasty, with the primary reason for poor outcomes being inappropriate patient selection confirmed by a 40% success rate in patients with two-level disc disease. The authors did not detail the degree of posterior facet degeneration, osteoporosis, or structural deformity preoperatively, which may have affected patient outcomes.

Lemaire[34] published their clinical results, which included 105 patients (154 prostheses) with a mean follow-up period of 51 months. Fifty-eight patients had single-level implants, 46 had a two-level replacement, and one patient underwent three-level arthroplasty. In contrast to the previously discussed studies, 79% of these patients had an excellent result, and 87% returned to work based on a Modified Stauffer-Coventry Classification. Sixty percent of patients returned to their previous work level, 27% had to modify their jobs to less demanding activity, and 13% were unemployed. Osteoporosis, overlying thoracolumbar kyphosis, and facet arthropathy were cited as key reasons for failure. Eleven (10%) complications occurred; half were vascular related (phlebitis, acute leg ischemia, or pulmonary embolism) and four cases were related to endplate failure or heterotopic ossification. The authors found that prosthesis malpositioning in the sagittal plane, as measured by a distance of more than 4 mm between the center of the prosthesis and center of the vertebral body on a lateral radiograph, correlated significantly with posterior facet pain if the prosthesis was placed too far anteriorly. They believed the implant was properly positioned when centered in the vertebral body.

Zeegers et al[63] examined the CHARITÉ Artificial Disc clinical results prospectively in 50 patients with a minimum 2-year follow-up (the first 50 of 350 patients to receive the implant). The authors demonstrated a 70% satisfactory clinical result in this cohort; however, twelve (24%) patients needed reoperation, and only three of these showed improvement. A total of 75 prostheses were implanted in the population over 3 years, all by the same surgeon. Twenty-nine patients had single-level surgery, 18 had two-level, and three patients had three-level device implantation. In contrast to the results from Cinotti et al,[9] Zeegers et al[63] found no differences in clinical outcomes in patients who had multilevel surgery. The ideal candidate for surgery (patients without previous surgery or other lumbar degenerative pathology) fared better than others, with 81% versus 66% satisfactory outcomes. Age less than 45 years also appeared to have a positive correlation with improved outcomes ($p < 0.05$). Eighty-one percent (35 of 43) of patients returned to some form of work; 43% returned to their original employment status. The average total hospital stay was 10 days, and 50% of patients wore a support belt for 12 weeks postoperatively. At the 2-year follow-up, patients retained 9 degrees (average) of segmental sagittal plane mobility. No significant implant migration (>2 mm) was noted. A disturbing factor with this study was the number of reoperations: 24 (48%) in 12 patients following the index surgery. Reoperations were performed at the segment with a prosthesis (n = 6), at other levels (n = 11), and as the result of complications (n = 7 in three patients). It is important to note that these were the first 50 patients in their series, highlighting a definite learning curve for technique, criteria, and patient selection. The authors cautioned that long-term follow-up of a larger cohort is necessary with optimal radiographic, clinical, and psychometric selection criteria adopted to improve outcomes.

Lemaire[34] presented a minimum 10-year clinical and radiologic follow-up of 100 patients following Charité intervertebral disc implantation. Sixty-two percent of patients had excellent results, 28% had good results; 80% of patients returned to the same level of work and 12% returned to lighter duties. Restoration and preservation of local lordosis and sagittal balance was maintained without evidence of cold flow polyethylene wear. These results appear encouraging regarding long-term outcomes of total disc replacement in the lumbar spine.

Recently results from the prospective, randomized, multicenter FDA-regulated study have been presented.[3,46] Blumenthal et al[3] reported the clinical results in 2004. The study involved 304 patients in a 2:1 ratio of patients who received the CHARITÉ Artificial Disc to patients who underwent anterior lumbar interbody fusion using cages. The VAS and Oswestry scores improved in both groups; however, the scores were significantly lower in patients who received the CHARITÉ Artificial Disc at most of the follow-up periods. Patient satisfaction was assessed during the 24-month follow-up period. The percentage of patients who were satisfied with their outcome was greater in the CHARITÉ group. Complications in the two groups were similar. The authors concluded that the CHARITÉ Artificial Disc performed as well as or better than anterior fusion for the treatment of single-level symptomatic disc degeneration that is unresponsive to nonoperative management. McAfee et al[46] presented the radiographic results. They found that the technical accuracy of positioning the device within the disc space was significantly related to the flexion-extension range of motion. Interestingly, the technical placement was also related to clinical outcome as assessed by Oswestry scores and VAS measures. At this time, the CHARITÉ Artificial Disc is the only disc prosthesis that has been approved by the FDA.

ProDisc

In the mid-1980s, Dr. Thierry Marnay[37,38] created the semiconstrained ProDisc I. His original study included 93 prostheses implanted into 64 patients from 1990 through 1993. At that point, the author stopped implanting any devices and followed patients clinically to assess their outcomes. Multiple follow-up abstracts have been constructed detailing patient outcomes; the latest was presented in 2002.[39] The author reported on 39 single-level cases, 21 two-level, and four 3-level cases. No devices had been explanted. The average follow-up was 8.6 years. No patients were lost during the follow-up period. The average VAS for back pain was 3.0, reduced from a mean of 8.6 preoperatively. The final VAS for leg pain was 1.9, reduced from 7.1 before implantation. Sixty-five percent of patients were "entirely satisfied" with their results, 28% were "satisfied," and 7% were "not satisfied." The average Oswestry score was 8.3 at the latest follow-up, and SF-36 and Beaujon scores had improved. Overall, 93% of patients were either "satisfied" or "entirely satisfied." Marnay did not address whether the multilevel cases performed better or worse than single-level implants. In another presentation, Huang et al[28] demonstrated motion preservation in this same group of patients with mean sagittal motion of 3.5, 4.0, 4.5, and 3.2 degrees at the L2-3, L3-4, L4-5, and L5-S1 levels, respectively.

Mayer et al[43] reported on the ProDisc I, with preliminary results of 34 patients receiving 37 implants. This was a prospective, nonrandomized, clinical multicenter study that included measuring VAS, Oswestry scores, SF-36, and numerous clinical and radiologic parameters. The average follow-up was 5.8 months. The authors reported improvements in VAS and Oswestry scores; however, statistical significance was not recorded. The mean hospital stay was 12 days and no implant loosening or migration was noted at the latest follow-up. Similar to Marnay's results, 60.9% of patients were "completely satisfied" with their outcomes, 21.7% were "satisfied," and the remaining 17.4% were not satisfied but stated they would undergo the procedure again if given the choice. In addition, 76% of patients had no back pain at the latest follow-up. Three complications occurred: one patient had nerve root irritation that eventually resolved after 3 weeks; in another patient, the polyethylene core dislocated anteriorly, and the implant was replaced without further untoward sequelae; the third patient had retrograde ejaculation present at 3-month follow-up. Overall, satisfactory clinical outcomes were achieved in about 80% of patients in this study.

As presented in Chapter 7, a prospective, randomized, FDA-regulated study designed to compare ProDisc to a standard anterior and posterolateral lumbar fusion (360 degrees) is ongoing in the United States. The preliminary results for the first 100 patients with a minimum 12-month follow-up were recorded. The safety and effectiveness of the ProDisc II were analyzed. Oswestry and the VAS scores improved significantly. Patient satisfaction was high. The authors concluded that total disc arthroplasty might be an attractive option to lumbar fusion for the surgical treatment of disabling mechanical low back pain secondary to lumbar disc disease. The collection of 2-year follow-up data is continuing.

AcroFlex Disc

The AcroFlex Disc is mentioned only for historic reasons. In the early 1990s, Enker et al[12] published their preliminary report (with 3-year follow-up) of the AcroFlex Artificial Disc (DePuy Spine, Inc, Raynham, MA). The implant comprises a hexane-based polyolefin rubber core vulcanized to two titanium endplates. Each endplate has four posts to improve porous ingrowth and stabile fixation. Of the six initial patients, four had satisfactory results. One patient had poor results. This patient was a 72-year-old woman who had undergone previous L5-S1 posterior lumbar interbody fusion with pedicle screw instrumentation for degenerative scoliosis; at 1 year the rubber core had fractured. The other failure was noted in a 51-year-old woman, who, despite adequate radiographic outcome at the 3-year follow-up, still had no relief of her preoperative pain. The authors noted that the study was limited because of small numbers, and further testing was necessary to draw any concrete conclusions from the limited follow-up. The latest version of the AcroFlex lumbar disc is an unconstrained design with porous coated titanium endplates. Regarding osseous ingrowth, data were similar to the ProDisc II. Bioactive endplate coating and prosthetic ingrowth had resulted in approximately 57% osteointegration using the AcroFlex lumbar prosthesis by 12 months in a baboon model.[10] Cunningham et al[10,11] also demonstrated improved range of motion in the AcroFlex-treated animals under axial rotation, flexion-extension, and lateral bending testing conditions at 6 months. By 12 months there was no significant difference between motion segments treated with autograft and fusion when compared with AcroFlex disc replacement. Interestingly, by 12 months, 60% of the baboons treated with the AcroFlex disc developed heterotopic ossification, primarily anterior to the prosthesis. In short, the AcroFlex lumbar disc appears promising based on a nonhuman primate model; however, clinical results with larger patient numbers are pending.

MAVERICK Disc

The MAVERICK prosthesis is a two-piece metal-on-metal design that allows motion through articulation between curved surfaces. Le Huec et al[35] recently presented the 24-month follow-up of 50 patients who received the implant at one or two disc levels. The authors reported significant improvement in pain scores, from 7.1 to 3.0, following the implantation of the prosthesis. The mean range of motion at the replaced levels was 6 degrees, ranging from 3 degrees to 12 degrees. In the United States, clinical trials were initiated in May 2003, in a study comparing the device to anterior fusion using cages and BMP (see Chapter 13).

FlexiCore Disc

The FlexiCore artificial disc is another metal-on-metal device. The FDA IDE study was initiated in 2003, and clinical data collection is ongoing.

Kineflex Disc

The Kineflex artificial disc, as described earlier, is a three-piece metal-on-metal device with a mobile metal core. The FDA IDE study begins in mid-2005.

Future Directions

We are in a very exciting time in the advancement of spine surgery. Disc replacement is the first step away from fusion. This situation is not unlike the development of total hip and knee replacement. Fusions of these joints provided acceptable results but did not restore normal function and were not without problems. Now total hip replacement is one of the most successful operations presently available. We must learn from history and carefully study the current results for these "first"-generation disc replacements, which are just the beginning. A long-term follow-up, beyond 2 years, will provide much-needed data with respect to wear, maintenance of motion, transition syndrome, subsidence, the ideal patients, and complications. These objective results will shape the next generation prostheses. Revision strategies for implant failure must be developed as total disc replacement continues to gain widespread acceptance for treating spinal disorders. Newer designs will likely employ alternative surgical approaches, because revision anterior surgery above L5-S1 or above the bifurcation of the great vessels is difficult.

For now, early clinical results must be treated with cautious optimism. As with all aspects of spinal surgery, patient selection, based on both physiologic and psychological criteria, is essential to optimizing patient outcomes. Careful adherence to surgical indications and proper surgical technique will also promote better clinical results. Total disc replacement is just the beginning of this truly remarkable era of functional restorative surgery. The story continues with facet joint replacement and nuclear replacement, which are discussed in other chapters. Finally, biologic solutions using gene therapy and stem cell treatments will be the ultimate treatment for our patients. The future of spine surgery will provide our patients with truly innovative treatments.

REFERENCES

1. Bao QB, Higham PA. Hydrogel bead intervertebral disc nucleus. US Patent No 5,192,326, Sept 9, 1993.
2. Baumgartner W. Intervertebral prosthesis. US Patent No 5,171,280, Dec 15, 1992.
3. Blumenthal S, McAfee P, Guyer R, et al. Randomized control trial of the Charité artificial disc vs. fusion for single level lumbar degenerative disc disease: A two-year follow-up study. Spinal Arthroplasty Society, Vienna, May 2004.
4. Bouvet JC. Prosthese destinée a restaurer une articulation entre deux os et application, notamment comme prosthèse de hanche et intervertébrale. French Patent No 2,761,878, Apr 11, 1997.
5. Bryan VE Jr. Cervical motion segment replacement. Eur Spine J 11(Suppl 2):S92-S97, 2002.
6. Buechel FF Sr, Buechel FF Jr, Pappas MJ, et al. Twenty-year evaluation of meniscal bearing and rotating platform knee replacements. Clin Orthop Relat Res 388:41-50, 2001.
7. Buttermann GR. Intervertebral prosthetic device. US Patent No 5827328, Oct 27, 1998.
8. Büttner-Janz K, Schellnack K, Zippel H, et al. Experience and results with the SB Charité lumbar intervertebral endoprosthesis. Z Klin Med 43:1785-1789, 1988.

9. Cinotti G, David T, Postacchini F. Results of disc prosthesis after a minimum follow-up of 2 years. Spine 21:995-1000, 1996.
10. Cunningham BW, Hallab N, Dmitriev AE, et al. Epidural application of spinal instrumentation particulate wear debris: An in-vivo animal model. Presented at the Third Annual Spine Arthroplasty Society Meeting, Scottsdale, Ariz, May 2003.
11. Cunningham BW, Lowery GL, Serhan HA, et al. Total disc replacement arthroplasty using the AcroFlex lumbar disc: A non-human primate model. Eur Spine J 11(Suppl 2):S115-S123, 2002.
12. Enker P, Steffee A, McMillian C, et al. Artificial disc replacement: Preliminary report with a 3-year minimum follow-up. Spine 18:1061-1070, 1993.
13. Errico T. SpineCore I & II Disc. Presented at the Dynamic Spine Stabilization Course, Plano, Texas, Oct 2002.
14. Fernström U. Arthroplasty with intercorporal endoprosthesis in herniated disc and in painful disc. Acta Chir Scand 357(Suppl):S154-S159, 1966.
15. Fitz WR. Artificial facet joint. US Patent No 5,571,191, Nov 5, 1996.
16. Gill SS, Walker C, van Hoeck J, et al. Artificial intervertebral joint permitting translational and rotational motion. US Patent No 611,637, Sept 5, 2000.
17. Graham D. Artificial disk. US Patent No 5,246,458, Sept 21, 1993.
18. Griffith SL, Shelokov AP, Büttner-Janz K, et al. A multicenter retrospective study of the clinical results of the LINK SB Charité intervertebral prosthesis: The initial European experience. Spine 19:1842-1849, 1994.
19. Guyer RD, Blumenthal SL. Preliminary United States experience with the SB Charité III artificial discs. In Büttner-Janz K, Hochschuler SH, McAfee PC, eds. The Artificial Disc. Berlin: Springer-Verlag, 2003, pp 139-145.
20. Guyer RD, McAfee PC, Hochschuler SH, et al. Prospective randomized study of the Charité artificial disc: Data from two investigational centers. Spine J 4(Suppl 6):S252-S259.
21. Hahnle UR, Weinberg IR, De Villiers M, et al. A new articulated lumbar disc prosthesis. Presented at the Third Annual Spine Arthroplasty Society Meeting, Scottsdale, Ariz, May 2003.
23. Hedman TP, Kostuik JP, Fernie GR, et al. Artificial spinal disc. US Patent No 4759769, July 26, 1988.
22. Hedman TP, Kostuik JP, Fernie GR, et al. Design of an intervertebral disc prosthesis. Spine 16(Suppl 6):S256-S260, 1991.
24. Hellier WG, Hedman TP, Kostuik JP. Wear studies for the development of an intervertebral disc prosthesis. Spine 17(Suppl 6):S86-S96, 1992.
25. Hilibrand AS, Carlson GD, Palumbo MA, et al. Radiculopathy and myelopathy at segments adjacent to the site of previous anterior cervical arthrodesis. J Bone Joint Surg Am 81:519-528, 1999.
26. Hilibrand AS, Yoo JU, Carlson GD, et al. The success of anterior cervical arthrodesis adjacent to a previous fusion. Spine 22:1574-1579, 1997.
27. Hochschuler SH, Ohnmeiss DD, Guyer RD, et al. Artificial disc: Preliminary results of a prospective study in the United States. Eur Spine J 11(Suppl 2):S106-S110, 2002.
28. Huang R, Girardi F, Cammisa F, et al. Long-term flexion-extension range of motion of the Prodisc I. Presented at the Annual Meeting of the North American Spine Society, Montreal, Canada, Oct 2002.
29. Ibo I, Pierotto E. Prosthesis of the cervical intervertebralis disk. US Patent No 5,755,796, May 26, 1998.
30. Keller A. Surgical instrument set. US Patent No 4,997,432, March 5, 1991.
31. Kostuik JP. Intervertebral disc replacement: Experimental study. Clin Orthop Relat Res 337:27-41, 1997.
32. Lehmann TR, Spratt KF, Tozzi JE, et al. Long-term follow-up of lower lumbar fusion patients. Spine 12:97-104, 1987.

33. Le Huec JC, Friesem T, Brayda-Bruno M, et al. Maverick total lumbar disc replacement prospective study. Preliminary report of 50 cases at 2 year follow-up. Spine Society of Europe, Porto, Portugal, May-June 2004.
34. Lemaire JP. SB Charite III intervertebral disc prosthesis clinical and radiological result with a series of 100 cases over 10 years follow-up. Presented at the Annual Meeting of the Spine Arthroplasty Society, Scottsdale, Ariz, May 2003.
35. Lemaire JP, Skalli W, Lavaste F, et al. Intervertebral disc prothesis. Results and prospects for the year 2000. Clin Orthop Relat Res 337:64-76, 1997.
36. Main JA, Wells ME, Keller TS. Vertebral prosthesis. US Patent No 4,932,975, June 12, 1990.
37. Marnay T. L'arthroplasty intervertébrale lombaire. Med Orthop 25:48-55, 1991.
38. Marnay T. Prosthesis for intervertebral discs and instruments for implanting it. US Patent No 5314477, May 24, 1994.
39. Marnay T. Lumbar disc replacement: 7- to 11-year results with ProDisc. Presented at the Annual Meeting of the North American Spine Society, Montreal, Canada, Oct 2002.
40. Martin JR. Vertebral joint facets prostheses, US Patent No 6,132,464, Oct 17, 2000.
41. Matthews HH, High W, McLay C, et al. Evaluation of wear debris in the rabbit's spine. Presented at the Annual Meeting of the Spine Arthroplasty Society, Scottsdale, Ariz, May 2003.
42. Matthews H, Le Huec JC, Bertagnoli R, et al. Design rationale and early multicenter evaluation of Maverick total disk arthroplasty. Presented at the Spinal Arthroplasty Society Meeting, Montreaux, Switzerland, May 2002.
43. Mayer HM, Wiechert K, Korge A, et al. Minimally invasive total disc replacement: Surgical technique and preliminary clinical results. Eur Spine J 11(Suppl 2):S124-S130, 2002.
44. Mazda K. Prothèse discale intervertébrale, French Patent No 2,694,882, Feb 25, 1994.
45. McAfee PC. In Kaech DL, Jinkins JR, eds. Spinal Restabilization Procedures. Amsterdam: Elsevier, 2002, pp 299-310.
46. McAfee P, Cunningham B, Hotsapple G, et al. A prospective randomized FDA study of the Charité disc replacement. A radiographic outcome analysis of 276 consecutive patients. Presented at the Annual Meeting of the International Society for the Study of the Lumbar Spine, Porto, Portugal, June 2004.
47. McAfee PC, Cunningham BW, Orbegoso CM, et al. Analysis of porous ingrowth in intervertebral disc prosthesis. Spine 28:332-340, 2003.
48. Mehdizadeh HM. Disc replacement prosthesis. US Patent No 6,231,609, May 15, 2001.
49. Mueller ME, Allgower M, Schneider R, eds. Manual of Internal Fixation, 3rd ed. Berlin: Springer-Verlag, 1995.
50. Nachemson A. Some mechanical properties of the lumbar intervertebral disc. Bull Hosp Joint Dis 23:130-142, 1962.
51. Nachemson A. The lumbar spine: An orthopaedic challenge. Spine 59-71, 1976.
52. Patil AA. Artificial intervertebral disc. US Patent No 4,309,777, Apr 8, 1982.
53. Pisharodi M. Artificial spinal prosthesis. US Patent No 5,123,926, June 23, 1992.
54. Salib RM, Pettine KA. Intervertebral disk arthroplasty. US Patent No 5,258,031, Nov 2, 1993.
55. Shelekov AP. Articulating spinal disc prosthesis. US Patent No 6,039,763, March 21, 2000.
56. Szpalski M, Gunzburg R, Mayer M. Spine arthroplasty: A historical review. Eur Spine J 11(Suppl 2):S65-S84, 2002.
57. Traynelis VC. Spinal arthroplasty. Neurosurg Focus 13:1-7, 2002.
58. Traynelis V, Haid R, Zdeblick T, et al. Clinical evolution of a metal-on-metal cervical disc prosthesis. Presented at the Annual Meeting of the Spine Arthroplasty Society, Scottsdale, Ariz, May 2003.
59. Weber BG. Zwischenwirbel Totaprothese. Swiss Patent No 624,573, Feb 1, 1978.

60. Weber BG. Zwischenwirbel Totaprothese. Swiss Patent No 640,131, Oct 3, 1979.
61. White AA, Panjabi MM. Clinical Biomechanics of the Spine. Philadelphia: JB Lippincott, 1978.
62. Yuan HA, Chih-L, Davidson JA, et al. Low wear artificial spinal disc, US Patent No 5,667,701, Oct 14, 1997.
63. Zeegers WS, Bohnen LMLJ, Laaper M, et al. Artificial disc replacement with the modular type SB Charité III: 2-year results in 50 prospectively studied patients. Eur Spine J 8:210-217, 1999.

CHAPTER

13

Total Disc Arthroplasty Using MAVERICK Total Disc Replacement

Hallett H. Mathews ▪ Lukas Eisermann
Jean-Charles LeHuec ▪ Tai Friesem

Restoration of the diseased spinal segment remains a fundamental surgical principle when surgery is required for advanced degenerative disease. Motion preservation fits well in the understanding of spine stabilization because mobilization can occur after restabilization of a diseased motion segment. Arthrodesis, dynamic stabilization, and mobile stabilization principles accurately define restabilization as a principle of restoration. Enhanced restoration by replacement arthroplasty of one or all three joints of a spinal segment can functionally restabilize a degenerative segment, allowing the patient to assume appropriate lordosis within the lumbar spine.

The rationale for developing total disc replacement is inherently understood by analyzing the function of the intervertebral disc. Healthy intervertebral discs function as the primary stabilizers of a functional spinal unit. Discs also protect the facets against shear and translational forces, function as load-sharing devices in axial and torsional load, and act as the primary shock absorber in a diseased motion segment. Approximately 80% of the load of the lumbar spine is borne anteriorly; therefore the appropriate load transfer is understood to be from anterior to posterior. This concept is an important consideration when designing an intervertebral disc replacement.

The work of designing the MAVERICK™ Total Disc Replacement (TDR) prosthesis began in the early 1990s. Drs. Richard Salib and Ken Pettine worked with Larry Boyd at Danek Medical on a ceramic-on-ceramic ball-and-socket disc replacement (Fig. 13-1). Important design characteristics for this prosthesis included a posterior center of rotation, a ball-and-socket design, and a two-piece design that would prevent any expulsion or dislocation.[1] Problems with

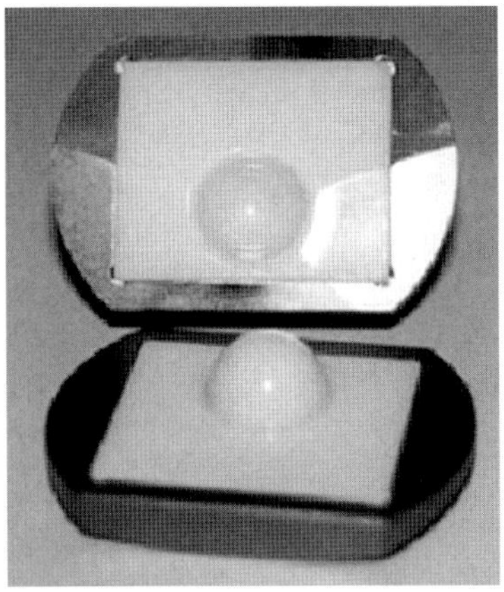

Fig. 13-1 The ceramic-on-ceramic lumbar disc proposed by Ken Pettine and Richard Salib. The device was prototyped by Medtronic Sofamor Danek and studied via finite element analysis and cadaveric studies at the University of Iowa.

manufacturing ceramic-on-ceramic ball-and-socket designs led to problems with this specific design, and it was considered a concept prosthesis for the future. Interest in developing anterior disc replacement systems reemerged in May 2001 when a team of investigators was formed to revisit the posterior center of rotation ball-and-socket design (Medtronic Sofamor Danek, Memphis, TN). Engineers and physicians were charged with the task of developing a prosthesis with unsurpassed durability and functional kinematics that would restore the basic function of the intact spinal unit. These pioneers worked to devise a simple surgical technique that most surgeons could adopt.

As the design rationale evolved from the initial work in the early 1990s, it became evident that a fixed posterior center of rotation could recreate the best biomechanical advantage for the intact functional spinal unit's instantaneous axis of rotation. This fixed center of rotation provides shear stability against translational forces, forces secondary to a diseased facet, and/or translational instability syndromes. Through facet unloading, the posterior center of rotation actually increases range of motion (compared to a central or anterior center of rotation), and decreases facet loads. These observations were made by Dooris et al[1] during their work in finite element analyses and cadaveric mechanical studies.

A cobalt-chrome-molybdenum on cobalt-chrome-molybdenum design was supported because these biomaterials undergo decreased wear and improve durability for younger patients. Hydroxyapatite coating on metal bone-contacting surfaces along with a keel would provide instant biomechanical and enhanced bony support against torsional loads at a very early time after implantation.

The biomechanical properties of a newly designed prosthesis required investigation. White and Panjabi suggested that a 1200-Newton load at 20 degrees of forward flexion is transmitted through a typical lumbar column. According to Nachemson (1981), this value should be 600 Newtons of load. Given the typical compressive load to failure capacity of cancellous bone, it could be calculated that a minimum bearing area of 675 mm^2 at the prosthesis-bone interface would be required to prevent bony failure. This conclusion helped to determine the footprint area of the small prosthesis and also provided the input values for mechanical device testing. At a safety factor of 3.3, the smallest prosthesis could be loaded to 10,000 Newtons, a worst-case scenario for a MAVERICK TDR prosthesis. This load was tested for 10 million loading cycles to verify that no mechanical device failures would occur.

Hedman et al suggested that a typical person undergoes approximately 125,000 significant bends per year and approximately 2,000,000 nonsignificant motions, such as walking strides. By developing a mathematical modeling method using significant bend testing and walking stride testing, it was possible to develop an accelerated test that used only significant bend cycles on the test machine to rapidly model clinical years of prosthetic usage with benchtop testing. Using the significant bends modeling test, approximately 10,000,000 cycles would equal 31.5 years of clinical use of the MAVERICK TDR prosthesis.

Wear considerations and durability are important design characteristics of the MAVERICK TDR prosthesis. MAVERICK annual wear calculations equal approximately 0.44 mm^3 per year. This value equals approximately 14 mm^3 of wear debris for a 31.5-year usage period. A typical metal-on-metal hip prosthesis would wear at an annual rate of 5 mm^3 and equal approximately 157.5 mm^3 of wear at 31.5 years. This value represents approximately 11 times the wear rate of a MAVERICK TDR prosthesis. In contrast, a metal-on-poly hip replacement wears 43 to 135 mm^3 per year, which is 97 to 322 times the amount of volumetric wear of a MAVERICK metal-on-metal prosthesis.

Allen and colleagues studied cobalt-chrome-molybdenum (CoCrMo) in vitro as well as concentrations of 0.01, 0.1, and 1.0 g/cm^3 of CoCrMo debris. The first two concentrations (0.01 and 0.1 g/cm^3) were well tolerated with no observable effects on alkaline phosphatase and osteocalcin expressions. When MAVERICK wear calculations are extrapolated into Allen's CoCrMo in vitro analysis, 0.1 g/cm^3 represent 61 years of clinical use and would be well tolerated according to this study parameter.

A review of the literature on total hip arthroplasty shows that 5 mm^3 of wear debris is generated per year for metal-on-metal hips without causing any osteolysis, excessive friction, foreign body reaction, or rejection. A total of 31.5 years of use of a metal-on-metal prosthesis would generate 157.5 mm^3 of debris. A total of 31.5 years of simulated use of a MAVERICK TDR prosthesis would generate 12 mm^3 of debris.[2]

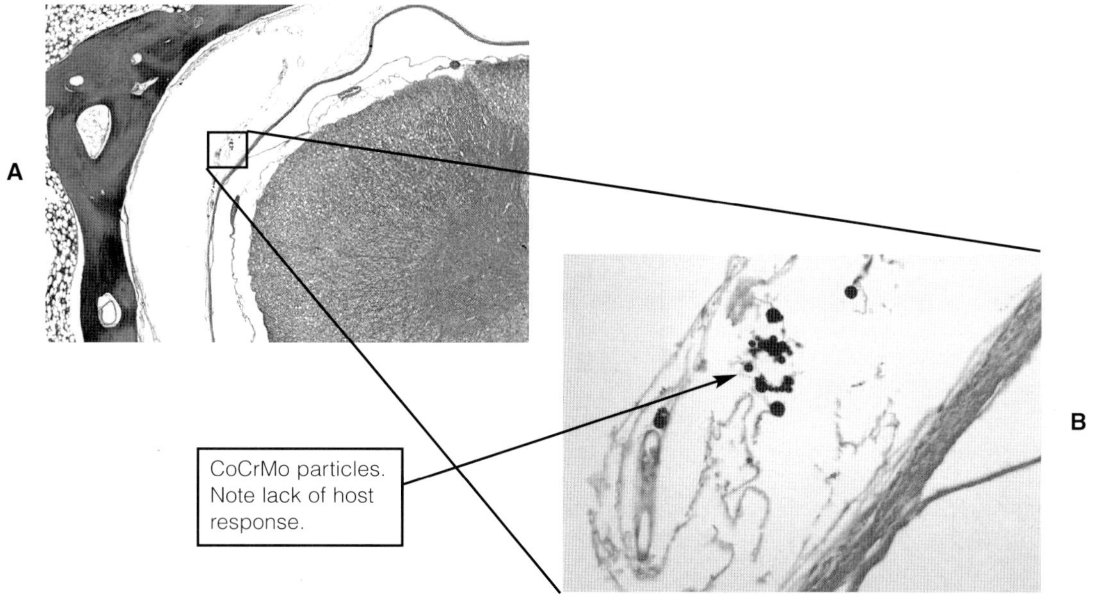

Fig. 13-2 **A** and **B,** Example of a typical tissue specimen showing cobalt-chrome-molybdenum debris in a rabbit's epidural space. The specimen shown was sacrificed 12 weeks after receiving an injection of wear debris.

Urban et al[5] discussed dissemination of wear particles to the liver, spleen, and abdominal lymph nodes in patients with hip or knee replacements. Their study suggested that particles were more commonly found in patients with failed arthroplasty. The concentration of metallic and polyethylene particles in the liver and spleen were relatively low for both types of particles, and no toxic side effects were apparent on histologic examination.

Nevertheless, when the MAVERICK TDR prosthesis was developed, a simulation of as much as 60 years of accumulated debris was injected in a single bolus into the epidural space in rabbits. The histologic reaction was surprisingly quiet, with no evidence of foreign body cells, macrophages, toxicity, or other deleterious effects. The blunt trauma from the needle appeared to be more damaging to the tissue than the metal particles[3] (Fig. 13-2).

Some concerns were raised that a prosthetic disc should act as a shock absorber. It was proposed that using a polyethylene insert, rather than a metal-on-metal articulation, may allow for some shock absorption or vibration damping. Although theoretical calculations did not support this hypothesis, primarily because of the thin cross-section required of the polymer insert, an experiment was performed to verify whether or not an effect could be obtained. A MAVERICK TDR prosthesis and a ProDisc (Synthes, Paoli, PA) were tested in shock and vibration loading, and outputs were compared. The measurable dif-

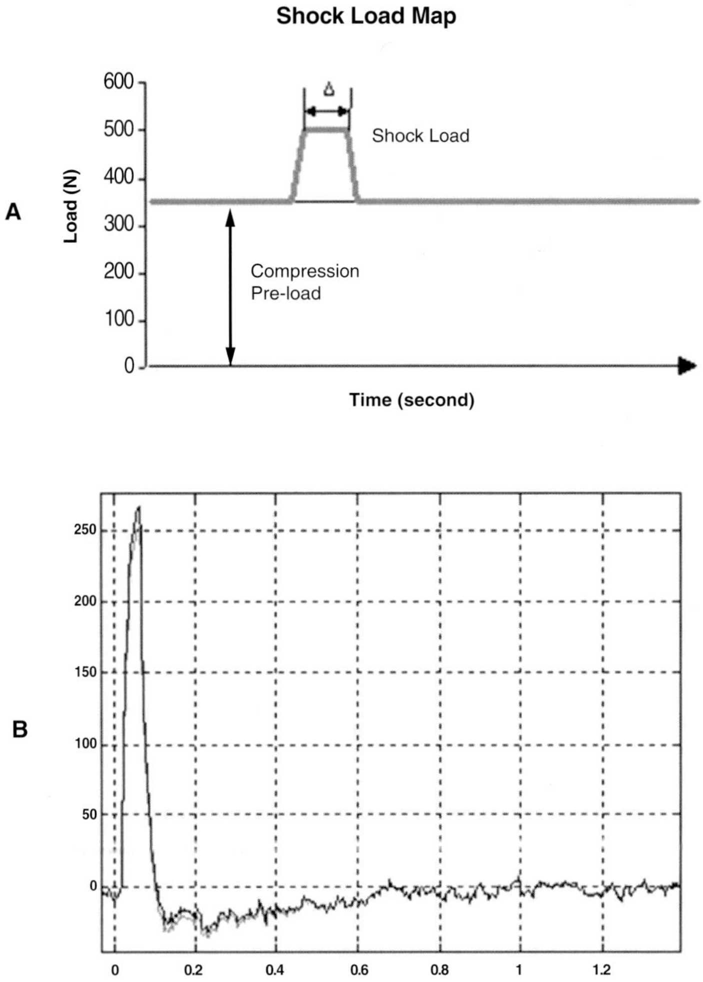

Fig. 13-3 A and **B,** A comparison of the shock absorptive capabilities of the MAVERICK TDR prosthesis and a design having a polyethylene locking insert. The devices exhibited equivalent behavior.

ferences were within the noise range of the instruments and hence were not definable as differences[4] (Figs. 13-3 and 13-4).

Cadaveric mechanical studies were required to evaluate the MAVERICK TDR prosthesis versus intact specimens. The MAVERICK TDR prosthesis was numerically, though not statistically, stiffer than the intact segment in compression, torsion, and flexion. In extension, segments implanted with the MAVERICK TDR prosthesis were numerically and statistically stiffer than the intact specimens. In lateral bending, the specimens with the MAVERICK TDR device were numerically but not statistically less stiff than the intact specimens. The MAVERICK TDR prosthesis also had similar ranges of motion in all modes examined[2] (Fig. 13-5).

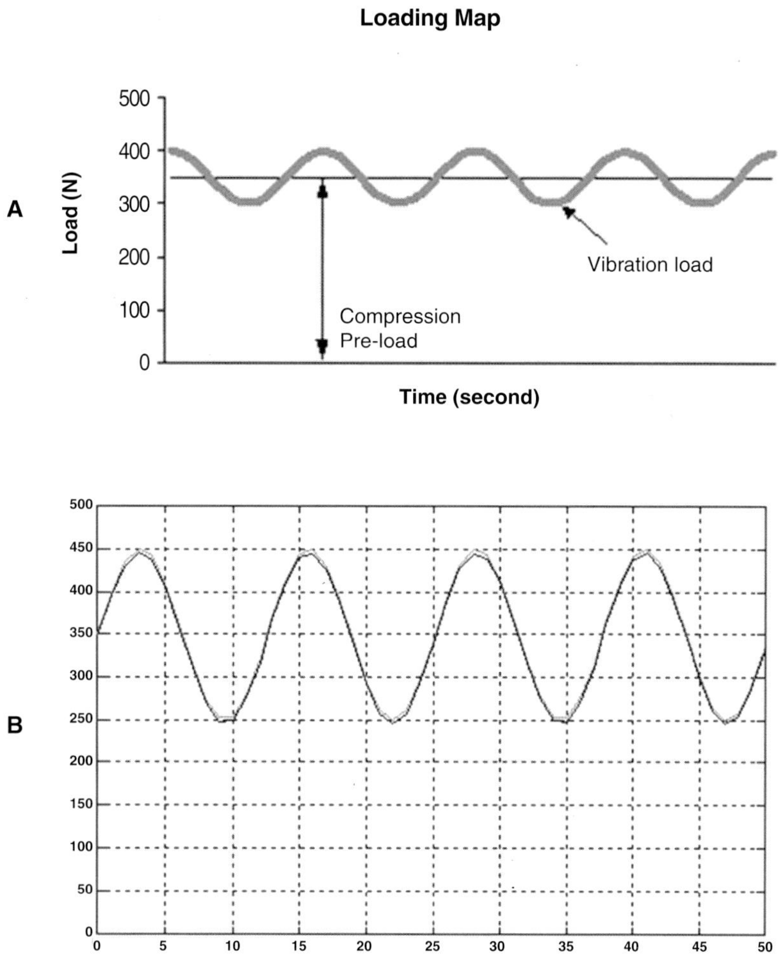

Fig. 13-4 A and **B,** A comparison of the vibration damping capabilities of the MAVERICK TDR prosthesis and a design having a polyethylene locking insert. The devices exhibited equivalent behavior.

Kinematics of the MAVERICK TDR prosthesis and any ball-and-cup total disc arthroplasty relate to the positioning of the center of rotation and potential facet loads that are translated based on the position of the center of rotation. Dooris et al[1] discussed the position of the center of rotation of a ball-and-cup prosthesis with relation to motion and facet loads on a finite element analysis model. By altering the center of rotation and applying an 800-Newton load to an anteriorly placed ball-and-socket design, approximately a 2.5 increase in facet loads could be encountered. However, this same force applied to a posterior center of rotation ball-and-socket total disc arthroplasty did not affect facet loads. Dooris et al[1] also found that motion was increased with the posterior center of rotation total disc arthroplasty rather than with an anteriorly placed ball-and-socket design. Restoration of the anterior longitudinal ligament was

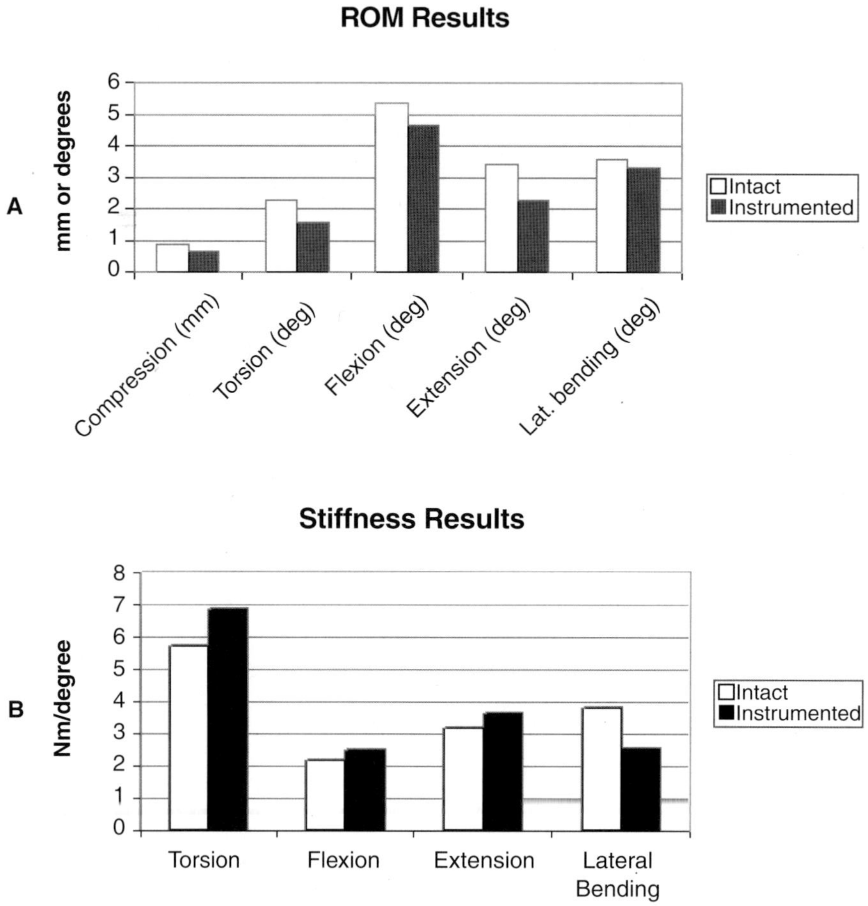

Fig. 13-5 A, Cadaveric stiffness and range-of-motion testing of the MAVERICK TDR device compared to intact cadaveric specimens under typical physiologic loading. **B,** Only stiffness in extension showed a statistical difference from intact to instrumented states.

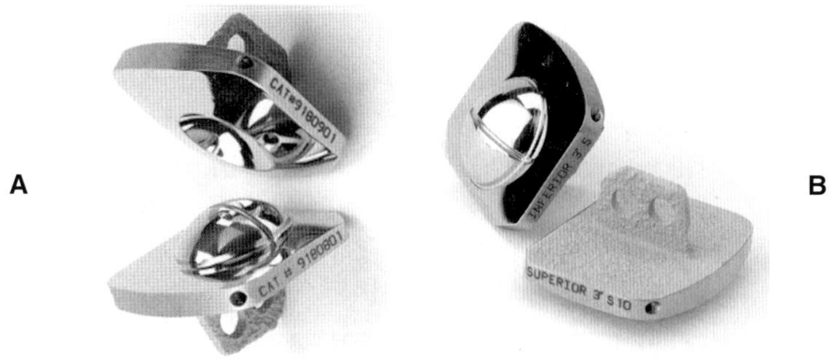

Fig. 13-6 **A** and **B,** The MAVERICK Total Disc Replacement prosthesis.

also shown to reduce pedicle stresses, facet loads, and extension rotation to near normal.

The Prosthetic Components

The MAVERICK Total Disc Arthroplasty System (Fig. 13-6) is designed to be a two-piece ball-and-socket replacement for the anterior column. Its posterior center of rotation mimics the location of the natural center of rotation of a typical asymptomatic disc, and places the balance and load transfer points in line with the neutral axis of the spine. The cobalt-chrome-molybdenum on cobalt-chrome-molybdenum design allows 16 degrees of motion in all planes and has a 1.5 mm coupled translation. The device does not allow for translational motion independent of rotation. According to Errico's classifications, it is a semiconstrained device.

The bone-implant interface surfaces are designed to have a thermally deposited hydroxyapatite coating over a roughened surface texture on both superior and inferior components to allow for rapid bony ingrowth of the prosthesis. Keel heights have been reduced since the development of the original MAVERICK prosthesis. Lower keel designs will more readily facilitate multilevel usage with fewer stress risers in the intermediate vertebral body.

Three overall endplate sizes are included for complete coverage of the endplate. Small, medium, and large sizes equal 25, 27, and 30 mm of anteroposterior coverage, and 32, 35, and 39 mm of mediolateral endplate coverage, respectively. The three posterior disc heights of 10, 12, and 14 mm are measured from the posterior aspect of the prosthesis, providing adequate versatility for all potential situations. The height of the prosthesis is determined after significant and complete posterior anular and ligamentous release during the mobilization of the diseased spinal unit.

Three angle configurations were initially available in the early MAVERICK designs. A series of insertional tools has been engineered that allows for the prosthesis to be inserted with 6, 9, or 12 degrees of angulation. The device will adapt to the angle at which the patient wishes to restabilize the spinal unit; lordosis will reflect the patient's rebalancing to the preferred conformation.

Indications

Patient selection criteria are the most important aspect of the insertion of any disc replacement device. Disc replacements currently represent only anterior column restorations, and the presence of significant posterior disease within the spinal canal needs to be considered before the application of any anterior disc replacement technology. The correlation of clinical symptoms with appropriate imaging studies, including magnetic resonance imaging (MRI) and discography, and evaluation by rehabilitative therapists helps to define the clinical syndrome, which anterior disc replacement can potentially alleviate.

The presence of a black disc alone does not support the indication for a total disc replacement. The clinical syndrome associated with anterior column insufficiency syndromes includes failure of conservative care management despite appropriate modifications of the patient's activities, and correlational findings from imaging studies. Together, these factors represent a clinical picture that supports the potential indication for a total disc replacement. Other indications for total disc replacement surgery may include:

- Degenerative disc disease and loss of disc height with dehydration
- Extensive modic changes within the disc space
- Intensive anular pathology, including high intensity zones and anular disruption and tears
- Degenerative disc disease with anular pathology, including disc fragment extrusion and/or containment within the anulus
- Degenerative disc disease or acute disc space collapse after previous open microdiscectomy using a facet-saving technique

Contraindications to total disc replacement surgery include:

- Multilevel pathology with an indeterminate source of pain
- Idiopathic lumbar scoliosis
- Translational instability syndrome including spondylolisthesis and spondylolysis
- Previous infection, tumors, or vertebral body dysmorphism
- Presence of stenosis, subarticular disease, and severe facet joint pathology
- Persistent epidural fibrosis from previous open decompression procedures

Preoperative Planning

Preoperative computed tomography (CT) templates should be used to evaluate the maximum footprint size of the device to achieve maximum endplate coverage. Particularly at L5-S1, it is important to determine the location of the nerves posterior to the S1 endplate, relative to the insertion of a posteriorly-based prosthesis. Sacral endplate anatomy can allow for passage of nerve roots more anteriorly than expected.

Patients who have had previous abdominal surgery and/or patients with morphology can also represent a relative contraindication in the preoperative planning phase. Previous intra- and retroperitoneal dissections may make access to the anterior lumbar spine quite difficult and represent a technical challenge. The use of access surgeons to assist spinal surgeons in this process is important because experience varies based on surgical training and difficulties of patient presentation.

Significant preoperative planning of total disc replacement surgery occurs well in advance of the surgical procedure, both in the office and in the operating room. The appropriate anesthesia and operative setups for anterior lumbar surgery represent significant concerns for surgeons in many operative settings. The anesthesia department should have backup personnel available 24 hours per day. Similarly, vascular or access surgeons should be on-call 24 hours per day should complications occur. The presence of an intensive care unit is important to ensure that patients are monitored effectively if surgical complications occur. Operating room equipment should include a radiolucent operating table with multiple positioning options and a high quality fluoroscopy unit.

Instrumentation for inserting the MAVERICK TDR system includes:

- A centering pin for fluoroscopic verification
- A template for anulotomy of the anterior longitudinal ligament
- Instruments to remove the endplate cartilage and disc material
- Posterior curettes and rongeurs
- Ligament elevators to elevate and release the posterior longitudinal ligament
- A disc space spreader
- Shim distractors
- Angled trials
- Footprint trials
- A four-in-one guide with 6-, 9-, and 12-degree angled plates
- Disc shaping chisels for superior and inferior components with keel chisels independently inserted or in conjunction with disc shaping chisels
- Prosthesis holder for insertion and prosthesis inserter

The operative technique involves using a transperitoneal or a retroperitoneal approach to the lumbar spine. Specific anatomic considerations are made preoperatively to determine the safest approach to the level of pathology. Many retractor systems are available to help reflect and stabilize anatomic structures while an anterior anulotomy is planned.

Whether a transperitoneal or retroperitoneal approach is performed, a safe approach to the lumbar spine involves delicate dissection of tissues. The tissues, including great vessels, must be protected as they are reflected away from the surgical field. This high level of protection must be maintained during the anterior disc removal and endplate preparation techniques. The use of good quality fluoroscopy allows the surgeon to see parallel endplates and pedicles, and allows for nonoblique right-angle imaging studies to verify the position of instruments, tissue removal, and positioning of the prosthesis during insertion.

The MAVERICK Total Disc Arthroplasty System stresses a precise anulotomy to maintain appropriate lateral anular supports. A template is used to resect the correct amount of anterior longitudinal ligament and anulus to allow the appropriate endplate coverage device to be inserted. After the anulotomy is performed in the center of the functional anulus, the endplates are prepared for cartilage removal. The lenticular nature of each endplate is inspected. This biconcavity may hinder posterior dissection and release of the anulus and ligamentous structures.

After complete removal of the disc and preparation of the endplates with curettage and endplate shavers and contouring equipment, the posterior anulus and longitudinal ligament become important structures to dissect. Posterior release of osteophytic bone, calcified ligament and anulus, and potential disc material allows remobilization of the spinal segment. Often the ligament is either released and/or resected during this process. Care is taken to avoid epidural bleeders. If necessary, thrombin-saturated Gelfoam or other clot-forming devices may be used for hemostasis.

After the appropriate release is performed, adequate disc height measurements may be obtained. The MAVERICK Total Disc Arthroplasty System uses a shim distractor to help calculate the appropriate height and lordosis before the use of a four-in-one guide. This templating-sizing device provides an early measurement of height and lordosis that may be required after remobilization of the spinal segment. The four-in-one guide verifies this process by actively distracting the disc space, allowing a keel cutter to be inserted both proximally and distally. This distraction is also required for potential endplate shaping in the corners of a lenticular disc space. Endplate shaping in these corners is an option and it is not required in all cases.

After keel cuts are performed using the four-in-one device, the prosthesis can be prepared on the back table. The appropriate lordosis can be determined. The lordosis must allow the prosthesis to be applied in the optimal balance for which the spinal segment has been prepared. Although the appropriate lordosis is determined as the spinal segment is released, final balance is established when the patient is ambulatory the next day.

The prosthesis is inserted in a one-step technique that allows the superior and inferior prosthesis to be inserted as it is mounted on an inserting device. This procedure can be monitored under lateral fluoroscopic control. Anteroposterior (AP) and lateral views of the prosthesis location are important to help determine final adjustments. Because this is a front-to-back insertion technique, lateral fluoroscopy is imperative to ensure that the prosthesis and center of rotation are appropriately placed in the posterior third of the vertebral body. This placement represents a fundamental advantage of the MAVERICK Total Disc Arthroplasty System, because this posterior center of rotation mimics the intact spinal center of rotation of the functional spinal unit.

Final AP and lateral fluoroscopic views are saved as hard copies, and closure of the transperitoneal or retroperitoneal approach is performed. An abdominal binder is often used to provide soft tissue support and patient comfort after surgery. Ice can be placed posteriorly and anteriorly to control soreness after the surgical procedure, especially during the mobilization process. The patient is often mobilized that evening or the day after surgery and recovers quite quickly. Incisional soreness is the limiting factor in how quickly patients recover and rehabilitate. Abdominal strengthening exercises are often begun within the first 3 weeks and patients often resume rigorous activity within 6 weeks of surgery. The presence of the interference fit and the keels of the prosthesis provide instant and complete control of rotation and translational motions. Hence recovery is fast, efficient, and activities of daily living can be regained quite quickly after MAVERICK TDR surgery.

Complications

Complications of anterior disc replacement initially involve the access through an anterior transperitoneal or retroperitoneal approach. These complications are well documented and access surgeons and spinal surgeons should become familiar with anterior lumbar surgery before beginning total disc replacement procedures.

Complications involving the use of total disc replacements have been reported by various authors. These complications include:

- Poor imaging that does not adequately define the pathology
- Inadequate experience of the operating surgeon and/or approach surgeon
- Poor fluoroscopic imaging that cannot be used to see the instruments
- Failure to identify the midline, thus causing incorrect placement of the prosthesis
- Inadequate discectomy and mobilization of the anulus and osteophytes, hampering the insertion and mobilization of the segment
- Exuberant canal exploration and risk of nerve injury
- Epidural bleeding and cerebrospinal fluid (CSF) leakage
- Overdistraction and overstuffing of the prosthesis height with endplate damage and joint reactive forces and subsidence of the superior endplate
- Failure to insert the prosthesis adequately, forcing the center of rotation to the middle of the disc
- Undersizing the endplate and causing subsidence
- Placing the prosthesis (and ball-and-socket) upside down
- The use of keel cuts and inadvertent foraminal extrusion of the osteotomes
- Excessive removal of bone from the posterior margin leading to subsidence of the prosthesis
- Injury to the iliac veins, ureter, or arterial structures
- Retroperitoneal injury to the hypogastric plexus
- Injury to the sympathetic nerves and other retroperitoneal structures

- Ileus secondary to narcotics administered during surgery or excessive bowel retraction
- Posterior osteophyte and/or wall fracture because of inadvertent posterior anular release, overstuffing the prosthesis, or placement of the prosthesis too far posteriorly
- Neuropathic pain secondary to motion and overdistraction in patients who have previously undergone microdiscectomy procedures and have developed epidural fibrosis

Clinical Results

A prospective multicenter study of the MAVERICK Total Disc Arthroplasty System was launched in January 2002. This study represents a consecutive series of patients with a minimum 2-year follow-up. Results were reported in June 2004 at EuroSpine. This study represents the best multicenter study performed outside of the U.S. Food and Drug Administration (FDA) IDE study.

All patients underwent surgery for single-level degenerative disc disease (DDD). The patients had to have symptomatic low back pain resistant to conservative care of more than 1 year. The effectiveness of the device was evaluated via visual analog scale (VAS) scores, Oswestry, the SF-36 Health Survey, and radiographic analysis of range of motion. All preoperative and postoperative complications were noted. According to an FDA mandate, to be considered successful by Oswestry criteria, 15 points of improvement were required. This method provides a measurement of efficacy over time. The initial series of 50 patients had degenerative discs at L4-5 and L5-S1. Efficacy of the procedure was measured at 6 months and again at 2 years using Oswestry and was 81% and 82%, respectively. There was no measurable subsidence greater than 2 mm. Mean range of motion was 6 degrees of flexion and 4 degrees of extension, and there were no explants in the series. There was one ureter injury secondary to the anterior approach to the spine.

In April 2003, MAVERICK began its FDA IDE study. This study officially closed in 2004 after reopening for late entry of control patients only. When the study was completed, over 577 patients were enrolled in 32 sites. A minimum 2-year follow-up was required before seeking FDA approval for the PMA application. This study was designed as an equivalence study using a control of a Wyeth INFUSE bone graft and LT-CAGE Lumber Tapered Fusion Device (Medtronic Sofamor Danek, Memphis, TN).

Before beginning the FDA IDE study in the United States, considerable planning was undertaken to choose the best control to evaluate standalone anterior interbody fusion techniques versus anterior motion preservation techniques, such as total disc arthroplasty. It was decided that the use of LT-CAGE/INFUSE bone graft represented the best FDA fusion data and prospective randomized IDE clinical series. The use of this control as a standard of care represents the most difficult barrier against which any disc replacement could be tested, and the truest comparison of anterior standalone static stabilization versus mobile stabilization devices.

Because of the preliminary nature of the FDA IDE data, only trends can currently be determined in establishing comparisons to existing IDE studies. Although the clinical data indicate that MAVERICK is trending better than previous FDA IDE static stabilizing device outcomes measured at 1 year, it cannot be assumed that this trend will continue during the second year. According to data collected at 1 year, the MAVERICK TDR prosthesis would pass the test established in the IDE study, making it at least equivalent to control patients with the LT-CAGE/INFUSE bone grafts, based on the outcome parameters designed in the IDE study. However, 1-year data are required for PMA approval, and extrapolation of these data cannot be considered scientifically valid at this point in the study.

Many believe that motion preservation outcome assessments will require a minimum of 10 years before true efficacy can be determined relative to our goal standard of static stabilization or arthrodesis. The correlation of motion preservation relative to adjacent level disease in patients undergoing fusion surgery versus mobilized patients cannot be determined at the 2-year juncture. Continued evaluation of all motion preservation systems will be required to determine whether motion preservation decreases problems with adjacent level degeneration.

Closing Thoughts

The MAVERICK Total Disc Arthroplasty System represents the first metal-on-metal, two-piece anterior lumbar total disc replacement system. As many arthroplasty systems become available for motion preservation, ease of use and durability become paramount in the selection of these devices for surgical application.

The MAVERICK system was designed for enhanced durability based on its metal-on-metal cobalt-chrome on cobalt-chrome design and its minimal wear debris. These features are critical because these devices will be implanted in young individuals with very active lifestyles. The prosthesis itself is not thought to be a likely mode of clinical failure, inasmuch as the prosthesis could be considered a lifelong implant because of its durability and design characteristics. Despite the accumulation of large volumes of debris in joints of patients who have undergone large joint arthroplasty, metal ion toxicity has never been significant. Minimal debris of metal-on-metal articulations in patients who have undergone lumbar disc replacement arthroplasty (for example, with the MAVERICK TDR prosthesis) represents the best balance of durability, less wear debris, and functional restoration of the spinal motion segment. Additionally, this device is encompassed in a two-piece keel design with rapid ingrowth and ease of insertion. It is this combination of functional biomechanics and favorable biomaterials that makes the MAVERICK TDR prosthesis a strong contender for a lifelong motion preservation process.

As we enter the era of motion preservation in total disc arthroplasty, we need to consider the possibility that we may be inserting a prosthesis that will not last the entire lifetime of the patient. Large joint revisions have been quite commonplace; however, experience with surgical revisitation of the anterior lumbar spine has been less than optimistic. Prostheses need to be designed to last the lifetime of the patient. Consideration must be given at the time of insertion relative to the patient's anticipated lifespan. There is variation among the currently used prostheses, and none fulfills all patient expectations of longevity and durability. The MAVERICK TDR prosthesis may represent the best option for younger, active patients.

REFERENCES

1. Dooris AP, Goel VK, Grosland NM, et al. Load-sharing between anterior and posterior elements in a lumbar motion segment implanted with an artificial disc. Spine 26:122-129, 2001.
2. Ferrara L. Cadaveric testing of MAVERICK vs. intact spine: Part of Medtronic internal test report summary. TS03-045.
3. Evaluation of wear debris in the rabbit spine. Medtonic Sofamor Danek report 0007B0010, Memphis, May 2003.
4. LeHuec JC, Kiaer T, Friesem T, et al. Shock absorption in lumbar disc prosthesis. A preliminary mechanical study. J Spinal Discord Tech 16:346-351, 2003.
5. Urban RM, Tomlinson DJ, Hall RJ, et al. Accumulation in liver and spleen of metal particles generated at nonbearing surfaces in hip arthroplasty. J Arthroplasty 19(Suppl 3):S94-S101, 2004.

CHAPTER

14

The Cervitech Porous Coated Motion Cervical Disc Replacement

Paul C. McAfee ▪ Bryan W. Cunningham
Luiz Pimenta ▪ Andrew Cappuccino

The indications for anterior cervical disc replacement are the same as for anterior cervical decompression: radiculopathy or myelopathy caused by either one or two levels of anterior cervical compression. Most surgeons would agree that a patient presenting with a compressive lesion causing arm weakness, paresthesia, and unremitting radicular pain, with or without lower extremity hyperactive reflexes, requires anterior cervical decompression. The only difference of opinion surgeons may have is what to do following anterior surgical spinal cord or nerve root decompression. The goals are to restore the intervertebral disc height and neuroforaminal height to prevent recurrence of neurologic compression.

Prevention of Symptomatic Adjacent Segment Disease

Robbins and Hilibrand[12] and Hilibrand et al[6] have focused attention on cervical adjacent segment disease. They chronicled 374 patients having a total of 409 anterior cervical arthrodeses followed for up to 21 years after Henry Bohlman performed a Smith-Robinson anterior cervical fusion. They found symptomatic adjacent segment disease occurring at a relatively constant incidence of 2.9% per year (range 0.0 to 4.8% per year). New disease was defined as new onset of myelopathy or radiculopathy significant enough to require surgery. Survivorship analysis projected that 25.6% of the patients (95% confidence interval, 20% to 32%) who had an anterior cervical arthrodesis would have new disease at an adjacent level within 10 years after the operation. The most likely levels to develop adjacent segment disease were C5-6 and C6-7.

Normal Patterns of Motion in the Lower Cervical Spine

White and Panjabi[14] outlined the normal kinematics of the lower cervical spine, the restoration of which is the goal of cervical arthroplasty. Coupling patterns are very important in the motion of the cervical spine—this would escape detection unless one used a 6 degrees of freedom load cell capable of simultaneous measurement of axial rotation, lateral bending moments, and compressive load with flexion-extension. Cunningham et al[5] have developed a pure moment biomechanical testing apparatus (Fig. 14-1) that is consistent with

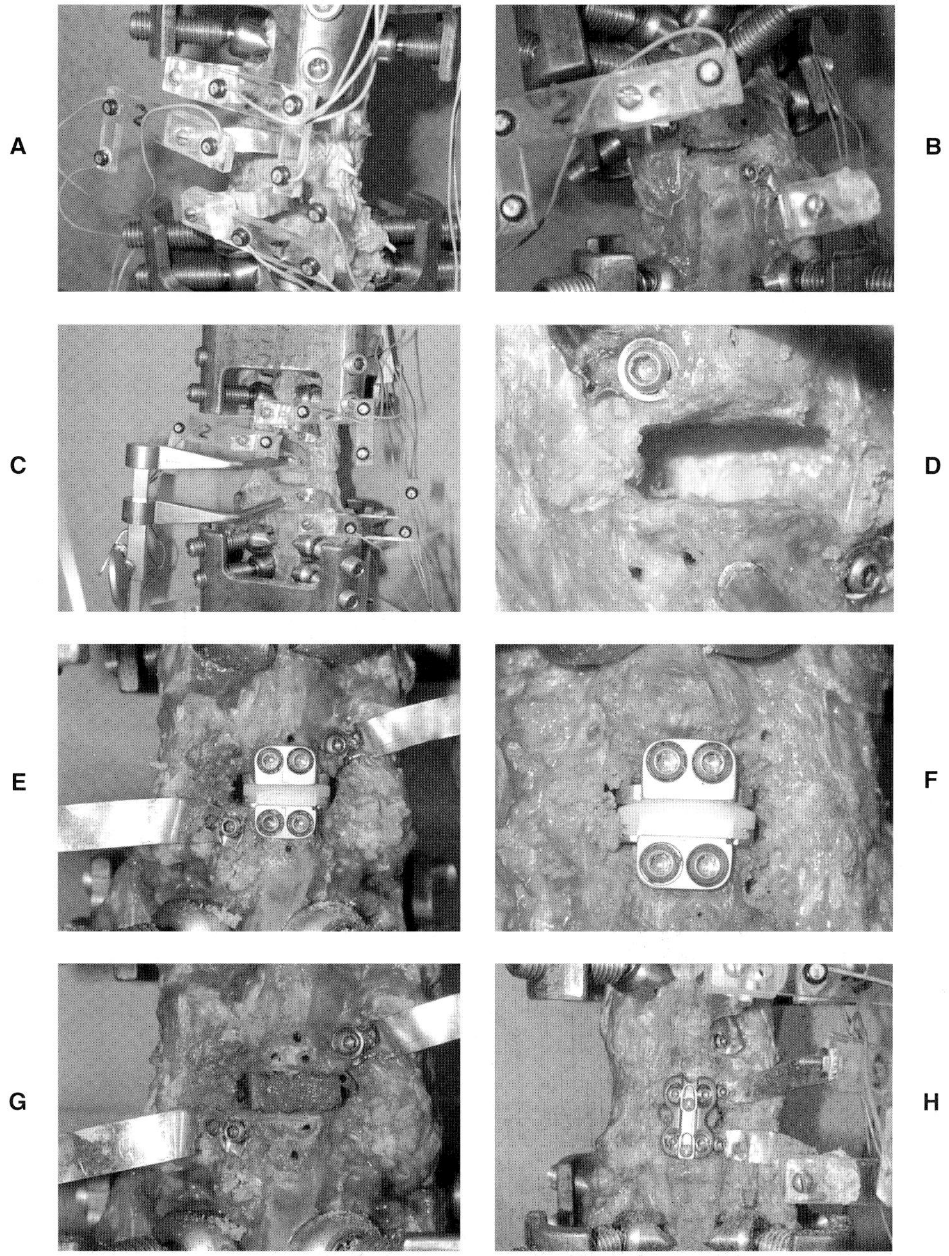

Fig. 14-1 Benchtop cadaver biomechanical testing using a 6 degrees of freedom unconstrained testing apparatus with the OptoTrak 3020. **A**, The cervical spine was mounted from C3 to C7 with orthogonal LEDs skeletally fixed to each vertebral level. **B**, Anterior discectomy at C5-6. Notice the narrowed disc space secondary to cervical spondylosis. **C**, Restoration of normal disc space height and visualization of the posterior longitudinal ligament is facilitated by the Caspar-type distractor at C5-6. **D**, A close-up view. For the third and fourth bars on the bar graph, the PLL was preserved. **E**, The fixed PCM cervical prosthesis. Notice that little extra reaming or external guideframes are required for acute solid fixation. Long-term fixation is added by hydroxyapatite (TiCaP) bony ingrowth, but it also provides an element of immediate stability through friction and a ridged-grooved surface. **F**, A close-up view of the fixed PCM prosthesis. **G**, Tricortical structural iliac allograft. **H**, Anterior translational (subsidence) plate with four screws and tricortical structural iliac allograft.

Panjabi's principles: (1) the uppermost vertebrae in the spinal column are not constrained and free to move, (2) pure moments are applied, (3) an OptoTrak 3020 video image analysis recorder measures skeletal markers on each independent spinal segment with light-emitting diodes (LEDs), (4) there is a skeletal three axis (x, y, and z) coordinate system attached to each cervical vertebral level, and (5) conventional anchoring of the lowest (C7) cervical vertebra to a biaxial load cell.

The coupling is such that with lateral bending the spinous processes rotate into the convexity of the curve. In lateral bending to the left, for example, the spinous processes go to the right. At C2 there are 2 degrees of coupled axial rotation for every 3 degrees of lateral bending, a ratio of 0.67. At the seventh cervical vertebra there is 1 degree of coupled axial rotation for every 7.5 degrees of lateral bending, a ratio of 0.13. The gradual change in the coupling ratio is related to the varying inclination of the facet joints and we believe synchronous motion of the cervical disc arthroplasty must be integrated with this relationship.

The representative ranges of motion for the normal C5-6 and C6-7 levels, according to White and Panjabi, are:

- *Combined flexion-extension:* Limits of ranges = 13 to 29 degrees, 6 to 26 degrees
- *One-side lateral bending:* 0 to 16 degrees, 0 to 17 degrees
- *One-side axial rotation:* 2 to 12 degrees, 2 to 10 degrees

The normal cervical range of motion can also be listed at C5-6 and C6-7 as total range of motion and neutral zone (deformations at low loads):

- *Flexion-extension:* ROM ± 10 degrees, neutral zone ± 5 degrees
- *Axial rotation:* ROM ± 7 degrees, neutral zone ± 4 degrees
- *Lateral bending:* ROM ± 11 degrees, neutral zone ± 4 degrees

Cunningham et al[5] measuring cadaveric cervical specimens with ranges of cervical spondylosis compared the range of motion in flexion-extension in the following seven constructs: (1) intact cervical C5-6 level, (2) anterior discectomy, (3) a low-profile Porous Coated Motion (PCM) prosthesis, (4) anterior cervical decompression-destabilization = anterior discectomy, anterior resection of posterior longitudinal ligament, and removal of posterior osteophytes, (5) a Porous Coated Motion prosthesis fixed with two screws in each component, (6) anterior tricortical structural allograft at C5-6, and (7) anterior translational type cervical plate with structural allograft. The mean and standard deviation of each construct (N = 6) is graphed in Fig. 14-2.

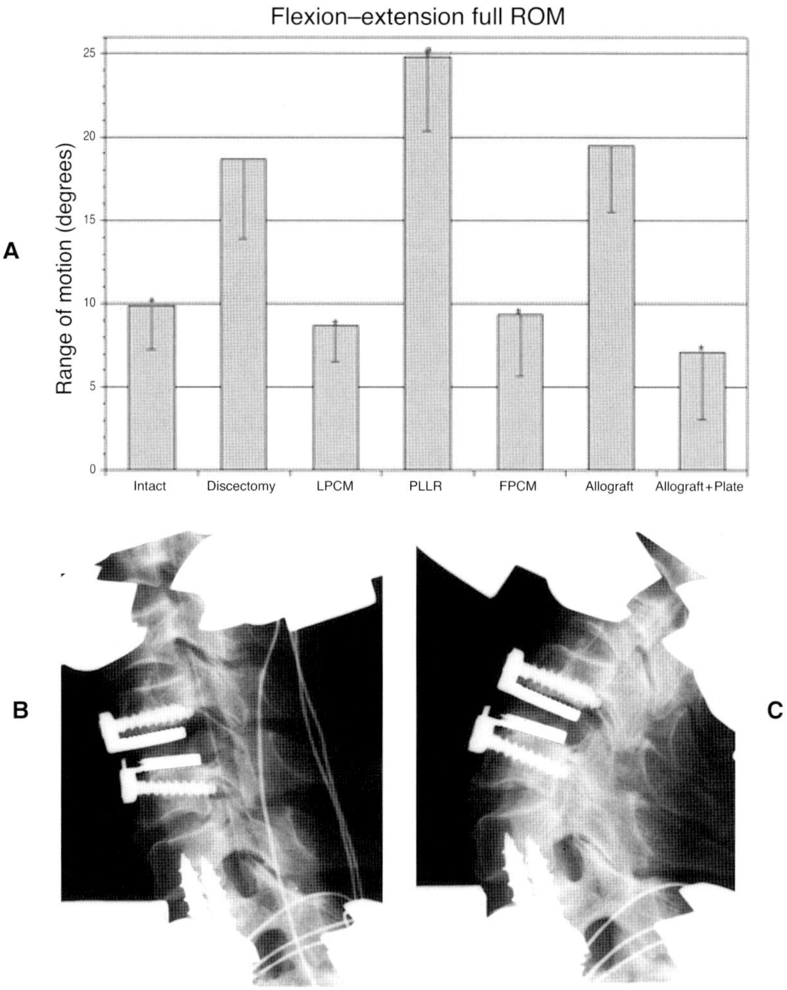

Fig. 14-2 **A**, Starting from the left, each bar represents (1) intact C5-6, (2) anterior discectomy, (3) a low-profile Porous Coated Motion prosthesis, (4) complete anterior decompression with resection of posterior longitudinal ligament, posterior osteophytes and complete discectomy, (5) a fixed Porous Coated Motion prosthesis with anterior flanges and two screws in each component, (6) anterior tricortical structural allograft, and (7) anterior translational plate with tricortical structural allograft. **B** and **C**, Lateral radiographs of the fixed Porous Coated Motion prosthesis demonstrating 10 degrees of flexion-extension motion.

Two Generic Types of Cervical Arthroplasties—the PLL Is the Key

There are two basic types of total knee replacements: posterior cruciate ligament (PCL)–preserving and PCL-sacrificing designs. In the cervical spine an analogous situation exists biomechanically depending on whether the posterior longitudinal ligament (PLL) needs to be removed as part of the spinal cord decompression part of the procedure—PLL-preserving and PLL sacrificing total cervical disc replacements. Buechal and Pappas[3] reported the difference between cruciate-sparing and cruciate-sacrificing total knee replacement prosthesis. The analogy for the PCM prosthesis is to use the low-profile version in cases where a press-fit joint surface replacement can be considered. The fixed version of the PCM anchored with cancellous screws could be considered in cases with myelopathy where the entire posterior aspect of the vertebral bodies needs to be removed with the posterior longitudinal ligament (Fig. 14-3). Our biomechanical studies have shown that the PLL does exert a stabilizing influence on the cervical spine—*fortunately, either the low-profile PCM version or the fixed version with screws can restore stability to the PLL-deficient spine*. The analogous situation exists with the Bristol prosthesis[4] (now evolving into the Prestige I and Prestige II versions), which has screws and a significant anterior profile anterior to the plane of the anterior longitudinal ligament (similar to the

A

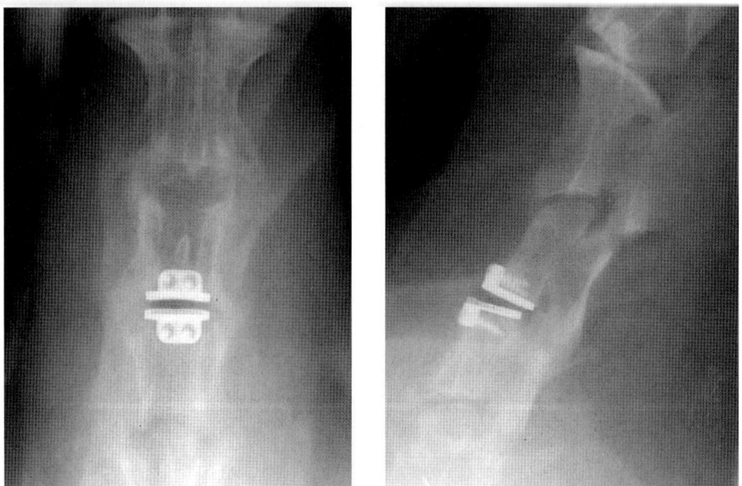

B

Fig. 14-3 The caprine model at C3-4 proved to be the best animal model (N = 12) to evaluate the porous ingrowth, lack of particulate wear debris, and safety of the PCM prosthesis. **A**, Anteroposterior radiograph of the fixed variety of the prosthesis in a goat at C3-4. **B**, Lateral radiograph demonstrates the extension view in a goat with 16 degrees of flexion-extension range of motion.

fixed PCM). The Bryan prosthesis,[2] with no anterior profile and comparatively more unstable in translation, is generically similar to the low-profile PCM. The key distinction would be the biomaterials used in the PCM are more traditional UHMWPE and cobalt chrome used in other conventional diarthrodial joint prostheses.

The Meaning of the Name "Porous Coated Motion"

The name "Porous Coated" highlights the superior ingrowth capabilities of the HA coated CHARITÉ Artificial Disc used worldwide since 1998. McAfee et al[10] measured the amount of bony ingrowth and calculated via a computerized microscopic imaging system called the Bioquant; histomorphometric analysis at the metal-bone interface (bone contact area/total endplate area) showed a mean ingrowth of 47.9% (standard deviation ± 8.12%). The total range of ingrowth was 35.5% to 58.8%.

Twenty-two mature baboons *(Papio cynocephalus)* weighing between 45 and 50 kg were used for this animal model of porous ingrowth. We did not want to use a scaled-down miniature prosthesis, so we used the largest available nonhuman primate model and implanted the size 1 HA-coated CHARITÉ Artificial Disc with 7.5 mm thick UHMWPE cores (i.e., human-sized implants). Using an anterior transperitoneal approach, a complete discectomy was performed at the L5-L6 level followed by implantation of the CHARITÉ HA-coated disc prosthesis.[8] The hydroxyapatite coating is electrochemically bonded to the implant surface and serves to optimize mineralized anchorage at the vertebral endplates. The endplates are composed of cobalt chrome and bear a primary coating of pure titanium with pore size 75 to 300 microns. The titanium coating consists of a special adhesive layer (<90 microns) and a cover layer (<180 microns). The procedure of electrochemical coating of hydroxyapatite retains the open cell structure of the underlying pure titanium coating for optimal implant bonding. The resulting electrochemical HA contoured surface is stronger than prostheses using plasma spray HA coating. The technical parameters of the porous surface are as follows:

Coating thickness	300 + 100 microns
Coating porosity	20% to 40%
Pore sizes	75 to 300 microns
Roughness Ra	35 microns
Roughness Rz	220 microns
Tensile strength	>45 MP

The bioactive coating has been available worldwide for the Charité SB III, excluding the United States, since 1998. It has been used for anchoring dental implants since 1995. The tradename TiCaP™ refers to this unique implant-

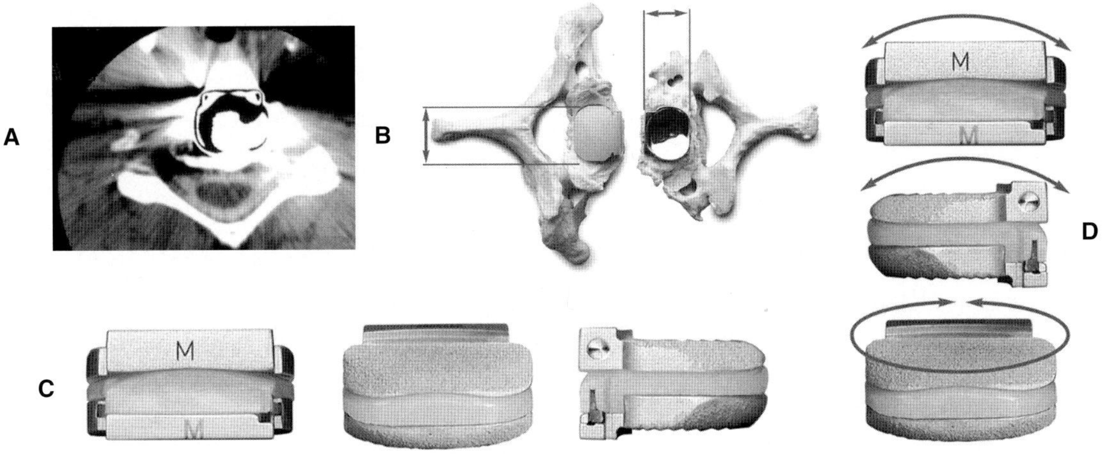

Fig. 14-4 **A**, Axial view of the PCM in a patient demonstrating that good imaging of the outline of the spinal cord is possible postoperatively despite this crosssection, which represents the largest mass of metal in the entire prosthesis. In other words, the principles of Charnley's low-friction arthroplasty are compatible with good postoperative assessment of the neurologic structures. **B**, The footprint of the PCM prosthesis extends laterally far enough to articulate with the lateral trabecular pillars of bone adjacent to the uncovertebral joints to prevent subsidence. Other circular prostheses with round footprints are inferior and demonstrate subsidence. **C**, The PCM is available in various heights from 6.5 mm up to 10 mm instead of mobile bearing prostheses which require obligatory reaming due to a minimum thickness of 10.5 mm. **D**, The PCM should be thought of as a "joint surface replacement" instead of a "total joint replacement," which demonstrates motion along Panjabi's 6 degrees of freedom motion pattern without excessive reaming of vertebral body bone.

coating, which is partially bioabsorbable. It starts out as calcium phosphate (CaP) (Figs. 14-4 and 14-5).

Motion in the name *porous coated motion* highlights the principles in Charnley's low-friction arthroplasty, where conservative decisions have been made in choosing time-honored biomaterials, UHMWPE and cobalt chrome alloy (see Fig. 14-4).

With every major design parameter of the Cervitech Porous Coated Motion™ prosthesis, the more conservative option was used:

1. The biomaterial, ultrahigh-molecular-weight polyethylene (UHMWPE) (7) (ISO 5834/2; ASTM 648) cast CoCrMo alloy (ISO 5832/IV; ASTM F75-82) articulating bearing surface (rather than metal-on-metal or ceramic-on-ceramic)
2. A mobile bearing design rather than a ball-and-socket design

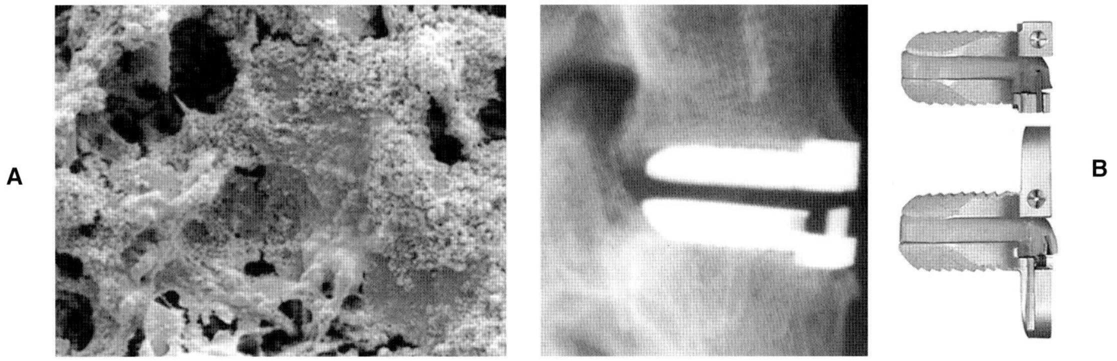

Fig. 14-5 **A**, The porous ingrowth surface of the PCM comprises two layers of titanium electrochemically coated with calcium phosphate in a 1:1 ratio. This is a TiCaP surface similar to the one used by the version of the CHARITÉ Artificial Disc marketed worldwide by Johnson & Johnson/DePuy Spine. This SEM illustration demonstrates an osteoblast growing into the TiCaP porous ingrowth surface after only 36 hours. **B**, This drawing demonstrates the ingrowth fixation within 3 months postoperatively. Both the "low-profile" and the "fixed-with-screws" versions of the PCM prosthesis come with the TiCaP coating as standard.

3. The metal-bone porous ingrowth surface
4. Compression-molded sheet polyethylene, standard gamma irradiation sterilized versus highly cross-linked polyethylene
5. The maximum preservation of vertebral body bone stock as opposed to cutting a groove into the middle of the vertebral body, insertion of a fin possibly requiring a corpectomy for revision

Basically, the same amount of bone resection required for anterior spinal cord decompression is sufficient for preparation of the PCM prosthesis, and excessive reaming or cumbersome fixation jigs are not required.

Excessive reaming may result in heterotopic ossification and "spontaneous" postoperative fusion across the vertebral levels bridged by the disc prosthesis.[9] Pointillart[11] also described a prosthesis in this category but encountered 8 of 10 patients with excessive pain and anterior osteophytes. It is uncertain whether the heterotopic ossification associated with the Bryan prosthesis reported at the 2002 Cervical Spine Research Society meeting is caused by reaming or results from inherent properties in the chemical stability of the polyether urethanes and polycarbonate urethanes. "However," noted Tanzi et al,[13] "biomedical uses for implantation in humans currently appear limited because of adverse effects, such as polymer degradation (hydrolytic, oxidative, and enzymatic) and calcification, as the body environment is a rather aggressive medium."

The first commercially available version of a lumbar disc prosthesis, designed by Karin Büttner-Janz and Kurt Schellnack, was manufactured of cobalt chrome and UHMWPE in Germany in 1987. This predates any other cobalt chrome disc replacement by more than 10 years. More than 20,000 Charité prostheses have been implanted worldwide—the second largest experience in the world was less than 800 cases. This background is important for understanding the conservative decision-making and durability of the specific prosthetic design of the PCM prosthesis.

The Bearing Surface

The articulating surface is cobalt-chrome alloy and high-density polyethylene, which has been used since 1987 in the lumbar disc prosthesis. The calculated wear rate of this type of UHMWPE is less than 0.152 mm per year. More favorable wear particulate and incidence of osteolysis has been described with highly crosslinked UHMWPE—crosslinked either with radiation or peroxidase. The early wear rates in hip simulators of this newer configuration of UHMWPE are improved (0.015 mm per year); however, the highly crosslinked variety has a greater chance of plastic deformation because of its reduced crystallinity, ultimate tensile strength, and, most important, the reduction of tensile elongation at fracture.[7] The PCM will continue to be manufactured out of the more traditional compression-molded sheet high density UHMWPE until longer term reports of other proven polyethylenes show less plastic deformation or "cold flow."

Metal-on-metal bearing surfaces show particulate with increased systemic distribution of smaller particulate, and remain class III as opposed to safer class II total hip devices. There is also a 0.5% reported incidence of hypersensitivity. This is why metal on metal systemically disbursed particulate debris creates a big "unknown" with regard to the Bristol cervical disc. Ceramic-on-ceramic total hip prostheses possess theoretical advantages over CoCr-UHMWPE with regard to wear rates. Unfortunately, the brittleness of the material has led to partial or total component fracture, especially in cases of component impingement. The practical demonstration of this is the fact that Zirconia femoral heads were recalled after more than 80 cases of catastrophic ceramic fracture, and that occurred with a totally constrained application in the hip joint, which has a fixed, one-point center of rotation.

Caprine Animal Model for Cervical Arthroplasty

Animal model testing was completed—12 goats undergoing disc replacement with the PCM cervical disc prosthesis at C3-4. The goats were followed for 6 months (see Fig. 14-3). There was no evidence of particulate debris, cytokines, cellular apoptosis, or membrane-bound TNF-α. The caprine model was used to test a variety of brands and models of cervical disc replacements using criteria analogous to the baboon lumbar spine for testing a lumbar disc replacement:

1. Anatomic dimensions between the caprine C3-4 intervertebral disc and the human C5-6 and C6-7 discs are similar.
2. There are similar ranges of motion in flexion-extension and axial compression. Axial rotation is more restricted in the goat because of larger uncovertebral joints, and the overall disc has more of a domelike shape than the human disc does.
3. Human-sized cervical disc replacements can be used in the goat at C3-4.
4. The caprine model represents a worst-case scenario with regard to evaluating the durability of the cervical prosthesis. The goats are ambulatory without a brace several hours after surgery. They butt heads with each other, violently shaking and extending their cervical spines, and they occasionally leap over 4-foot stockade fences, becoming completely airborne.

Anderson et al[1] also used the caprine model to investigate the wear debris associated with the Bryan cervical disc prosthesis. In two of three goats followed 6 months postoperatively, they found polarizable foreign material, and partially polarizable intracellular granular material was found exterior to the dura mater and in macrophages in periprosthetic tissues. The significance of this wear debris cannot be determined unless cytokines are specifically looked for.

In more than 12 goats with the PCM device there were no significant perioperative complications in the animal model: no loosening, no osteolysis, and no translational instabilities at 6 months postoperatively (see Fig. 14-3).

Clinical Experience

In a series of 27 PCM prostheses implanted in 20 patients, there were no significant perioperative complications, with all 20 patients' length of stay less than 2 days; eight of the cases were performed on an outpatient basis. Preoperatively, seven of the patients presented with myelopathies, 12 with radiculopathies, and one with discogenic pain. Sixteen of the patients underwent the prosthesis insertion as a primary procedure and four of the patients had prosthesis insertions adjacent to prior anterior cervical fusions, one with a prior titanium cervical cage directly above the index arthroplasty. Seven cases were performed as two-level implantations, and this did not appear to detract from the clinical results. Fig. 14-6 demonstrates a three-level implantation in a patient with myelopathy.

A 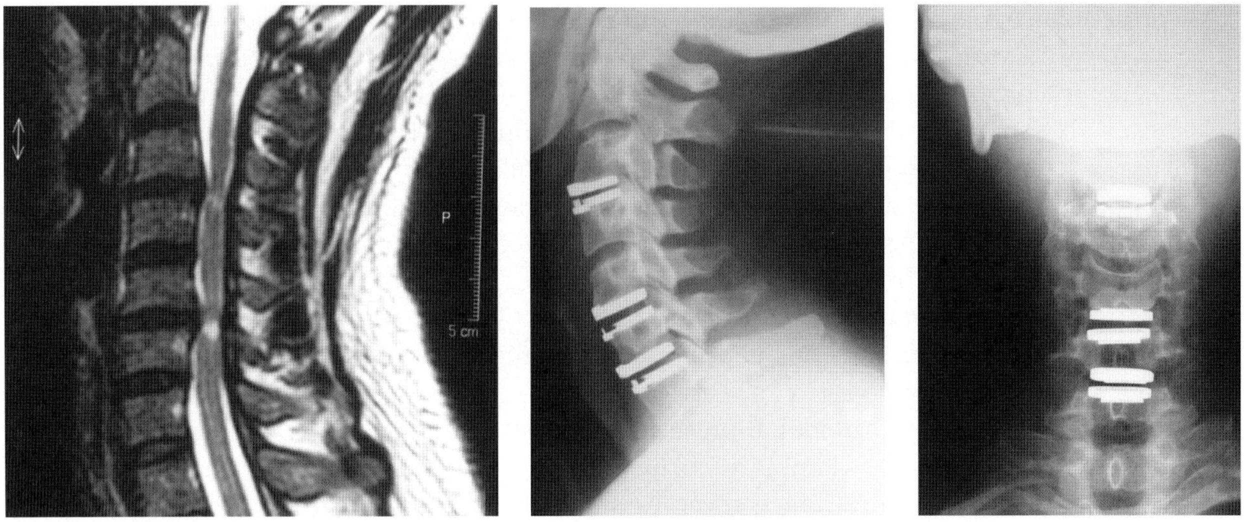 B

Fig. 14-6 A triple-level PCM arthroplasty. **A**, This 40-year-old man presented with myelopathy with bilateral arm weakness and hyperactive lower extremity reflexes. The preoperative MRI indicates three-level anterior spinal cord compression from herniated discs, and at C5-6 there is evidence of myelomalacia. Also apparent on the MRI are ischemic changes in the spinal cord, to a lesser degree at the C3-4 level. **B**, After undergoing three-level anterior spinal decompression, the patient had PCM triple-level implantations at C3-4, C5-6, and C6-7. EBL = 100 cc; the length of the surgery was 150 minutes for the decompression and the spinal reconstruction and the length of hospital stay was 1 day. The patient experienced a full neurologic recovery over the next 2 weeks, with full return of upper extremity strength. His outcomes, from preoperative to 18 months postoperatively, improved as follows: NDI, 28 to 12; VAS, 5 to 0, and Odom's criteria, good. Notice that in contrast to a three-level spinal arthrodesis, each of the three arthroplasty levels behave biomechanically as independent vertebral levels, so the lever arm and stress concentration at the ends of the spinal reconstruction do not negatively affect the clinical outcome or accentuate any complications.

The PCM prosthesis design does not require a cumbersome external frame or complicated reaming, as evidenced by the fact that two of the cases were performed totally endoscopically through a 20 mm anterior cervical cannula (Fig. 14-7).

Postoperatively all patients were neurologically normal. Based on Odom's criteria, the results in five patients were good and in 15 patients were excellent (Fig. 14-8).

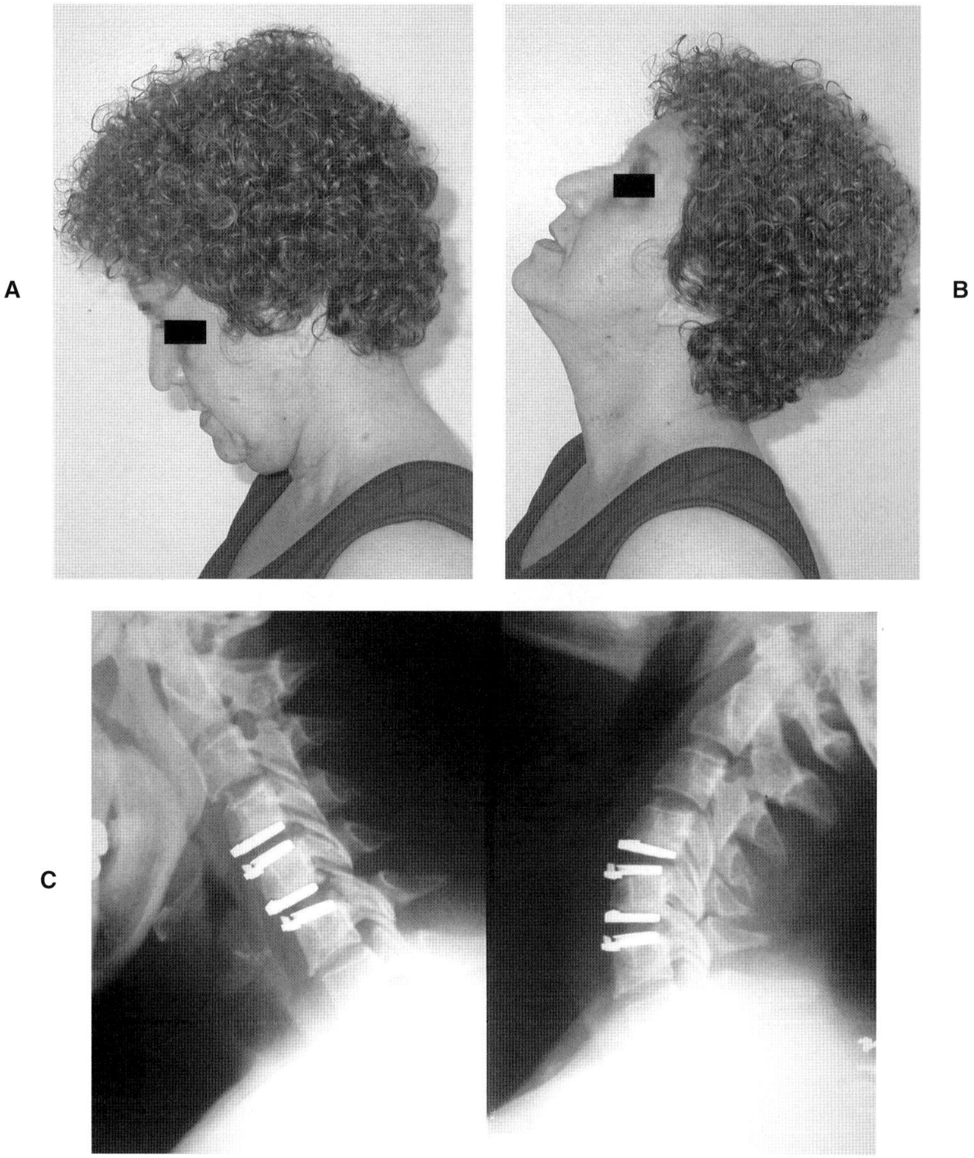

Fig. 14-7 Low-profile PCM prosthesis. **A**, Postoperative flexion and **B**, extension clinical photograph of a 49-year-old woman 3 months after a two-level low-profile PCM procedure at C5-6 and C6-7. C, The corresponding flexion and extension cervical spine radiographs demonstrate 10 degrees of motion at each level and slight physiologic translation at the extremes of motion. The patient had complete relief of left arm weakness and radiculopathy.

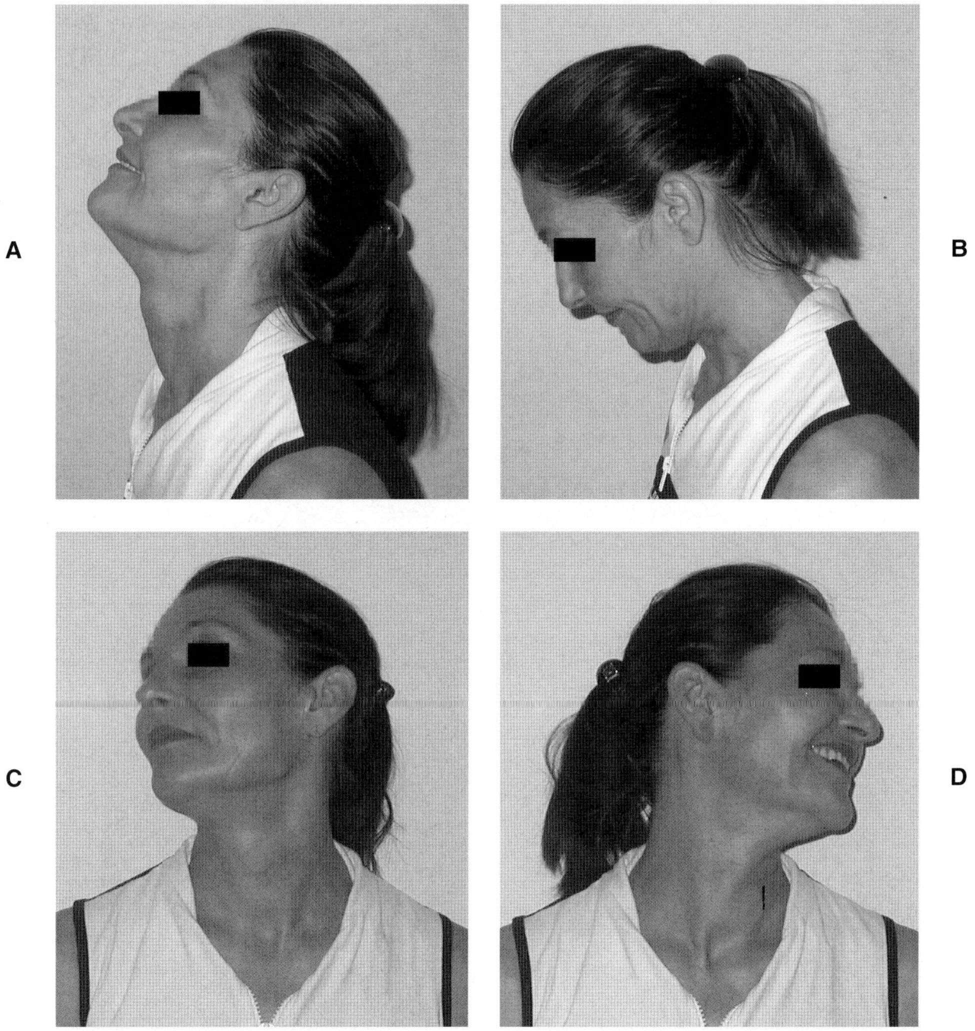

Fig. 14-8 Fixed PCM prosthesis. **A**, This 42-year-old woman presented with an HNP at C5-6 and myelopathy. The photo demonstrates normal cervical extension 3 months following insertion of a PCM prosthesis insertion and cervical decompression. **B**, Normal flexion. The patient was completely recovered neurologically and returned to aerobic fitness activities. **C** and **D**, Cervical rotation and lateral bending were normal three months postoperatively.

E

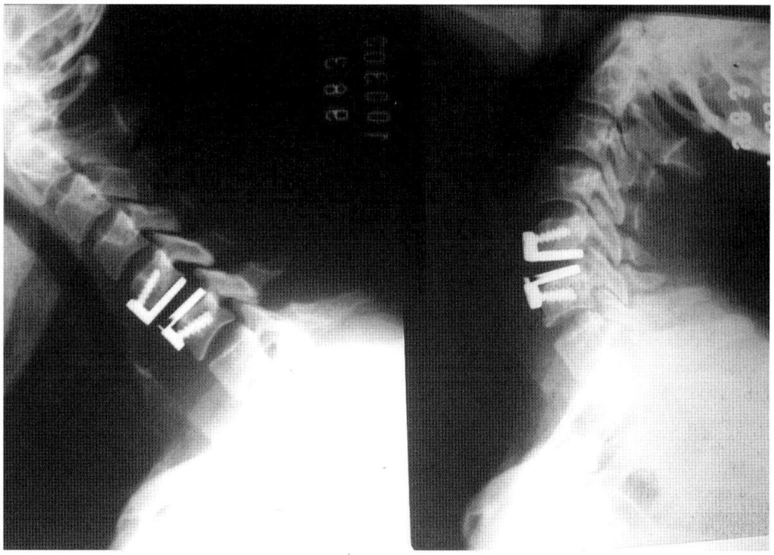

Fig. 14-8—cont'd E, Lateral flexion and extension radiographs of the PCM prosthesis document good prosthesis fixation, 12 degrees of flexion-extension motion, and no excessive translation despite the extensive osteophyte and posterior longitudinal ligament removal during the surgical decompression. At this writing, more than 2 years postoperatively, the patient is entirely neurologically intact and asymptomatic.

Conclusion

In summary, the porous coated motion-preserving anterior cervical disc replacement restores normal neuroforaminal height and can preserve cervical motion. The procedure can be safely performed in an outpatient surgery setting. Endoscopic techniques can be used through a 20 mm diameter trochar, if desired, for both parameters—the low-profile and fixed-with-screws versions of the PCM prosthetic design. Depending on the biomechanical parameters, the PCM prosthesis can be placed press-fit (see Fig. 14-7) or fixed (see Fig. 14-8) with three-dimensional fixation and in each of two biomechanical situations, depending on the flexion-extension or lateral bending stability.

REFERENCES

1. Anderson PA, Rosler DM, Rouleau, JP, et al. Evaluation of the inflammatory response to the Bryan™ Cervical Disc Prosthesis in a caprine model. Presented at the Annual Meeting of the Spine Society of Europe, Nantes, France, Sept 2002.
2. Bryan VE. Cervical motion segment replacement. Eur Spine J 11:S92-S97, 2002.
3. Buechel FF, Pappas MJ. Long-term survivorship analysis of cruciate-sparing versus cruciate-sacrificing knee prosthesis using meniscal bearings. Clin Orthop 260:162-169, 1990.

4. Cummins BH, Robertson JT, Gill SS. Surgical experience with an implanted artificial cervical joint. J Neurosurg 88:943-948, 1998.
5. Cunningham BW, Gordon JD, Dmietriev AE, et al. Biomechanical evaluation of total disc arthroplasty: An in-vitro human cadaveric model. Presented at the Annual Meeting of the International Meeting on Advanced Spine Techniques, Montreaux, Switzerland, May 2002.
6. Hilibrand AS, Carlson GD, Palumbo MA, et al. Radiculopathy and myelopathy at segments adjacent to the site of a previous anterior cervical arthrodesis. J Bone Joint Surg Am 81:519-528, 1999.
7. Lewis GL. Properties of crosslinked ultra-high-molecular-weight polyethylene. Biomaterials 22:371-401, 2001.
8. McAfee PC. Artificial disc prosthesis: The Link SB Charité. In Kaech DL, Jinkins JR, eds. Spinal Restabilization Procedures. Amsterdam: Elsevier Science BV, 2002, pp 299-310.
9. McAfee PC, Cunningham BW, Devine JD, et al. Classification of heterotopic ossification (HO) in artificial disc replacement. Presented at the Annual Meeting of the North American Spine Society, Montreal, Canada, Oct 2002.
10. McAfee PC, Cunningham BW, Orbegoso CM, et al. Analysis of porous ingrowth in intervertebral disc prostheses. A non-human primate model. Spine 28:332-340, 2003.
11. Pointillart V. Cervical disc prosthesis in humans. Spine 26:90-92, 2001.
12. Robbins MM, Hilibrand AS. Post-arthrodesis adjacent segment degeneration. In Vaccaro A, Anderson DG, Crawford A, Benzel E, Regan J, eds. Complications of Pediatric and Adult Spinal Surgery. In press.
13. Tanzi MC, Mantovani D, Petrini P, et al. Chemical stability of polyether urethanes versus polycarbonate urethanes. Biomaterials 18:550-559, 1997.
14. White AA, Panjabi MM. Kinematics of the spine. In White AA, Panjabi MM, eds. Clinical Biomechanics of the Spine. Philadelphia: JB Lippincott, 1990, pp 86-125.

CHAPTER

15

Cervical Arthroplasty With a Multifunctional Prosthesis

Vincent Bryan

As a result of degenerative disc disease (DDD), the spine loses cushion and motion. To the office worker or homemaker, the actual loss of cushioning and/or motion in a cervical functional spine unit (FSU) may be less disabling than the pain that may accompany the functional loss in the degenerating segment. On the other hand, to a heavy equipment operator, a long-distance truck driver, a wallpaper hanger, or a concert violinist, the loss of cushioning and/or motion in the cervical FSU may be professionally incapacitating. To a biomechanical engineer, the loss of elasticity and motion represents a condition that exposes the adjacent FSUs to increased stress. To a physiologist, the loss of cushioning and motion signals the progressive decline in the nutrient pump mechanism for disc nutrition and repair, whereas to a pathologist, the loss of elasticity, cushioning, and motion is seen as part of a progressively cascading degenerative process.

However, to date, many surgeons consider cushioning and motion to be expendable functions if postoperative symptomatic relief and stable cervical spine units can be achieved. Altered function, unattended kinematics, and biomechanical deficits have been ignored, for the most part, because symptoms in most patients showed improvement in the short run after surgical fusion. These surgical management goals and outcomes, although not ideal, have been taught and accepted. When posterior surgical approaches for intractable symptoms of radiculopathy and/or myelopathy were found to not lend themselves to all cases with acceptable risk, attention turned to anterior approaches in the 1950s and 1960s. To lessen the probability of mechanical instability after anterior discectomy, improve lordosis, provide distraction to narrowed neuroforamina, and unload the facets, surgical fusion after anterior discectomy with the use of bone grafts became popular. Subsequently a variety of means of internal fixation were added as well. Little regard was given to the patient's functional losses, the increased adjacent FSU concerns of the biomechanical engineer, or the pathologist's cascading degenerative process, despite the reality that the degenerative disc process was, in fact, being surgically accelerated to its end stage as a result of this 1-hour operation.

For both the patient with surgical radiculopathy and the operating surgeon treating the condition, success in the past has been equated with the alleviation of symptoms. Symptoms were primarily of a sensorimotor type—pain, numbness, tingling, and weakness. Outcome assessment at 6 to 12 weeks was usually sufficient to determine whether symptomatic relief had been obtained after a surgical decompression procedure, regardless of the approach. The addition of surgical fusion to the operative procedure required a prolongation of the outcome assessment period to 12 to 24 months to determine whether surgical fusion had been achieved. Within that time period, fusion outcome was usually quite good, although it should be noted that in some published series[6,9] this addition of internal fixation was only able to produce modest gains in patients' overall symptomatic relief despite improved fusion rates. Any concern about motion loss was dismissed after it was found that overall cervical range of motion after single-level fusion was often the same as it had been before surgery.

During the 1990s, in an effort to improve the percentage of patients experiencing good symptomatic relief, a fundamental philosophical change in surgical indications evolved. Previously, the rule of thumb had been to limit the operation to the symptomatic level, for example, the level from which the radicular or myelopathic symptoms emanated. Because a significant number of patients undergoing anterior cervical discectomy and fusion (ACDF) procedures had degenerative changes at adjacent levels that might then or in the future give rise to axial symptoms, the adjacent degenerative level was often operated on at the same time. As a result, more FSUs were rendered motionless, thereby increasing even further the stress at adjacent levels.

Although the trend was toward increasing the number of cervical levels being surgically fused anteriorly, some investigators and surgeons, evaluating outcome results after more than 24 months, were becoming increasingly aware of possible long-term deleterious effects of fusion.[1,5,7,8] This led to a host of new, less invasive anterior approaches ranging from a return to discectomy without surgical fusion to anterolateral and endoscopic microdiscectomies, as well as renewed interest in posterior discectomy. Although these nonfusion approaches did not increase the amount of stress on adjacent levels, they also did not repair the nutritional pump or rectify the already compromised biomechanics of the FSU.

The possibility of multifunctional cervical arthroplasty offers exciting new options for treating patients with DDD while preserving motion and restoring cushioning. The remainder of this chapter will discuss the rationale for cervical arthroplasty as well as the development of prosthetic devices and will present early clinical results.

Spinal Degeneration as a Disease

It has been argued that the spinal DDD process and the normal aging process are one and the same. If that were the case, the rationale would support the notion that symptomatic relief alone is all that is necessary, and the Hippocratic concept of treating the whole patient might not apply. However, Goffin et al[4] performed a retrospective radiographic analysis of 120 patients who had undergone an ACDF procedure for radiculopathy. Thirty-seven patients (average age 31.5 years) were operated on after trauma, whereas 83 (average age 42.5 years) were operated on for degenerative disease or other radiculopathic conditions. These investigators observed the same degree of radiographically demonstrated adjacent-level disease (92%) in both groups. This strongly suggests that the development of adjacent-level degeneration was influenced primarily by the surgical fusion as opposed to the normal aging process.

The term *disease* at times implies pathologic cells, systems gone awry, or other equally ominous concepts. But equating DDD with the aging process seems to have diminished the alarm usually associated with the term disease. If one were to consider the rate of change in the degenerative disc process as the factor that elevates the process to that of a disease, is that sufficient cause for concern? Certainly the rate of aging in patients with progeria provides more than ample reason to consider the rate of change to be the significant factor. Usually the rate of a person's spinal disc degeneration is not known. However, when the degeneration has become accelerated to the point that symptoms first occur, it should be considered as having been validated as a disease by this occurrence; for example, the degeneration rate exceeds that of the general population of similar age.

Rationale for Cervical Arthroplasty

To develop a rational basis on which to consider indications for cervical spine arthroplasty, it is helpful to review the fundamental premises on which arguments favoring cervical arthroplasty are constructed. First, the degenerative disc process is defined as having achieved the status of DDD at the time of the onset of clinical symptoms, which in effect means the process has declared itself as being on the "fast track" outside the normal range. Second, the degenerative disc process may place increasing stress on the affected as well as the adjacent FSUs, resulting in accelerated degeneration. Third, DDD is a progressively destructive process that is the result of both biomechanical and physiologic changes in the FSU. Finally, any process, whether natural or iatrogenic, that advances the degenerative process, such as surgical fusion (which is biomechanically detrimental), or diminishes the effectiveness of the nucleus, such as discectomy (which is physiologically detrimental), is counterproductive in the long run. Given these premises, it is anticipated that if cervical spine arthroplasty can provide a more nearly normal range of motion, elasticity, axis of rotation, and load-bearing, the long-term biomechanical consequences associated with DDD will be lessened. If cervical spine arthroplasty permits function without a dependency on normal intervertebral disc physiology, such as the nutrient pump mechanism, the long-term physiologic consequences associated with DDD will be lessened.

As surgeons we should be prepared to think beyond the patient's symptoms and assess outcomes over periods of 5, 10, or 20 years, or even a lifetime, before selecting a surgical procedure. If we do not, there is little reason to consider cervical arthroplasty as a treatment option. On the other hand, having acknowledged that the degenerative disc process becomes symptomatic, then only by restoration and/or maintenance of more nearly normal function and biomechanics can the rate of degeneration be brought in line with that of the general population. Spinal arthroplasty, therefore, becomes critical to the surgical armamentarium.

Prosthetic Device Development: Design Considerations, Objectives, and Solutions

To address the functional loss associated with symptomatic DDD, prosthetic features should include elements allowing for a full range of motion and cushioning, a variable instantaneous axis of rotation, preferably posterior and inferior to the center point of the intervertebral disc space, appropriate load-bearing in the anterior column, intrinsic stability, durability, safety, and biocompatibility. To realize these considerations, motion objectives were established including the following (Fig. 15-1):

1. Eleven degrees of flexion, extension, and lateral bending; 2 mm translation
2. Unconstrained through normal range of motion
3. Motions through normal range of motion determined by soft tissue and facet interactions
4. Provide for coupled motions
5. Provide for normal spinal biomechanics including a variable instantaneous axis of rotation

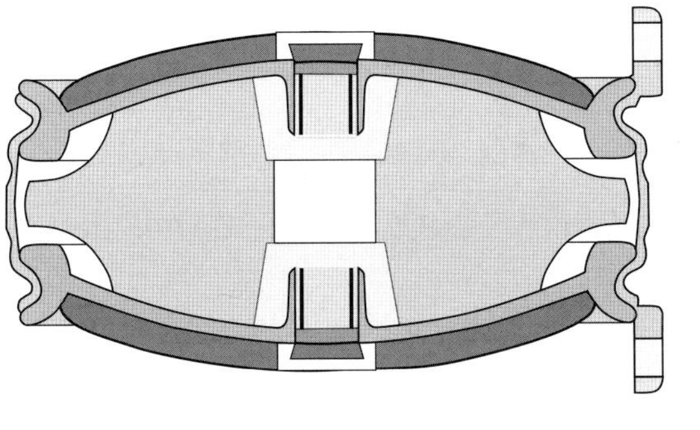

Fig. 15-1 The concavoconvex opposing surfaces of the nucleus and shells provide for coupled motions of flexion, extension, or lateral bending with translation. It is not until the normal full range of motion is exceeded that internal constraints limit further motion of the device.

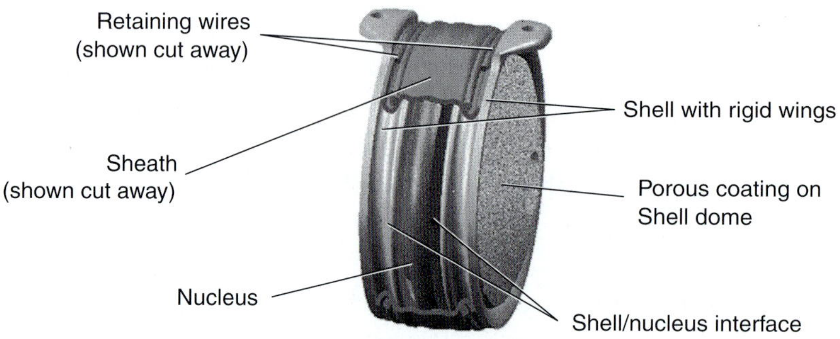

Fig. 15-2 The nucleus is a composite construct of highly durable low-surface-friction elastomer, which freely slides on the highly polished and lubricated interior surface of the shells.

Elasticity and Durability

A means of reducing stress introduced at times of abrupt, jarring loads that occur in rapid succession (e.g., when driving on a badly rutted road) was required. More commonly referred to as the shock absorption function of the disc, materials and/or mechanical means of providing damping and elasticity were necessary. Some elastomeric materials possess properties appropriate for the loads typically found in the cervical spine. However, because the articulation and elastic deformation of polymeric materials can result in wear of the material, it is critical to select or modify a biocompatible material that is extremely durable and possesses all of the aforementioned characteristics as well as the following (Fig. 15-2):

- Composite nucleus construction resistive to abrasive wear while providing elasticity more like the natural disc
- Low friction and thus reduced wear

Safety and Stability

Given the potential consequences on nearby neurologic, vascular, or other adjacent soft tissue structures, and the issues of device or vertebral subluxation, device stability and vertebral stability are essential safety features that need to be considered from the time of insertion. There should be immediate and long-term stability at the following:

- Shell-bone interface
- Shell-nucleus interface
- Adjacent vertebral interface

To accomplish the short- and long-term stability objectives, the device design should incorporate the following:

- Adjacent, form-fitting, concavoconvex shell and bone interfaces using maximized surface areas and cortical bone contact points to provide immediate stability

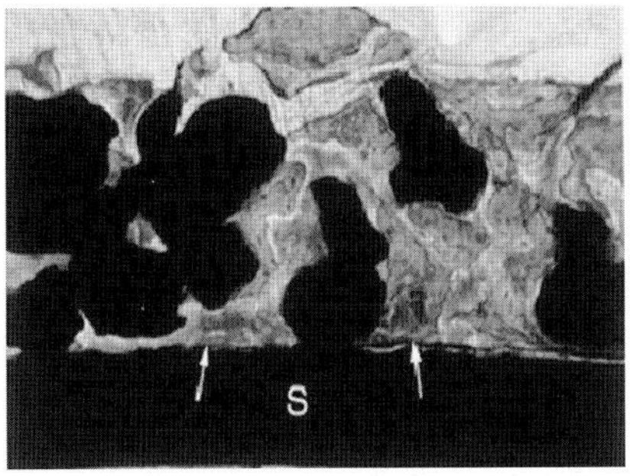

Fig. 15-3 Photomicrograph demonstrating new bone ingrowth (fluorochrome labeling technique) into the interstices of the titanium *(black)* porous surface at 3 months in a chimpanzee.

- Porous ingrowth surface for long-term stability
- Internal central and peripheral device constraints limiting extreme motion
- Friction, lubricated, diarthrodial joint-like shell-nucleus interface
- Preservation of critical FSU soft tissue and bony structures

Fig. 15-3 shows bone ingrowth into the interstices of the porous surface 3 months after implantation.

Biocompatibility

Any material placed into a biologic environment for an extended period of time must be well tolerated, producing neither an allergic nor inflammatory response that could lead to rejection or clinical symptoms. Thus it is helpful to use materials with a long history of biocompatibility in the human body:

- All metallic materials should have a history of use in orthopedic devices.
- All polymer materials should have a history of use in other devices (e.g., cardiovascular devices or devices that have been extensively tested in vivo).
- All materials should have established compatibility in a biologic environment.

Placement and Performance

Although the design features described above are fundamental to the prosthesis itself, the performance of the device is also related to the accuracy of its position in the disc space. Where the precise placement of a bone graft or other fixation device may not be essential to achieving a satisfactory surgical fusion, the imprecise placement of a functional disc prosthesis may result in undesirable biomechanical consequences and may influence the longevity of the prosthesis.

Uniquely specialized instrumentation is required to achieve localization in the disc space and provide for maximum surface area, good cortical contact, an acceptable instantaneous axis of rotation, correct angulation, and centering. Visualized anterior vertebral and soft tissue anatomy is often misleading in establishing a true midline position because of degenerative and congenital variability. Radiographic means of positioning, being subject to the same limitations, may lead to incorrect placement of the device. Internal disc space measurements have proved to be more reliable and also help ensure the safety of critical anatomic structures (Fig. 15-4).

After the position in the disc space has been precisely determined, specialized power cutting tools are used to create shallow concavities in the opposing endplates of the adjacent vertebral bodies, each milled at a separate angle to account for the anterior open angle of the normal intervertebral disc space while

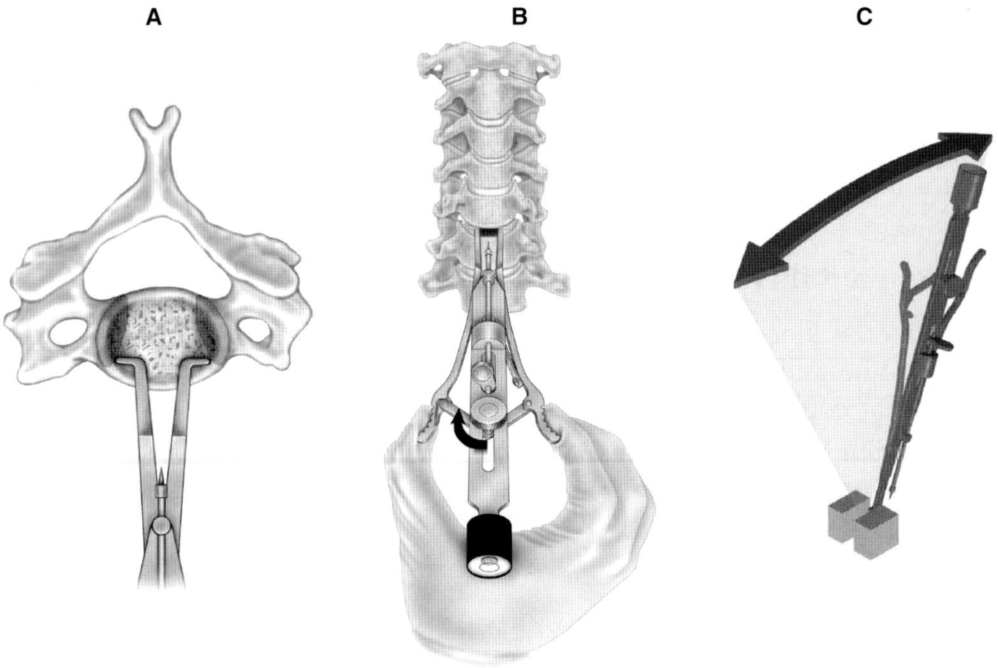

Fig. 15-4 A-C, Transverse centering tool used to establish the interior midpoint from right to left.

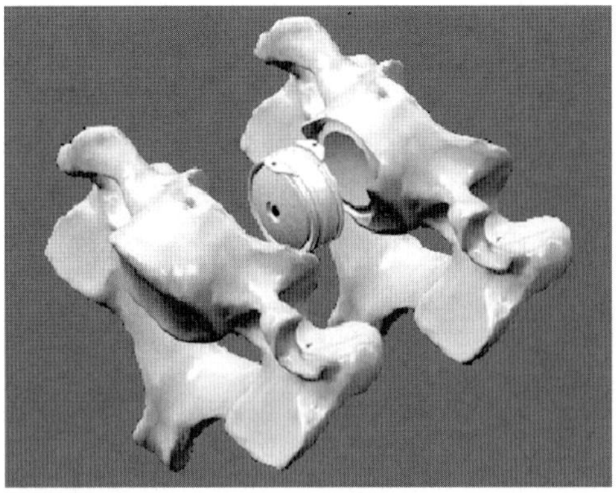

Fig. 15-5 Precision localization and milling can achieve, with a high degree of consistency, an ideally positioned prosthesis bed in both vertebrae to ensure stability in the short and long run, safety, good functionality, and maximum durability.

at the same time creating the immediate stability of a mortis and tenon joint for each shell (Fig. 15-5).

Summary

Through prosthesis and specialized precision instrumentation designs, the principle objectives that provide for full range of motion cushioning, short- and long-term stability and durability have been achieved. It remained for bench, simulator, animal, and finally clinical testing to determine safety, functionality, extent of durability, and surgeon factors.

Preclinical Testing

Physical Testing

Bench testing has been conducted on components, subassemblies, and actual and simulated final devices. The following testing was conducted to establish that the Bryan prosthesis meets design specifications (Fig. 15-6). The preclinical physical testing consisted of the following series of tests:

1. Porous coating
   - Metallurgical analysis of materials
   - Mechanical testing of the shell surface porous coating
   - Microstructure analysis of the shell surface coating
   - Frictional torque assessment
2. Shells and seal plugs
   - Fatigue testing of the coated shells
   - Fatigue testing of the shell post
   - Seal plug pressure test
3. Nucleus, sheath, and retaining wire
   - Durability testing
   - Static torsion testing
   - Static compression of the nucleus
   - Compression fatigue of the nucleus
   - Creep test of the nucleus
   - Static tension test

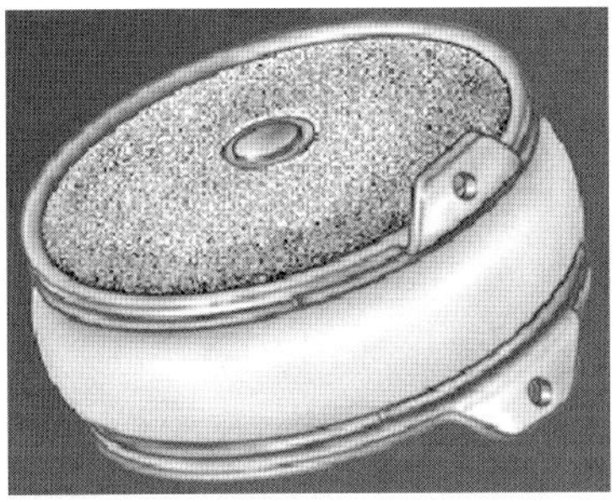

Fig. 15-6 The Bryan Cervical Disc prosthesis, studied extensively on the bench and in animal and clinical trials.

4. Prosthesis
   - Shear testing of the Bryan prosthesis in a cadaveric model
   - Expulsion testing of the Bryan prosthesis

Animal Studies

Animal studies were conducted in the cervical spines of adult chimpanzees. The cervical spine chimpanzee model was selected because (1) the size and shape of the disc space are comparable to the human cervical spine, allowing adequate evaluation of the device and of the surgical tooling and procedure associated with the device, and (2) the biomechanics of the chimpanzee cervical FSU are similar to those in humans.

The preclinical animal study demonstrated that the safety acceptance criteria of the surgical procedure, instrumentation system, and prosthesis had been met. All prostheses functioned as intended, providing for shared motion and a demonstrated range of motion. All devices exhibited good acute and chronic stability. No frank dislocations or gross migration of components were observed in an animal model with high activity levels. The functional components of the primary prosthesis (shells and nucleus) performed as intended and exhibited no significant deterioration. No significant debris was found in the internal portion of the device. However, there were several observations that prompted the incorporation of modifications into the device and the instrumentation, primarily related to improving the likelihood of obtaining biologic ingrowth and reducing wear associated with fixation portions of the device.

Benefits

The major benefit of decompression and fusion in the surgical treatment of cervical DDD is the reduction or elimination of neurologic signs and symptoms, as well as a reduction in pain. However, these procedures lead to a loss in the range of motion of the FSU at the treated level. Recent literature indicates that this treatment produces a predisposition to progressive disease at adjacent intervertebral disc space levels leading to recurrent pain and disability.

The major benefits of surgically treating cervical DDD using the Bryan prosthesis are as follows:

- Relief from pain is similar to that seen with current methods of treatment.
- The prosthesis is designed to provide for range of motion equal to or greater than fusion, which should reduce the progression of disease at adjacent levels.
- The nucleus of the prosthesis is made of compliant material, which will more closely match the mechanical performance of the natural disc than will the currently available disc spacers, such as bone.

- The device is configured to restore and/or maintain near-normal intervertebral disc space height and biomechanics.

Clinical Results

The Bryan Cervical Disc System (Medtronic, Inc., Minneapolis, MN) and associated instrumentation have been the subject of a controlled prospective single-level clinical investigation since January 2000 (Tables 15-1 and 15-2). These

Table 15-1 Patient Demographics

Patients implanted (N = 101)

Age range (yr)	26 to 79					
Sex	Male (n = 42)				Female (n = 59)	
Clinical diagnosis*	Radiculopathy (n = 94)				Myelopathy (n = 13)	
Primary etiology*	HR† (n = 75)	HM‡ (n = 10)	SR§ (n = 31)	SM¶ (n = 7)		
Duration of patient symptoms	6 wk (n = 6)	3 mo (n = 18)	6 mo (n = 24)	1 yr (n = 17)	2 yr (n = 16)	>2 yr (n = 20)
No. of levels implanted	C3-C4 (n = 0)	C4-C5 (n = 11)	C5-C6 (n = 42)	C6-C7 (n = 48)		
Size of prostheses implanted	14 mm (n = 24)	15 mm (n = 22)	16 mm (n = 25)	17 mm (n = 21)	18 mm (n = 9)	
Follow-up period completed	2 yr (n = 27)	1 yr (n = 68)	6 mo (n = 2)	3 mo (n = 4)		

*Several patients presented with multiple diagnoses and/or etiology.
†Disc herniation with radiculopathy (HR).
‡Disc herniation with myelopathy (HM).
§Spondylotic radiculopathy (SR).
¶Spondylotic myelopathy (SM).

Table 15-2 Summary of First Two Years' Clinical Follow-up (Patients Implanted N = 101)

Follow-up	Sample Size	Clinical Success (%)	Excellent (%)	Good (%)	Fair (%)	Poor (%)
2 yr	26	92	73 (n = 19)	0 (n = 0)	19 (n = 5)	8 (n = 2)
1 yr	85	85	70 (n = 59)	7 (n = 6)	8 (n = 7)	15 (n = 13)
6 mo	87	90	70 (n = 61)	7 (n = 6)	13 (n = 11)	10 (n = 9)
3 mo	86	90	62 (n = 53)	10 (n = 9)	18 (n = 15)	10 (n = 9)

data have been published in *Neurosurgery*[3] and are referenced in the *European Spine Journal*.[2] Neurologic and patient-based pain and function assessments are available for 26 patients at 2-year follow-up and 85 patients at 1-year follow-up. The device is currently not available in the United States, and a clinical investigation to establish its safety and effectiveness is ongoing. Following is a summary of European data evaluated as of August 16, 2002.

Twenty-four (92%) of 26 patients evaluated at 2-year follow-up and 72 (85%) of 85 patients evaluated at 1-year follow-up were scored as clinical successes (i.e., Odom's classification of excellent, good, or fair). The data clearly show that properly placed devices do not migrate and that segmental motion at the treated level is present. The implantation of the device produces an alleviation of neurologic signs and symptoms. Symptoms have shown continued improvement up through the 2-year follow-up period. To date, the implantation procedure has been shown to be safe and patients recover quickly. Restrictive postoperative management has not been necessary.

Adverse Events and Adverse Device Effects

One intraoperative adverse event was reported; bleeding from the anchor hole was reported after removal of the anchor post. The anchor post is placed in the vertebral body to facilitate placement of the device and is removed at the end of the implant procedure. The bleeding was readily controlled using bone wax, and the patient was subsequently released without further incident. No blood transfusion was required.

Two postoperative adverse events were associated with performing surgery at the wrong cervical level in one patient. After the initial implantation at the wrong level, there was a report of unresolved pain that was corrected by follow-up surgery at the targeted level. A report of dysphonia (hoarseness), a minor complication anticipated in anterior cervical surgery, resolved postoperatively.

There have been three reports of unresolved pain (i.e., pain present before surgery was still present after surgery). One patient reported pain in the right shoulder, right arm, and sternum region approximately 6 months after surgery. The follow-up neurologic examination did not demonstrate any significant signs and magnetic resonance imaging ruled out any remaining disc fragments at the implant level. The investigator prescribed antiinflammatory drugs, physical therapy, and intermittent use of a soft cervical collar. To date the pain has not resolved. In the investigator's opinion, this adverse event is possibly, but not likely, related to the prosthesis. Another patient remarked about unresolved shoulder pain at the 3-month follow-up visit. However, the pain was resolved by the 12-month follow-up. A third patient underwent surgery to correct a radiculopathy that existed before the implant at the level immediately below the implant level. The investigator stated that the condition existed preoperatively and was not caused by or exacerbated by the Bryan prosthesis.

One surgical intervention at the target space occurred approximately 26 hours after surgery. A standard drainage catheter had loosened and ceased draining. Subsequently, the patient experienced pain and shortness of breath. The reoperation revealed a hematoma, which was evacuated, and no active bleeding was detected. The intervention was uneventful and the patient responded well. In the investigator's opinion, this adverse event was not related to the prosthesis.

An additional surgical intervention followed a patient's report of pain subsequent to the 3-month follow-up visit. According to the investigator, the patient was doing well during the initial postoperative period but then developed intense recurrent brachialgia in the right arm. The surgeon suggested that the initial surgical decompression was not sufficient, and a posterior decompression was performed without involvement of the device. The nerve root was totally decompressed and the patient was discharged from the hospital with good general health status, with the radicular pain decreased but not totally gone.

To date there have been no device failures or device explants reported in the clinical study.

Flexion/Extension

Postoperative Cobb angles for flexion/extension of the FSU at the implant level demonstrate motion of the device in flexion/extension. These range-of-motion measurements are obtained actively, that is, patients are instructed to move their heads as much as possible.

At 2 years, 26 (96%) of 27 patients demonstrated flexion/extension range of motion equal to or greater than 2 degrees. One patient had a measured range of motion of 1 degree; the device is implanted at C6-7, making assessment of the motion difficult. It was not possible to fully assess the preoperative motion in this patient. The range of motion for patients at 2 years averages just over 9.4 degrees, with a standard deviation of 5.2 degrees.

At 1 year, 78 (88%) of 89 patients demonstrated a flexion/extension range of motion of at least 2 degrees. The range of motion for patients at 1 year averaged 8.0 degrees, with a standard deviation of 5.3 degrees. One patient had decreased range of motion at 1 year relative to range of motion at 6 months. The motion measured 10, 6, 7, and 1 degree at 6 weeks, 3 months, 6 months, and 1 year, respectively. Paravertebral ossification may be present in this patient, but the movement of the head at 1 year is more limited than at 6 months, making it difficult to determine whether patient compliance or ossification is responsible for the decrease.

Device Position

Device positioning is measured in lateral radiographs at each follow-up visit to ensure that clinical results are not due to device instability:

- Subsidence: Measurable subsidence has not been observed in any of the patients.
- Anteroposterior device migration: Migration greater than 3.5 mm, the threshold for the study, has not been observed in any of the patients.

However, one patient has a reported cephalic shell migration of 2 to 3 mm in the anterior direction. The shell has stabilized in this position. The migration appears to have been caused by an instrument failure that resulted in incomplete milling of the endplate to accommodate the device. This instrument failure was observed in several of the early implant cases. Subsequently the instrument has been redesigned. Although no other patients in that group have displayed similar movement, analysis of the 2-year follow-up radiographs confirmed that a full concavity was not milled in some of the initial surgeries. This patient's clinical results have remained consistently excellent through the 12- and 24-month follow-up periods.

Lateral Bending

Lateral bending range-of-motion measurements were obtained from patients reaching the 3-month and 24-month follow-up periods. Nineteen (90%) of 21 patients measured at 24 months demonstrated left and right lateral bending equal to or greater than 2 degrees. The range of motion for patients at 2 years averaged 6.1 degrees, with a standard deviation of 3.4 degrees.

At the 3-month follow-up, 44 (92%) of 48 patients demonstrated left and right lateral bending greater than 2 degrees. The range of motion measured 6.5 degrees, with a standard deviation of 4 degrees.

Quality-of-Life Results

SF-36 Health Survey results for all patients who reached 12 months and/or 24 months are averaged. Table 15-3 presents values for each period in the SF-36 Physical Component Summary (PCS) and Mental Component Summary (MCS) scores, which use United States population means to establish normalized scores. All PCS/MCS scores are norm based, with the general population mean equal to 50 and the standard deviation equal to 10. At 2 years after implants were placed, patients' averaged PCS scores were just under the United States mean (49.0), a 35% improvement over the averaged preoperative scores. At 2 years after implants were placed, patients with the Bryan prosthesis meet or exceed the United States population means for PCS and MCS scores.

TABLE 15-3 COMPARISON OF SF-36 SUMMARY SCORES* (AVERAGE WITH ONE SD)

		Preoperative	6 mo	12 mo	24 mo
Physical component summary (PCS)	Bryan Cervical Disc	36.3 ± 6.4	45.5 ± 10.4	46.8 ± 10.1	49.0 ± 10.3
	BAK cervical cage	≅33 ± 9	≅53 ± 11	≅44 ± 11	≅43 ± 11
	ACDF	≅34 ± 10	≅43 ± 12	≅43 ± 9	≅44 ± 9
Mental component summary (PCS)	Bryan Cervical Disc	40.8 ± 12.0	52.1 ± 10.4	50.1 ± 12.4	54.3 ± 9.7
	BAK cervical cage	≅43 ± 12	≅52 ± 11	≅52 ± 11	≅53 ± 9
	ACDF	≅41 ± 13	≅49 ± 12	≅47 ± 13	≅49 ± 12

Figures provided for the Bagby and Kuslich (BAK) cervical cage and ACDF groups are approximations based on bar charts presented in the journal article.
*Average ± 1 standard deviation.

Ongoing Clinical Studies

Two-Level Treatment

The clinical study in Europe was expanded in January 2001 to allow the addition of patients who were treated for two adjacent levels of DDD. To date 39 patients participating in the study have had implants placed.

Radiostereometric Analysis

A substudy of 10 patients in the single-level European clinical study is being conducted in Göteborg, Sweden to assess the ingrowth stability of the Bryan prosthesis using radiostereometric analysis and to analyze the effectiveness of the device in range of motion. Early ingrowth stability of an implant has been suggested as an indicator for long-term clinical success.

Dynamic Fluoroscopy Study

This substudy is part of a three-arm prospective study in which dynamic fluoroscopy data are being collected from patients with Bryan implants at a single center participating in the European clinical study.

CONCLUSION

Cervical spine arthroplasty presents a unique and complicated set of challenges for the designer and surgeon alike. These include multifunctional design, specialized testing with nonstandardized parameters, precision instrumentation, unique surgical technique, and a change in the surgeon's focus from procedures offering symptomatic relief alone to short- and long-term management of spinal degenerative disease. With the development of the multifunctional prosthesis described earlier, after extensive testing including simulators, animal studies (with both primates and quadrupeds) and European clinical trials, safety and efficacy have been achieved. Issues of importance including subsidence, instability, durability, screw failure or dislodgment, ingrowth, biocompatibility, spontaneous fusion, axial pain, facet arthropathy, and so forth have been successfully addressed. Multilevel operations have been formally evaluated in additional clinical studies with soon-to-be-published data showing results similar to single-level arthroplasty. Paravertebral ossification issues have been evaluated with comparisons made between cervical arthroplasty cohorts with and without nonsteroidal antiinflammatory drugs (NSAIDs) leading to recommendations for postoperative use of prophylactic NSAIDs, as in large-joint arthroplasty. New studies are being designed and implemented to investigate the long-term prophylactic benefits that retained and/or restored motion and cushioning of a diseased FSU have on the afflicted as well as the adjacent segments.

The importance of responsibly and safely advancing the field of functional reconstruction of the spine requires that the fundamentals of good science not be overlooked. It is essential after having clearly demonstrated safety and efficacy through extensive bench and animal testing that a prompt path to coding and reimbursement by agencies, carriers, and hospitals reflect acknowledgment of the immediate and the biomechanical prophylactic benefits offered by functional cervical spine reconstruction. Thereafter, following successful clinical trials and FDA confirmation, prosthetic cervical disc devices may begin to affect the natural history of DDD.

REFERENCES

1. Brumley J. Report for the Rocky Mountain Musculoskeletal Laboratory, Denver, Colorado.
2. Bryan V. Cervical motion segment replacement. European Spine J 11:S92-S97, 2002.
3. Goffin J, Casey A, Kehr P, et al. Preliminary clinical experience with the Bryan Cervical Disc Prosthesis. Neurosurgery 51:840-847, 2002.
4. Goffin J, Geusens E, Vantomme N, et al. Long-term follow-up after interbody fusion of the cervical spine. Presented at the Annual Meeting of the Cervical Spine Research Society, Charleston, SC, Nov-Dec 2000.
5. Goffin J, van Loon J, Van Calenbergh F, et al. Long-term results after anterior cervical fusion and osteosynthetic stabilization for fractures and/or dislocations of the cervical spine. J Spinal Disord 8:500-508, 1995.
6. Grob D, Peyer JV, Dvorak J. The use of plate fixation in anterior surgery of the degenerative cervical spine: A comparative prospective clinical study. Eur Spine J 10:408-413, 2001.
7. Hilibrand A, Carlson G, Palumbo M, et al. Radiculopathy and myelopathy at segments adjacent to the site of a previous anterior cervical arthrodesis. J Bone Joint Surg Am 81:519-528, 1999.
8. Pospiech J, Stolke D, Wilke H, et al. Intradiscal pressure recordings in the cervical spine. Neurosurgery 44:379-385, 1999.
9. Wang JC, McDonough PW, Endow K, et al. The effect of cervical plating on single-level anterior cervical discectomy and fusion. J Spinal Disord 12:467-471, 1999.

CHAPTER

16

Total Facet Replacement

Mark Reiley

This chapter attempts to apply the principles of total joint replacement that have been learned over the past 30 years, to degenerative problems of the posterior lumbar spine. Those problems, which include lateral recess stenosis, foraminal stenosis, central stenosis, degenerative spondylolisthesis, and pars interarticularis impingement syndrome, can be directly or indirectly related to arthrosed facet joints. Many of these diagnoses overlap with one another or are different aspects of the same problem, which is the loss of adequate anterior shear control. This does not mean that discogenic causes of low back pain and nerve root entrapment are hereby eliminated from consideration. Nor does this theory diminish the importance of the disc as an integral part of the three-joint complex of the spine. Concentrating primarily on the facets merely shifts the etiologic focus of degenerative pathology to the most destructive forces on any mobile system: the shear forces.

Facet Anatomy and Function

The lumbar facet joints have been thoroughly studied. Much is known about their loading, biomechanical function, time-related anatomic changes, tropism and asymmetry, modes of articular wear, and soft tissue attachments.* In its most narrow analysis, the facet joint is designed to function as an anterior shear stop (Fig. 16-1).

Facet joints prevent anterior shear forces from destroying the disc, which is primarily designed to absorb compressive loads. In fact, the disc is so well designed for its purpose that it is essentially impossible to injure the anulus with purely compressive loads.[35] The facet joints also control varying amounts of rotation and limit flexion of the lumbar spine,[36,39-42] but their most important function is to protect the disc from parallel force vectors.

*References 1-7, 9-13, 15, 19-21, 24, 25, 27, 29-31, 33, 35, 37, 39-43, 48, 50, 51.

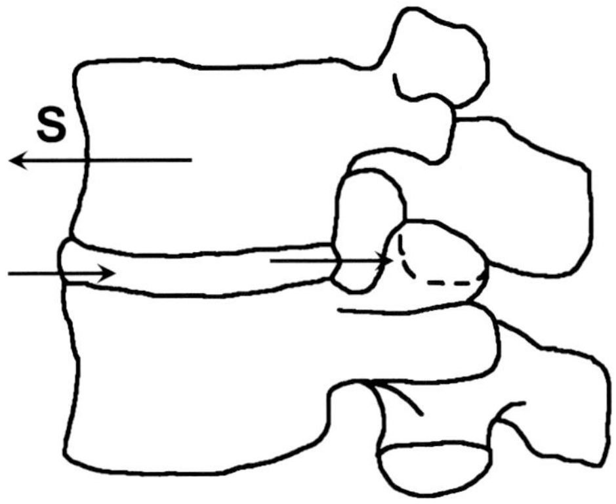

Fig. 16-1 At its most narrow analysis, the facet joint is designed to function as an anterior shear stop.

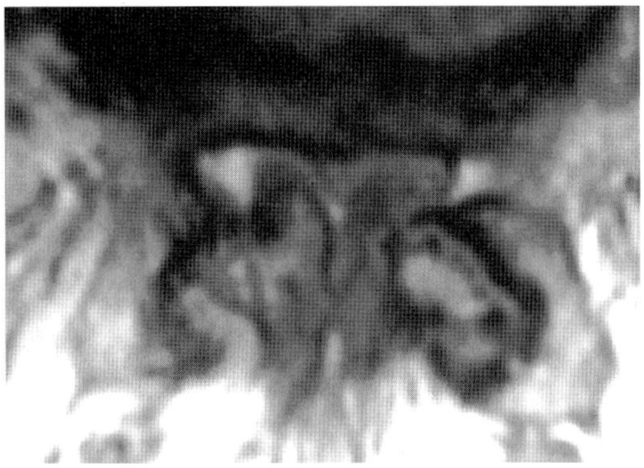

Fig. 16-2 Radiograph showing encroachment of osteophytes upon neural elements. Both central and lateral stenosis are illustrated.

Viewed in this simplified manner, it becomes clear why degeneration of the lumbar apophyseal joints can produce so much spine pathology. The loss of even 1 mm of cartilage thickness within the facet joint allows a significant increase in anterior-posterior translational motion to occur. This increased motion causes repeated strain of the multifidus muscle and facet capsule ligaments, increases the shear load on the disc as well as the posterior and the anterior longitudinal ligaments, and allows the neural foramen and lateral recess to collapse with flexion and extension of the spine. At the same time, cartilage wear stimulates spur formation in all directions around the facet joint, as cartilage degeneration typically does in all degenerative synovial joints. These osteophytes further encroach upon the neural elements, increasing both central and lateral stenoses, and the osteophytes act as their own source of pain when they impinge on each other or the pars interarticularis. Degeneration can continue until facet subluxation occurs, producing further stenosis (Fig. 16-2).

Concomitant with the five degenerative changes that occur in the apophyseal joints (loss of articular cartilage, spur formation, loss of control of anterior shear forces, facet subluxation, and increased anterior-posterior translation), the facets also undergo disadvantageous morphologic changes with aging.

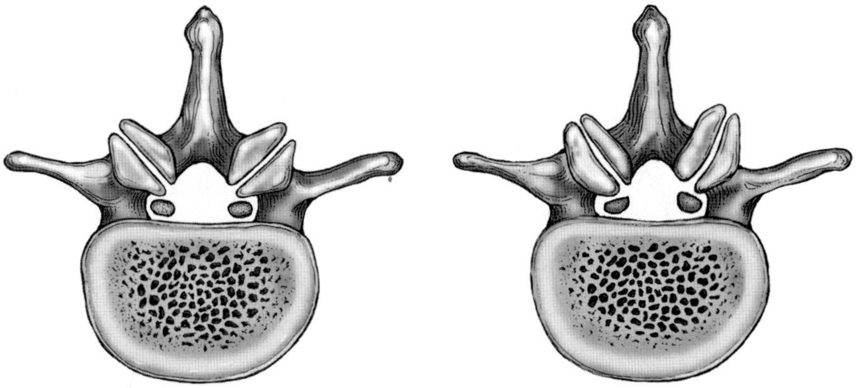

Fig. 16-3 In adult spines the lumbar facets usually have a small anteromedial coronal component and a large posterior sagittal component. The facets become more sagittally aligned as the spine ages.

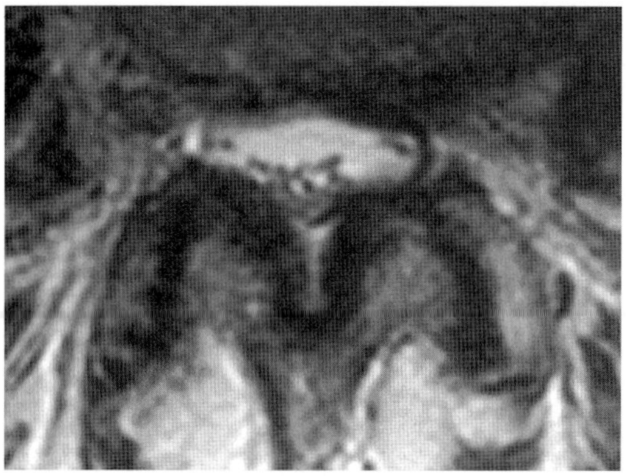

Fig. 16-4. Sagitally aligned lumbar facet in an adult.

These changes in morphology further undermine the spine's ability to withstand shear forces. In infants the facets are primarily coronally oriented.[32] In adults the lumbar facets generally have a small anteromedial coronal component and a large posterior sagittal component (Fig. 16-3). Thus, as the spine ages, the facet becomes more and more sagittally aligned with a smaller and smaller coronal component (Fig. 16-4), and it is this coronal part of the facet joint that controls shear forces.[39] In an excellent presentation using finite element analysis, DuPont verified how the shear forces across the disc increase as the facets are directed more and more sagittally.

There is at least one additional force working on the lumbar facet joint. Depending on the position of the spine, the facets absorb 0% (in full flexion) to 33% (in full extension) of the compressive (axial) load at a given level.[22,29] An incompetent, degenerative facet joint can no longer absorb its share of the

A 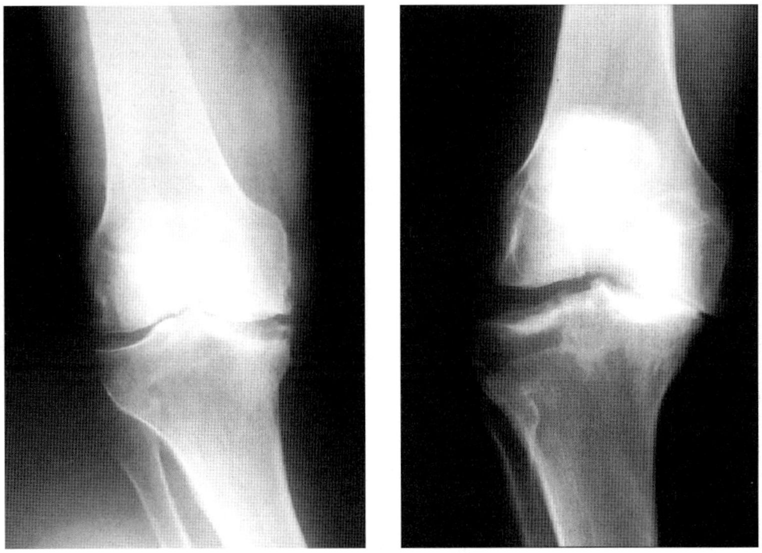 B

Fig. 16-5 **A,** Anteroposterior and **B,** 30-degree AP weight-bearing radiographs are helpful in detecting cartilage wear and/or joint laxity in the knee.

compressive loads, which can further stenose the neural foramen in an up-down direction, especially with the spine in extension.

Radiologic Diagnosis

However, although excellent radiologic tools exist, including the CT, CT myelogram, and the MRI, we still have not developed the spinal equivalent of the weight-bearing AP view, or rather the 30-degree AP weight-bearing view of the knee (Fig. 16-5) to detect either cartilage wear and/or joint laxity. Similar positional views of other joints of the extremities, such as weight-bearing AP and lateral views of the feet and the 30-degree angle view of the shoulder, have been developed to aid in making appropriate diagnoses.

MRI and CT scans of the spine are extremely informative, but most are performed with the patient in a simple supine position; however, most patients do not have back pain when lying down. It seems sensible to develop a technique that applies some extension to the lumbar spine, and perhaps some axial loading, to more accurately assess the functional capacity of the facet joints. Flexion and extension films are not always used in the spine, and even when used require patient cooperation. It may be easier to run a second sequence on an MRI with a pillow beneath the lumbar spine to obtain a comparison extension view.

Some harness devices are being developed to obtain weight-bearing extension views of the lumbar spine, but these are not yet generally available. Also, CT

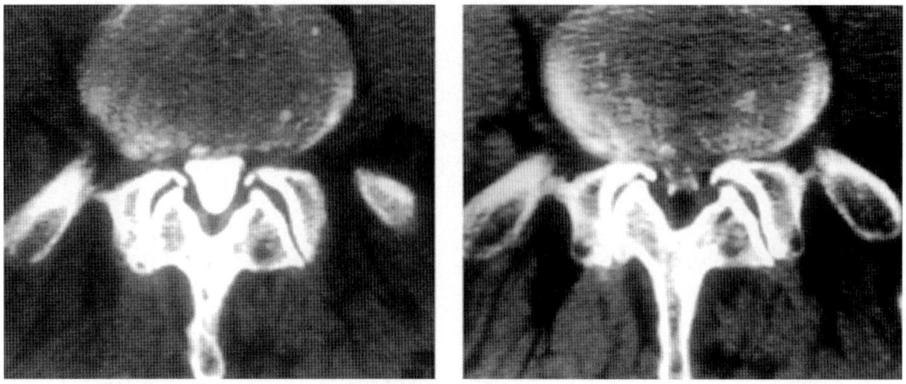

Fig. 16-6 CT scan showing positional lateral recess stenosis.

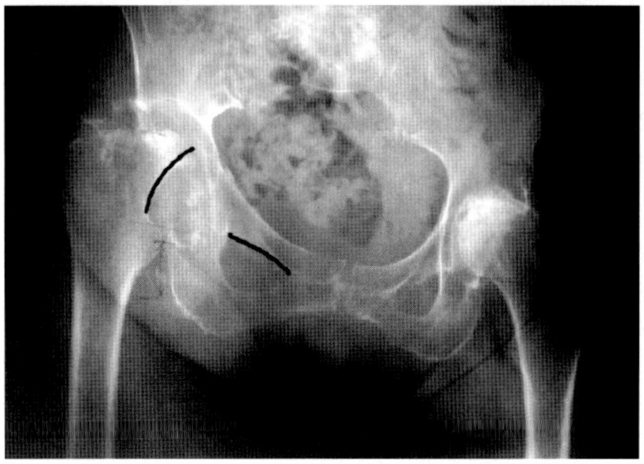

Fig. 16-7 Shenton's line, a continuation of the arc of the femoral neck with the arc of the superior pubic ramus.

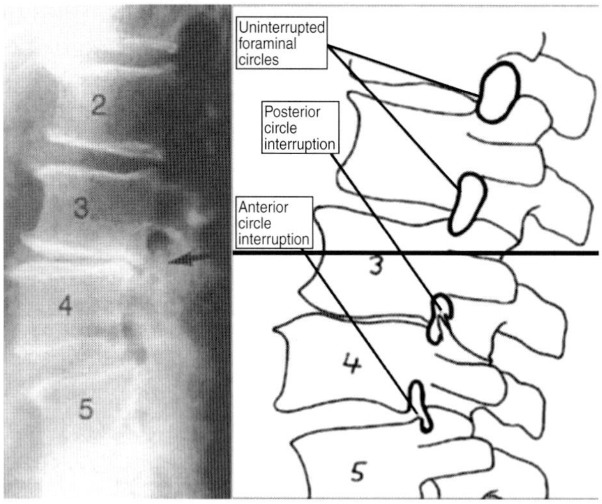

Fig. 16-8 A radiologic example of interrupted spatial relationships of both the posterior and anterior circles in the intervertebral foramina. At L3-4 the proximal end of the superior articular facet intrudes into the hemicircle formed by the pedicle and the inferior facet. At L4-5 the superior endplate intrudes into the intervertebral foramen. This results in facet joint degeneration and joint instability.

scan techniques have been developed to demonstrate positional lateral recess stenosis (Fig. 16-6). Upright MRI scanning may prove useful in demonstrating the pathoanatomy of the weight-bearing facet joint.

Until better techniques are developed to improve the radiologic diagnosis of facet instability, before the surgeon considers a total facet replacement, it may be useful to radiographically study the intervertebral foraminal opening for broken lines, as is done in hip pathology. This radiologic sign would be analogous to Shenton's line (Fig. 16-7), which is a continuation of the arc of the femoral neck with the arc of the superior pubic ramus. When the line is unbroken, the hip is located and biomechanics are considered optimal.

One radiologic sign that could be used to determine whether the spatial relationships have been interrupted in the intervertebral foramina is to follow the arc of the pedicle inferiorly along the inferior articular process and onto the arc of the superior articular process and finally onto the lateral view of the spine. If this circle is unbroken, that is, if the line is smooth (Fig. 16-8), then the foraminal space, at least in a static film, is probably adequate from a bony standpoint. If the proximal end of the superior articular facet or the superior spurs of the inferior articular surface intrude into the hemicircle formed by the pedicle and the inferior facet, the broken foraminal line would indicate facet joint degeneration and instability. This could be performed simply with flexion and extension films, and is a more subtle sign than measuring the number of millimeters of spondylolisthesis. The intrusion sign of the superior endplate into the intervertebral foramen may also aid in diagnosis. Fig. 16-8 illustrates both abnormalities, the former at L3-4 and the latter at L4-5.

Current Treatment for Posterior Lumbar Degeneration

Currently there are three types of operative procedures to treat lumbar degeneration:

1. The surgeon can perform a decompressive debridement of the soft tissue and bony elements (including the ligamentum flavum, part or all of the lamina and the spinous process, a portion of the pars interarticularis, and up to 50% of the facet joint) that are involved in the stenotic process.
2. The surgeon can perform a debridement type of procedure for the stenotic pathology combined with a fusion type of procedure, be it anterior, posterior, combined, posterolateral, instrumented, or noninstrumented.
3. The surgeon can perform one of the newer extension-stop procedures using a "stiff rope" or an interspinous process block. However, it should be noted that stiff ropes and interspinous process extension blocks are currently under investigation for treatment of the degenerative spine. Follow-up so far has been only short term, and the future utility of these devices has yet to be determined.

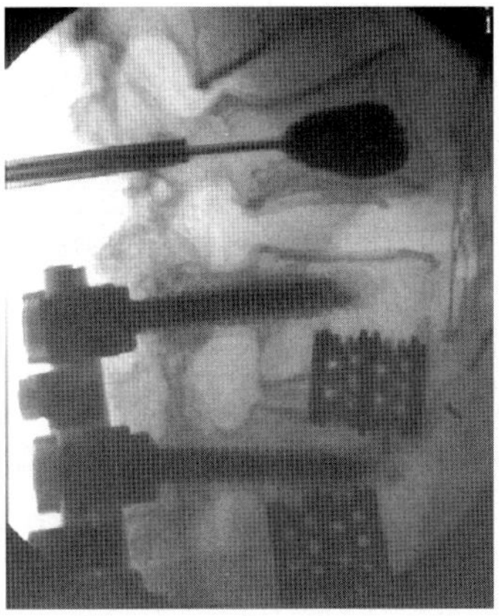

Fig. 16-9 Juxtasegmental complication after decompression and arthrodesis with internal fixation.

Disc replacement is primarily for isolated disc pathology and is not indicated for patients with posterior degenerative disease. However, some manufacturers, either inadvertently or deliberately, have designed total discs with a single point of rotation. This type of total disc system would force the anterior column of the spine to control shear forces, which is not the function of the disc; it is the purview of the facets to control forces parallel to the disc.

All these operations have their successes and failures. Wide decompressive laminectomy has been shown to have good results at 4 years' follow-up in 57% to 85% of cases.[17,18,23,38] Postoperative problems and complications include segmental instability, recurrent spinal stenosis, continued back pain, infection, neural injury, and dural tears.[45,50]

Decompression and arthrodesis together are the mainstay of treatment for degenerative spine diseases. Numerous fusion techniques and appliances are available and the operation has improved to the point where a successful radiographic fusion is the rule. However, as Vaccaro and Ball have said, "Though the majority of studies have shown that the radiographic fusion success rate is improved with the addition of internal fixation, the benefits in the majority of degenerative spinal disorders is unclear in terms of patient function."[45] Some of the complications from this operative procedure include a 3% infection rate,[47] continued pain, juxtasegmental instability or fracture (Fig. 16-9), failed fusion, and failed hardware.

Total Facet Replacement

There are basically six prime directives for any total joint system. These guidelines encompass principles that will provide the best results for patients and therefore also for surgeons:

1. Save as much bone as possible.
2. Achieve maximum bony contact with the implant.
3. Make the surgery as easy as possible.

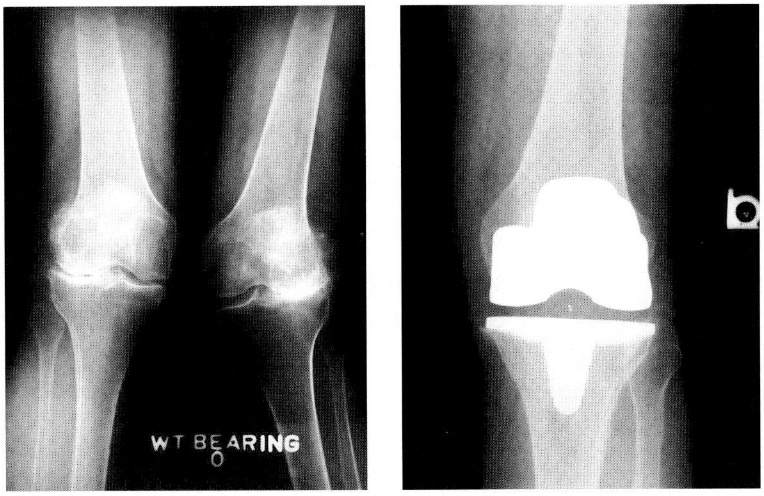

Fig. 16-10 Total knee replacement showing joint realignment.

4. Properly align the joint.
5. Achieve solid, immediate fixation.
6. Produce a durable prosthesis.

In keeping with these directives, and after multiple cadaver studies, I believe that for optimal nerve root decompression, prosthetic fixation, and appropriate facet joint realignment, the surgical resection should include complete resection of both the inferior and superior articular processes, along with all osteophytes and the ligamentum flavum. It may not be possible to save the posterior facet capsule. At present it appears unlikely that a portion of the facet joint capsule can be saved, but it is probably not necessary for stability. In addition, some sort of joint capsular structure may form around the new facet joint postoperatively, as it does following total hip replacement.

Also, other aspects of wide decompression laminectomy described in the literature may not be needed. It is unnecessary to perform extensive laminectomy, except for the attachment of the inferior articular process. This is because in most cases if the facet joint is properly realigned, both in terms of direction and thickness, the lamina will no longer be an impinging component of the stenosis. So too would it be unnecessary to resect part of the pars interarticularis. If the pars is compressing the nerve root, the subjacent facet is by definition degenerative and functioning improperly; thus, this joint below the pars would need to be replaced and realigned also.

This realignment is a major theoretical component of total facet replacement. It is well known from total joint replacement that merely resurfacing the joint is frequently not enough. This is particularly true in total knee replacements (Fig. 16-10) and in total ankle replacements. A large part of the problem of degenerative arthritis in the extremities is either varus or valgus malalignment.

Total joint replacement not only resurfaces the joint, it also realigns the joint into a more functional position. Many degenerative facet joints are similarly malaligned, most often in a sagittal direction, which adds to their poor control of anterior shear forces. It is both simple and necessary to place a new facet in any desired direction; optimally, the sagittally directed facet joints should be corrected to a more coronal direction.

Another consideration in lower extremity total joint replacement is leg-length discrepancy. Unequal leg length can be corrected with total hip arthroplasty. This ability to add length to a joint system is crucial for adding volume to the spinal canal and intervertebral foramina. By reestablishing a proper distance relationship in the posterior arch, neural elements can be completely decompressed without removing unnecessary bone.

Spinous process and interspinous ligament resection may or may not be necessary depending on the bone quality. If the bone quality is poor, then it is likely that the prosthesis will need some sort of a stabilizing bar. If the bone quality is good, then a transverse stabilizing support may not be necessary.

Diagnoses Theoretically Treatable With Total Facet Replacement

Because many pain syndromes arise from the degenerative facet joint, it makes conceptual sense to restore function and anatomy to that joint, as we do for many failed synovial joints in the extremities. Theoretically, facet replacement would solve many of the following problems that afflict the lumbar spine:

1. It is well known that facet arthritis alone can give rise to low back pain. This has been well examined and facet injections have been routinely performed with good short term relief[26] (Fig. 16-11). However, with the exception of antiinflammatories and flexion exercises of the trunk, little

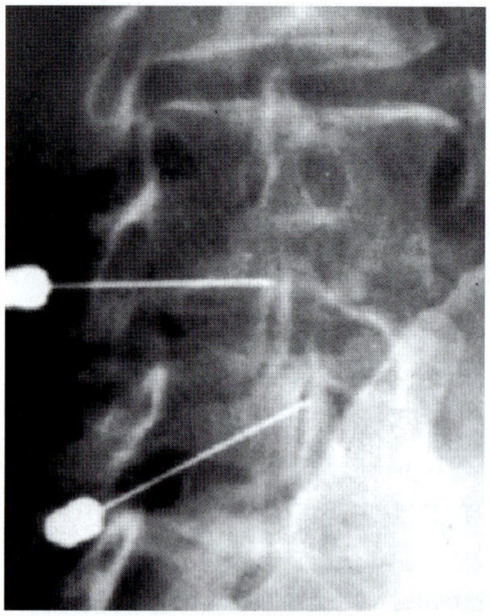

Fig. 16-11 Facet injections have been used for short-term pain relief.

other treatment is available for this problem. Facet replacement would resurface the joint and relieve the pain from joint synovitis and the articular wear.

2. Total removal of the facet joint followed by replacement would allow complete resection of all osteophytes that stenose nerve roots medially and laterally, and those spurs that cause pars impingement. As with facet arthritis, because the spine is a complex three-joint system intertwined with nerve roots, it is not always easy to know in which patients this is a source of pain.
3. It is not unusual when preserving a facet joint during decompressive laminectomy to debride bone around a nerve root with incomplete visualization (when undercutting the pars and facet joints) as it passes beneath the joint. This can give rise to dural tears, the incidence of which has been reported to be as high as 13.7%.[47] Removing the facet joint completely, as one would do in total facet replacement, would allow decompression of all nerve roots under direct vision, which may lower the incidence of dural tears and nerve root injury. In addition, by focusing on the bony obstruction from the facet joint, it is unnecessary to remove the lamina, the spinous process, part of the pars interarticularis, or the undersurface of the pedicle of the superior vertebra.
4. It would be possible to realign the facet joint into a more coronal position, similar to that of a younger spine (see Fig. 16-3). Current estimates from the literature suggest that the optimal coronal angle for L5-S1 is 54 degrees; the suggested coronal angle for L4-L5 is 42 degrees. Higher joints in the lumbar spine have lesser amounts of coronal angulation to allow for more rotation at those levels.
5. Because a facet joint of essentially any thickness can be made, it would be possible to construct a joint that would realign the foraminal space and widen the spinal canal. It is possible that an incompetent anulus or anterior longitudinal ligament would allow retrolisthesis; excessive retrolisthesis may be a contraindication to total facet replacement.
6. In addition, at times the pedicle lengths are different from side to side (Fig. 16-12) perhaps because pedicular asymmetry adds to degenerative

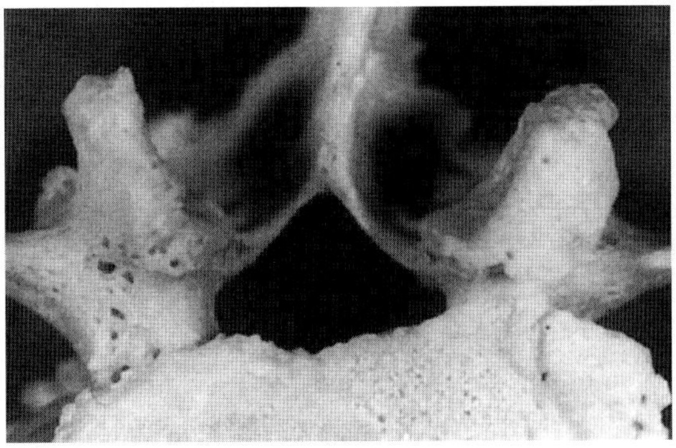

Fig. 16-12 Pedicular asymmetry.

scoliosis. Because it is possible to construct a facet joint of variable thicknesses, it would also be possible to lengthen the pedicle on either side.

7. If the disc has suffered severe degeneration and has lost much of its height, it is definitely possible to construct a facet joint of an appropriate angle so that it can participate in axial load sharing. This, however, may cause too much stress on the artificial facet system, resulting in premature loosening of the prosthesis.
8. It may be possible to correct part of a degenerative spondylolisthesis. Certainly, a long-term, fixed spondylolisthesis would probably not be reducible, but it may be possible to reduce the mobile portion seen on flexion and extension radiographs of the spine.

Complications

Many of the same complications seen in total joint replacements of the extremities can occur in total joint replacement of facets. Briefly, those surgical complications can be divided into three categories: intraoperative, postoperative, and late failure types of complications. Within these categories are osseous fracture, vascular injury, nerve injury, implant mismatch, dislocation of the prostheses, infection, implant loosening, implant breakage, joint surface wear, and multiple joint failure requiring complex joint revision. These anticipated medical complications will be discussed later in this text.

Intraoperative Complications

The most common intraoperative complication of total joint reconstruction is malposition of the prosthesis, but that will be discussed under dislocation, which is a postoperative complication. The second most common intraoperative complication is osseous fracture. In total hip replacement the femoral shaft is frequently fractured or split when a surgeon tries to fit a femoral canal with a slightly oversized femoral stem using an uncemented prosthesis. This complication is usually treated with a long stem prosthesis and cerclage wiring; sometimes an onlay bone graft is required if bone stock is deficient (Fig. 16-13).

Femoral shaft fractures that occur during total hip replacement would be analogous to splitting the pedicle with stem placement down the pedicle. A pedicular split would be a complex problem to treat. It is unlikely that cerclage wires will be a useful tool in the spine because of the close proximity of nerve roots to the pedicle. A fracture of the pedicle is likely to require cement fixation of the stem in the vertebral body. The pedicle fracture would heal with the stem in place, even in the presence of cement.

Vascular injuries are uncommon in total hip and knee arthroplasties, but are devastating.[32] In the hip the external iliac artery or the femoral artery can be damaged either with sharp instruments or with hardened spicules of cement. Immediate surgical attention is required, but even so part of the extremity can be lost because the bleeding from the vessel is not readily apparent during surgery and is usually discovered postoperatively. In the spine it is anticipated that on occasion the common iliac arteries or the aorta could be injured by protruding stems or by the leakage of cement anteriorly. Although no arterial complications have been reported from cement extravasation in kyphoplasty, late false aneurysms have been reported in the external iliac arteries months after intrapelvic extravasation of cement.

In total hip replacement the sciatic nerve is the most frequently injured nerve. On very rare occasions it is cut, but usually it only suffers a neuropraxia. In the spine, nerve root injury is a major concern. However, an appropriately designed implant that allows for complete visualization of the nerve roots will lessen the risk.

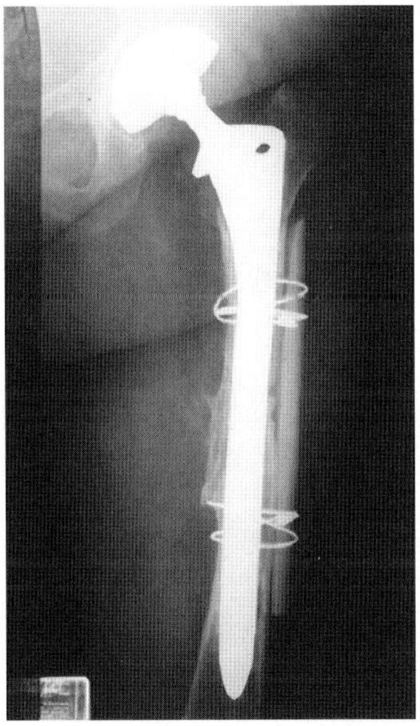

Fig. 16-13 Bone fracture of the upper femoral shaft. The bone was stabilized with a long stem prosthesis and cerclage wiring.

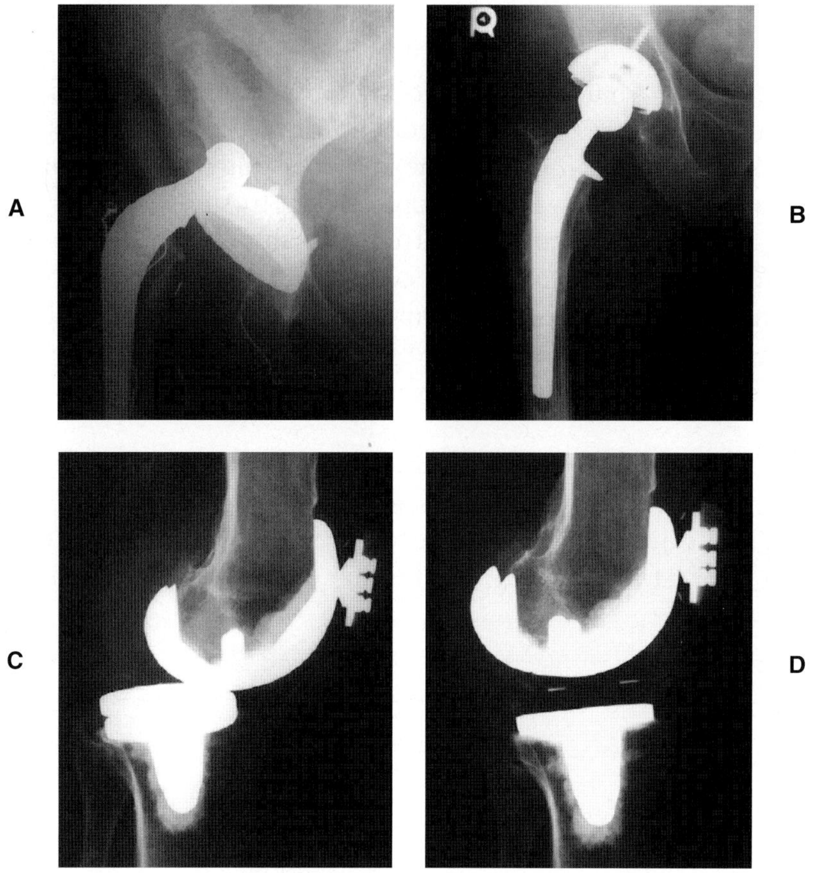

Fig. 16-14 In the early postoperative period dislocation of the joint system can occur in both the hip (**A** and **B**) and in the knee (**C** and **D**).

Early Postoperative Complications

Dislocation occurs in nearly all total joint systems. Whether it is a total knee, total hip, or total shoulder that has been dislocated, it is necessary to diagnose the cause of the dislocation before surgical correction is initiated. Hip dislocations (Fig. 16-14, *A*) can occur from incorrect version of the femoral component or the acetabular component, incorrect femoral neck length, incompetent hip abductors, vertical placement of the acetabular component, prosthetic mismatch (Fig. 16-14, *B*), or a noncompliant patient. Total knee dislocations (Fig. 16-14, *C* and *D*) can occur with undersized components, incompetent extensor mechanisms, or incompetent ligaments.

Just as a total hip can be unstable either anteriorly or posteriorly, it is anticipated that total facet joint replacements will be able to dislocate either in flexion or in rotation. The articular surfaces of the facet are modified appropriately to lessen the risk of dislocation in all directions, but it is prudent to limit range of motion of the spine during the first 6 weeks postoperatively. It is routine to limit motion for 6 weeks after a total hip replacement to allow some sort of new capsular structure to form and mature. After 6 weeks most patients who have undergone total hip replacement surgery are allowed complete freedom of motion except for hyperflexion.

Total joint infection can be an overwhelming problem for both the patient and the surgeon. It is extremely time consuming and expensive to manage, both medically and surgically. An infected total hip replacement can cost up to $50,000 to treat. In the best of circumstances, it can be managed with prolonged antibiotics administered at the patient's home or in a skilled nursing facility. Depending on the bacterial organism, one-, two-, or three-stage operations may be necessary to manage the problem surgically; on other occasions the patient may need to have the hip joint permanently removed.

An infected total knee is equally difficult to manage, sometimes requiring removal of the implant, followed by arthrodesis. Rarely, after multiple surgical failures a patient with a septic prosthesis will be treated with an above-knee amputation.

The current laminectomy/fusion infection rate is 3%,[47] which is unacceptable for joint replacement. At the present time, most total joint surgeons use clean air rooms, with either laminar flow, ultraviolet lights, and/or space suits, to perform joint replacements. Ultraviolet lights are extremely effective at killing all bacteria and viruses, and are much less expensive to install than laminar flow systems. However, they do not function well when the humidity is greater than 70%. In addition, preoperative and postoperative antibiotics are routinely given to all patients who have undergone total hip replacement surgery. It is estimated that the infection rate for the index total hip replacement is approximately 0.4%; it is hoped that total facet replacement surgeons will adopt some of the same techniques to prevent bacterial infection.

It should be noted that 50% of total joint infections occur 1 year or more after surgery. This is felt to be caused by dental work, dental infections, skin infections or heart infections. All patients receiving a total joint replacement of any joint need prophylactic antibiotics when they go to the dentist for the rest of their lives.

Late Complications of Total Joint Replacements

Aseptic prosthetic loosening is the most common late complication in total joint arthroplasty requiring surgical intervention.[49] It occurs in both cemented and uncemented implants. Many theories have been suggested to explain the cause of loosening including cement fatigue, malaligned implants, and pros-

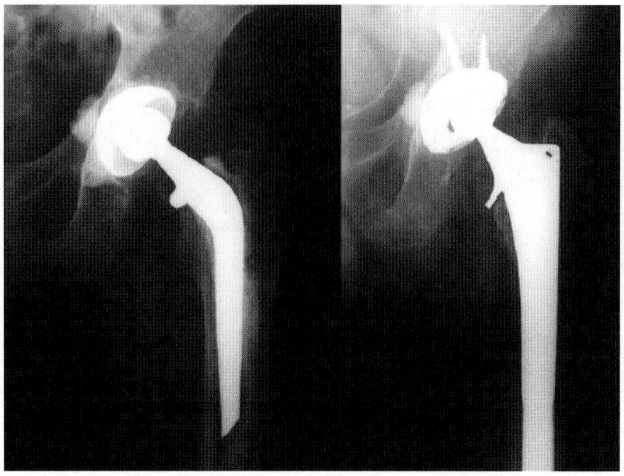

Fig. 16-15 Lateral radiographs showing the loosening of a cemented total joint system. Note the dark spaces between the prosthesis of the femur and the cement.

thetic design. Many surgeons now believe that aseptic loosening is caused by wear debris,[16] which will be discussed below. Fig. 16-15 shows many of the radiographic findings when a cemented total joint becomes loose. Note in the figure the dark spaces between the prosthesis of the femur and the cement. Frequently it is necessary to test the acetabular component intraoperatively to assess aseptic loosening.

Bearing Surface Failure

The original bearing surface for total hip replacement in the early 1960s was Teflon. Although frictionless, Teflon had terrible wear properties and produced an enormous amount of wear debris. Hip revisions had to be performed in most of these patients within 6 months.

Since that time, it has been discovered that the materials used for the bearing surfaces in a total joint replacement have a major influence on the long-term survival of a prosthesis. Certain types of material couplings for joint surfaces produce more wear debris than others. Particulate debris generated from the wear of prosthetic components produces the inflammatory osteolysis that has been implicated as the mechanism for aseptic loosening. Although wear debris from any joint coupling material (metal-metal, ceramic-ceramic, and ceramic-polyethylene) can cause an inflammatory response that leads to loosening, polyethylene wear has been recognized as the primary source of this debris.[16] Dowd et al[8] have shown a direct correlation between prosthetic wear rates and osteolysis.

Despite this, the gold standard for all total surfaces has been some sort of metal against some form of polyethylene. Several types of polyethylene formulas have

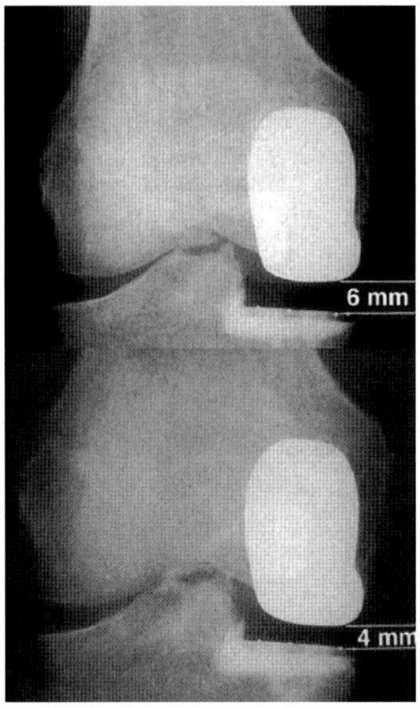

Fig. 16-16 The appropriate thickness of polyethylene in total joint systems has been studied. In total knee replacements a tibial tray of less than 9 mm has very poor longevity as illustrated here.

been studied over the years, and the wear life of each has been improved with various alterations in the curing process (decreasing the polyethylene oxidation) and with ionizing radiation (to increase the polyethylene cross-linking). In addition, titanium was found to be a poor surface for a bearing because of poor wear characteristics; now the preferred material for the femoral head is cobalt-chrome-molybdenum alloy and it has been so for years. The appropriate thickness of the polyethylene has also been studied. For instance, it has been shown that in a total knee replacement, a tibial tray of less than 9 mm has very poor longevity (Fig. 16-16). The exact thickness of polyethylene needed to handle the weight-bearing stresses in a facet joint is currently being studied. Size will be an important factor in the design of a total facet arthroplasty, more so than in the major weight-bearing joints of the extremities.

Alternate bearing surfaces have also been explored for decades. The ceramic-ceramic joint, the ceramic-polyethylene joint, and the metal-metal joint have all been used with success. In general, it has been found that ceramic surfaces are excellent because they are hard, inert, have a low coefficient of friction, and have high wettability. Hip simulator trials have shown that ceramic-on-polyethylene couplings demonstrate up to twenty times less wear than cobalt-chrome alloy-polyethylene couplings. Clinical trials have also shown less prosthetic wear with ceramic-polyethylene coupling.[44] In the laboratory the least wear has been found to occur with zirconium-polyethylene rather than with alumina-polyethylene.[46]

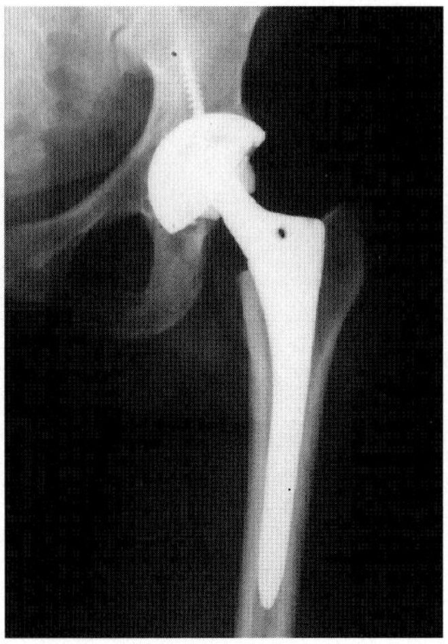

Fig. 16-17 A ceramic-polyethylene joint. If the polyethylene component is treated with ionizing radiation, the wear from the joint has been estimated at approximately 15 microns per year.

Ceramic-on-ceramic couplings have shown 100 times less wear than metal-polyethylene coupling.[34] It is estimated that the wear from a ceramic-polyethylene joint (Fig. 16-17) is about 15 microns per year, if the polyethylene component is appropriately treated with ionizing radiation. The wear for a ceramic-ceramic joint may be as low as 2 microns per year. The metal-metal wear is more difficult to estimate because the ionic debris is not released at a constant rate. Much more debris is released in the first 2 years than in subsequent years. In all total joint prostheses wear is a function of the geometry of the joint, the joint motion, and amount of use; these numbers are always rough estimates.

It should be noted that most wear data for weight-bearing surfaces have been found from studies of hip simulators or in clinical series of total hip replacements. This is unfortunate for total facet replacement, because the motions of the facet joint are more similar to a knee than to a hip. Very few wear data have been extracted from knee simulators, because the motion is very difficult to mimic. Ceramic-ceramic total knee systems are just being introduced in the orthopedic market, and little will be known of their results for several years.

Prosthetic Fracture

Prosthetic fracture was not uncommon years ago early in the era of total hip replacement. This was because the femoral stem was made of stainless steel, which has poor fatigue strength. Today femoral stems are made of "superalloys," cobalt-chrome and either pure titanium or titanium alloy. Even so, femoral stem breakage is still seen. Stem fracture at 5 years usually indicates that the stem has only been fixed distally with cement. Fracture at 7 years usually indicates the possibility of a flaw in the stem (Fig. 16-18).

Stem fractures are very likely to occur with total facet replacement. If the stems can be thick enough, the fixation uniform enough, and shear forces kept

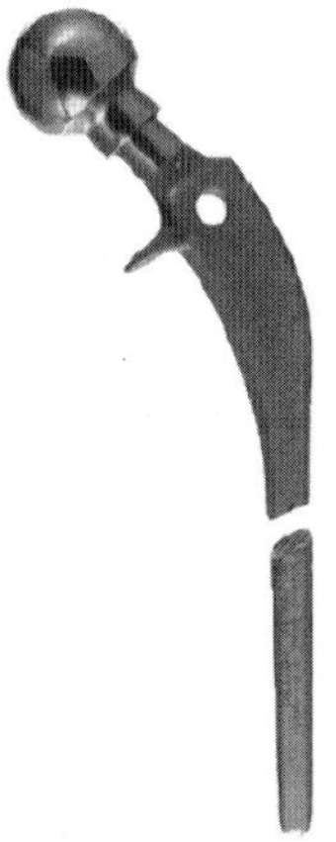

Fig. 16-18 Femoral stem breakage.

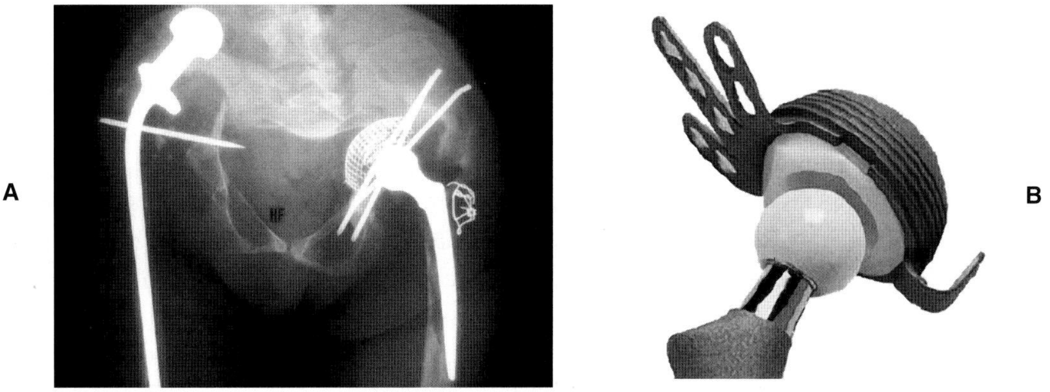

Fig. 16-19 A, Cup protusion seen on an AP radiograph. **B,** Hardware used for total hip replacement.

to a minimum, then the risk of stem breakage will be reduced. Because the salvage of a broken stem, cemented or not, is difficult, we need to design a system that reduces these risks.

Cup Protrusion

Cup protrusion or acetabular protrusion occurs in patients with rheumatoid arthritis and in patients in whom too much bone has been removed from the medial wall of the acetabulum (Fig. 16-19, *A*). It is less difficult to manage surgically now because of the extensive hardware available (Fig. 16-19, *B*).

It is extremely likely that this problem will occur at the level of the superior articular facet because this part of the joint is most analogous to the acetabulum. Protrusion of the superior articular half of the joint may require spine fusion for surgical salvage.

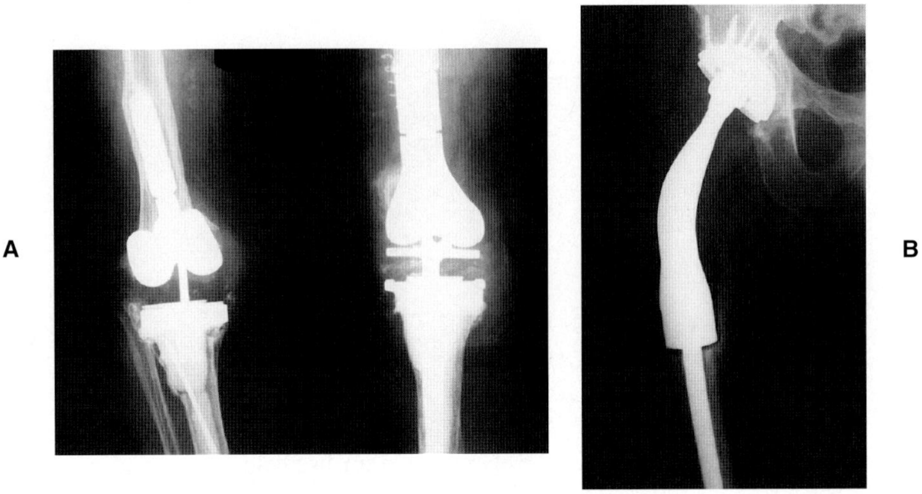

Fig. 16-20 Multiple revisions are possible in both **A,** knees and **B,** hips.

Multiple Revision Surgery

As time goes by, more and more total joints fail, and they can fail repeatedly. When multiple joint revisions are done, more and more bone loss occurs. In joints such as the knee (Fig. 16-20, *A*) and the hip (Fig. 16-20, *B*) the surgeon has many available options to replace bone with metal. It is even possible to replace major bone loss with femoral allografts. The spine will probably not allow this kind of total metal replacement because of the large amount of cancellous bone intertwined with ligaments and discs.

CONCLUSION

From total joint replacement of the extremities to total facet replacement is a short leap. Thirty-five years of laboratory and clinical studies have produced an enormous database for spine surgeons. Information on fixation techniques, metal alloys, complex prosthetic constructions, and bearing surfaces will enable surgeons of the future to implant total joint systems with much more confidence than early total joint surgeons did. The results of facet replacement will be better for most patients than with spine fusion, just as joint replacement is better than fusion in the extremities. It is also likely that patients will be saved a great deal of trouble in terms of expected complications because of the experience gathered from 30 years of total joint arthroplasty.

REFERENCES

1. Adams MA, Hutton WC. The mechanical function of the lumbar apophyseal joints. Spine 8:327-330, 1983.
2. Adams MA, Hutton WC, Scott JR. The resistance to flexion of the lumbar intervertebral joint. Spine 5:245-253, 1980.

3. Adams MA, McNally DS, Dolan P. "Stress" distributions inside intervertebral discs. The effects of age and degeneration. J Bone Joint Surg Br 78:965-972, 1996.
4. Badgley C. The articular facets in relation to low back pain and sciatic radiation. J Bone Joint Surg Am 23:481-496, 1941.
5. Berlemann U, Jeszenszky DJ, Buhler DW, et al. Facet joint remodeling in degenerative spondylolisthesis: An investigation of joint orientation and tropism. Eur Spine J 7:376-380, 1998.
6. Boden SD, Martin C, Rudolph R, et al. Increase of motion between lumbar vertebrae after excision of the capsule and cartilage of the facets. A cadaver study. J Bone Joint Surg Am 76:1847-1853, 1994.
7. Butler D, Tratimow JH, Anderson GB, et al. Discs degenerate before facets. Spine 15:111-131, 1990.
8. Dowd JE, Sychterz CJ, Young AM, et al. Characterization of long-term femoral-head-penetration rates: Association with and prediction of osteolysis. J Bone Joint Surg Am 82:1102-1107, 2000.
9. Farfan HF. Mechanical Disorders of the Low Back. Philadelphia: Lea & Febiger, 1973.
10. Farfan HF, Cossette JW, Robertson HG, et al. The effects of torsion on the lumbar intervertebral joints: The role of torsion in the production of disc degeneration. J Bone Joint Surg Am 52:468-497, 1970.
11. Farfan HF, Huberdeau RM, Dubow HF. Lumbar intervertebral disc degeneration: A postmortem study. J Bone Joint Surg Am 54:492-510, 1972.
12. Fujiwara A, Lim TH, Howard S, et al. The effect of disc degeneration and facet joint osteoarthritis on the segmental flexibility of the lumbar spine. Spine 25:3036-3043, 2000.
13. Grogan J, Nowicki BH, Schmidt TA, et al. Lumber facet joint tropism does not accelerate degeneration of the facet joints. Am J Neuroradiol 18:1325-1329, 1997.
14. Herno A, Airaksinen O, Saari T. Long-term results of surgical treatment of lumbar spinal stenosis. Spine 18:1471-1474, 1993.
15. Hickey RF, Tregonning GD. Denervation of spinal facet joints for treatment of chronic low back pain. N Z Med J 85:96-99, 1997.
16. Jacobs JJ, Shanbhag A, Giant TT, et al. Wear debris in total joint replacement. J Am Acad Orthop Surg 2:212-220, 1994.
17. Katz JN, Lipson SJ, Brick GW, et al. Clinical correlates of patient satisfaction after laminectomy for degenerative lumbar spinal stenosis. Spine 20:1155-1160, 1995.
18. Katz JN, Lipson SJ, Larson MG, et al. The outcome of decompressive laminectomy for degenerative lumbar stenosis. J Bone Joint Surg Am 73:809-816, 1991.
19. Kirkaldy-Willis WH, Farfan HF. Instability of the lumbar spine. Clin Orthop 165:110-123, 1982.
20. Koeller W, Muchlhaus S, Meier W, et al. Biomechanical properties of human intervertebral discs subjected to axial dynamic compression-influence of age and degeneration. J Biomech 19:807-816, 1986.
21. Lewin T. Osteoarthritis in lumbar synovial joints: A morphological study. Acta Orthop Scand 73:1-112, 1964.
22. Lin HS, Liu YK, Adams KH. Mechanical response of the lumbar intervertebral joint under physiologic (complex) loading. J Bone Joint Surg Am 60:41-55, 1978.
23. Lipson SJ. Spinal stenosis. Rheum Dis Clin North Am 73:809-816, 1991.
24. Lorenz M, Patwardhan A, Vanderby R Jr. Load-bearing characteristics of lumbar facets in normal and surgically altered spinal segments. Spine 8:122-129, 1983.
25. Malmivaara A, Videman T, Kuosma E, et al. Facet joint orientation, facet and costovertebral joint osteoarthrosis, disc degeneration, vertebral body osteophytosis, and Schmorl's nodes in the thoracolumbar junctional region of cadaveric spines. Spine 12:458-463, 1987.
26. Mooney V, Robertson J. The facet syndrome. Clin Orthop 115:149-156, 1976.

27. Panjabi MM, Oxland T, Takata K, et al. Articular facets of the human spine. Quantitative three-dimensional anatomy. Spine 18:1298-1310, 1983.
28. Panjabi MM, Oxland TR, Yamamoto I, et al. Mechanical behavior of the human lumbar and lumbosacral spine as shown by three-dimensional load-displacement curves. J Bone Joint Surg Am 76:413-424, 1994.
29. Panjabi MM, Yamamoto I, Oxland TR, et al. How does posture affect coupling in the lumbar spine? Spine 14:1002-1011, 1989.
30. Prosad P, King AI. An experimentally validated dynamic model of the spine. J Appl Mech 41:546-550, 1974.
31. Reichmann S. The postnatal development of form and orientation of the lumbar intervertebral joint surfaces. Z Anat Entwicklung 133:102-103, 1971.
32. Reiley MA, Bond D, Branick RI, et al. Vascular complications following total hip arthroplasty: A review of the literature and a report of two cases. Clin Orthop 186:23-28, 1984.
33. Scoles PV, Linton AE, Latimer B, et al. Vertebral body and posterior element morphology: The normal spine in middle life. Spine 13:1082-1086, 1988.
34. Semlitsch M, Lehmann M, Weber H, et al. New prospects for a prolonged functional lifespan of artificial hip joints by using the material combination polyethylene/aluminum oxide ceramic/metal. J Biomed Mater Res 11:537-552, 1977.
35. Shealy CN. Facet denervation in the management of back and sciatic pain. Clin Orthop 115:157-164, 1976.
36. Shirazi-adl SA, Shrivastava SC, Ahmed AM. Stress analysis of the lumbar disc-body unit in compression: A three-dimensional nonlinear finite element study. Spine 9:120-134, 1984.
37. Simkin PA, Graney DO, Feichtner JJ. Roman arches, human joints and disease: Differences between convex and concave sides of joints. Arthritis Rheum 23:1308-1311, 1980.
38. Spengler DM. Degenerative stenosis of the lumbar spine. J Bone Joint Surg Am 69:82-86, 1987.
39. Taylor JR, Twomey LT. Sagittal and horizontal plane movement of the human lumbar vertebral column in cadavers and in the living. Rheumatol Rehabil 19:223-232, 1980.
40. Taylor JR, Twomey LT. Age changes in lumbar zygapophyseal joints. Observations on structure and function. Spine 11:739-745, 1986.
41. Twomey LT, Taylor JR. Sagittal movements of the human lumbar vertebral column: A quantitative study of the role of the posterior vertebral elements. Arch Phys Med Rehabil 64:322-325, 1983.
42. Twomey LT, Taylor JR. Age changes in the lumbar articular triad. Aust J Physiother 31:106-112, 1984.
43. Twomey L, Taylor J, Furniss B. Age changes in the bone density and structure of the lumbar vertebral column. J Anat 136:15-25, 1983.
44. Urban JA, Garvin KL, Boese CK, et al. Ceramic-on-polyethylene bearing surfaces in total hip arthroplasty, seventeen to twenty-one-year results. J Bone Joint Surg Am 83:1688-1694, 2001.
45. Vaccaro AR, Ball ST. Indications for instrumentation in degenerative lumbar spinal disorders. Orthopedics 23:260-271, 2000.
46. Wang A, Essner A. Three-body wear of UHMWPE acetabular cups by PMMA particles against CoCr, alumina and zirconia heads in a hip joint simulator. Wear 250:212-216, 2001.
47. Wang JC, Bohlman HH, Riew KD. Dural tears secondary to operations on the lumbar spine: Management and results after a two-year-minimum follow-up of eighty-eight patients. J Bone Joint Surg Am 80:1728-1732, 1998.
48. White AA, Panjabi MM. Clinical Biomechanics of the Spine. Philadelphia: JB Lippincott, 1978, pp 236-242.

49. Wright T, Goodman S. Implant Wear: The Future of Total Joint Replacement. Rosemont, Ill: Academy of Orthopaedic Surgeons, 1995.
50. Yang KH, Kind AL. Mechanism of facet load transmission as a hypothesis for low back pain. Spine 9:557-565, 1984.
51. Zinreich SJ, et al. Computed tomography of the spine. In Frymoyer JW et al, eds. The Adult Spine: Principles and Practice, vol 1, 2nd ed. Philadelphia: Lippincott-Raven, 1997, pp 467-522.

PART IV

FUTURE CONSIDERATIONS

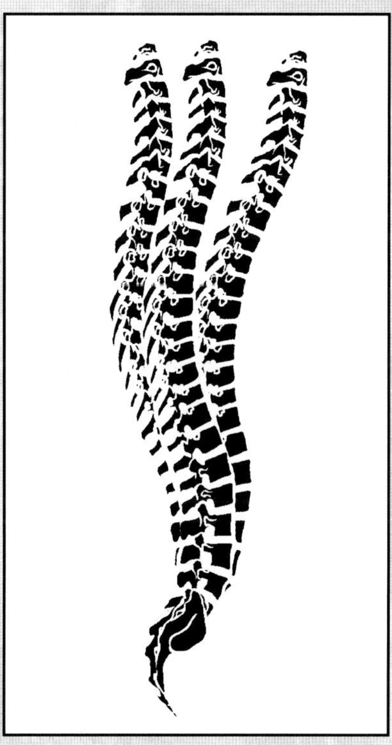

CHAPTER

17

Biologic Disc Repair

Koichi Masuda ▪ Howard S. An

Pathogenesis of Lumbar Disc Disease

Although the exact pathogenesis is unknown, degenerative disc disease is mechanically induced and biologically mediated. Aging does play a role in its development, but lumbar disc degeneration is more commonly found in the highly loaded lower lumbar spine. Repetitive loading, especially when associated with a torsional component, is an important biomechanical parameter of intervertebral disc (IVD) degeneration. For example, cases of IVDs with more advanced degeneration are less stiff and thus are less resistant to torsional and flexor-extensor stresses compared with normal IVDs.[61]

The IVD consists of an outer anulus fibrosus (AF), which is rich in collagens that account for its tensile strength, and an inner nucleus pulposus (NP), which contains large proteoglycans (PGs) that retain water for resisting compression loading. Biologically, cells in both the AF and NP maintain a balance between anabolism and catabolism, or steady-state metabolism, of their extracellular matrices (ECMs), and are modulated by a variety of substances including cytokines, and enzymes, their inhibitors, and growth factors such as insulin-like growth factor (IGF), transforming growth factor β (TGF-β), and bone morphogenetic proteins (BMPs).[55,72] The catabolic process, or breakdown of the matrix, is mediated by various enzymes, such as matrix metalloproteinases (MMPs),[21,27,28,33,63] and cytokines.[29] Disc degeneration is thought to result from an imbalance between the anabolic and catabolic processes, or the loss of steady-state metabolism that is maintained in the normal disc.

Nutrition is another factor in the pathogenesis of disc disease. The disc requires proper nutrition, mainly by diffusion from the vertebral bodies and endplates. Therefore trauma, cigarette smoking, and other factors that affect the endplates may affect diffusion and compromise the nutrition of the disc cells.[47] Further studies are also needed to elucidate the mechanism of pain in degenerative disc disease. Because pain is not necessarily correlated with morphologic or biomechanical changes in the disc, structural restoration of the disc by mechanical or biologic means does not necessarily relieve pain.

Biochemistry of the Intervertebral Disc

The metabolism of the cells that produce and maintain the ECM of both the NP and AF is not well understood.[12] The ECM of the NP, which is very similar to that found in articular cartilage,[26] is synthesized and maintained throughout adult life by relatively few cells. In the adult human, most NP cells are chondrocyte-like, whereas NP cells in the young have a significant number of large notochordal cells.[74] There is also a significant difference in the population of these two cell types among species.[24] For example, in the dog, more than 75% of NP cells are chondrocyte-like, with a significant number of large notochordal cells present, especially before adulthood.[36] It is not known if both NP cell types synthesize the large-molecular-weight hydrophilic PG, called *aggrecan,* that constitutes the most abundant molecule in the tissue.[1] As in articular cartilage, these aggrecan molecules interact extracellularly with long linear strands of hyaluronan (HA), forming aggregates that become entangled in a fibrillar network made up principally of type II collagen.[73] The swelling, fluid- and ion-transport properties, and intrinsic mechanical properties of the collagen-aggrecan solid matrix govern the deformational behavior of the NP. The collagen network gives the tissue tensile strength and hinders expansion of the viscoelastic, underhydrated, aggrecan molecules that provide compressive stiffness and enable the tissue to undergo reversible deformation. The AF contains a relatively homogeneous population of chondrocyte-like cells[36] that synthesize a matrix richer in collagen and poorer in PG than cells from the NP, although the presence of different populations of cells[12,58] and zonal differences in matrix metabolism are suggested.[24,35,78] It is important to note that some of the cells synthesize PG and collagen molecules not normally found in significant amounts in cartilage.[43,73,82] The AF is thus usually classified as a fibrocartilage: it is built for strength rather than to provide reversible deformation.

The progressive loss of the PG content of the IVD, with subsequent dehydration of the NP, has been implicated in the pathogenesis of disc degeneration.[9] The biochemistry of the disc plays an important role in its mechanical properties.[76,77] The NP is able to maintain its fluid pressure to balance the high external loads on the IVD because of the abundance of negatively charged PGs. This molecular meshwork of PGs entrapped in a collagen network endows the

IVD with both compressive stiffness and tensile strength. One of the biologic strategies for IVD repair is to enhance the synthesis of PGs and collagen, which may restore biomechanical function of the matrix.

Within the disc, the synthesis of PGs by chondrocytes embedded in the ECM decreases markedly with age and degeneration.* Several cytokines (i.e., interleukin-1, [IL-1]) and proteinases (i.e., stromelysin and other MMPs) were detected in degenerated or herniated discs.[21,27,28,33,63] Interleukin-1α also stimulates the production of some of the MMPs, nitric oxide, and prostaglandin E_2 by normal IVD cells[29] while inhibiting PG synthesis.[62] These inflammatory cytokines and proteases may be candidates for causing disc degradation. Another strategy for the biologic treatment of disc degeneration is to halt or counteract these cytokines by delivering inhibitors or other substances that block their enzymatic or catabolic activities. For example, IL-1 receptor antagonist (IL-1 Ra) has been investigated as a candidate to block IL-1 function in the IVD.[35,79]

Conventional Treatment for Degenerative Lumbar Disorders

The majority of patients with degenerative lumbar disorders can be managed with conservative treatment that emphasizes adequate pain control using nonnarcotic analgesics and antiinflammatory medications, along with proper exercise to improve cardiovascular fitness and to strengthen the abdominal muscles, back extensors, and lower-extremity muscles. After the diagnosis of a herniated disc or stenosis, surgery should be performed only after conservative treatment has failed. For a successful outcome when surgery is required, proper indications and the selection of the appropriate procedure are critical. Many operations for radiculopathy can be performed in a minimally invasive manner on an outpatient basis with high success rates.[2,3] Alternative treatment methods for the herniated disc include laser discectomy, chemonucleolysis, and endoscopic discectomy, among others. However, these procedures offer few advantages over outpatient microdiscectomy and generally have inferior success rates. Even though microdiscectomy to relieve radiculopathy achieves over 90% good to excellent results, the herniated IVD, with time, continues to undergo degeneration and chronic low back pain may become a significant disability.

Lumbar spinal fusion, with or without instrumentation, has a high success rate if performed on patients with deformities or documented instabilities such as spondylolisthesis and scoliosis. However, surgical procedures for low back pain without radiculopathy have less predictable outcomes; therefore these procedures, especially spinal fusion, should be considered only as last resorts. Fur-

*References 4, 8, 9, 16, 32, 35, 44, 46, 57.

thermore, there are a number of drawbacks to spinal fusion. First, the ability of the bone to heal or "fuse" varies; the average success rate of a lumbar spinal fusion is approximately 75% to 80%. Unfortunately, the failure of fusion may be associated with continued symptoms. Second, a spinal fusion at one or more levels causes stiffness and decreased motion of the spine. Third, having a spinal fusion at one or more levels will cause more stress to be transferred to adjacent levels; transferred stress may cause new problems to develop at other levels, leading to additional back surgery.

For these reasons, numerous investigators are working on alternative treatments to spinal fusion, including intradiscal electrothermal therapy (IDET),[59] disc prostheses,[30,31,84] and biologic repair. Although IDET may relieve discogenic pain, it does not restore structure or the biologic matrices of the disc. This book focuses on the development of various disc prostheses. However, disc replacement requires a surgical procedure and has associated potential surgical morbidities. In addition to the potential complications associated with undergoing any surgery using general anesthesia, complications associated with artificial disc replacement may include breakage of the metal plate, dislocation of the implant, and infection. Like joint replacement surgery, artificial implants may fail over time because of wear of the materials and loosening of the implants. Therefore long-term studies that track the life span of the implants are needed.

Strategies for Biologic Treatment of Degenerative Disc Disease

The biologic repair or regeneration of the IVD may be made feasible by the injection of growth factors, such as the BMPs, or the transplantation of cells transfected with therapeutic genes by viral or nonviral gene therapy. Molecular biology will also help identify candidate genes responsible for disc degeneration and repair. Tissue engineering of the IVD may help treat lumbar disc disease biologically rather than by surgery. In this discussion we will focus on recent developments in biologic treatments, including advances in tissue engineering methods, for degenerative disc disease.

Biologic Therapies: Limitations and Strategies Based on Stages of Degeneration

Depending on the stage of disc degeneration, biologic repair or regeneration is associated with some inherent limitations. The cells or tissues in the NP and AF will not survive if proper nutrition is not available[47,75]; therefore biologic therapies will not work in very severe stages of disc degeneration with disc space collapse and endplate sclerosis. Also, regarding the biomechanical properties associated with advanced disc degeneration if the stability of the motion segment is significantly compromised because of severe disc degeneration or facet joint osteoarthritis, biologic therapies such as growth factor injection and cell or tissue transplantation may not be sufficient to overcome the mechanical problems. However, biologic treatments in combination with some types of minimally invasive procedures may be able to restore biomechanical function.

After the severity of disc degeneration is assessed, a spectrum of biologic treatment strategies is available. In the early stages of IVD degeneration, the injection of a sufficient dose of an appropriate growth factor may be therapeutic. However, for later stages of IVD degeneration with large NP or AF defects, tissue engineering methods, including transplantation of cells or tissue, may be required. In addition, these tissue engineering methods may be combined with gene therapy strategies to express therapeutic genes for a prolonged period of time in vivo.

Stages of Degeneration and Treatment Modalities

Early-Stage Treatment

The production of PGs and collagen by cells within the disc is stimulated by IGF, TGF-β, BMPs, and other growth factors.[39,55,72] Specifically, the growth factor, osteogenic protein-1 (OP-1), also known as *BMP-7,* stimulates the synthesis and accumulation of matrix macromolecules, such as PGs, collagen, and HA, by IVD cells in a dose-dependent manner.[39] These results were confirmed in vivo in an experiment in which OP-1 was injected into a rabbit IVD. The intradiscal administration of OP-1 in vivo in the normal rabbit increased the disc height and the PG content of the NP when compared with the saline injection group.[65] Based on these preliminary data, it was hypothesized that the injection of the protein, OP-1, either as a single or repeated injection, would induce regeneration of an IVD exhibiting early stage degeneration.

Intermediate-Stage Treatment

A disc that has a more advanced stage of degeneration may require a prolonged exposure to growth factors to restore biochemical composition. For this purpose, the use of gene therapy, which stimulates IVD cells over a prolonged period of time, has been developed.

Gene therapy is relatively new to musculoskeletal research. The approach for development of gene therapies for heritable diseases is (1) to identify the defective gene(s) causing the disease and (2) to supplement the patient's defective gene(s) by introducing the corresponding functional gene(s). In the case of acquired diseases, the gene therapy approach is slightly different. The first step is to identify genes encoding molecules that provide a therapeutic effect; the second step is to transfer these genes into the cells of the patient such that the therapeutic benefit is manifested. Most gene therapy studies in the musculoskeletal area use the latter approach although the former approach may have potential applications in the treatment of genetic diseases such as chondrodysplasia caused by a mutation in cartilage-derived morphogenetic protein-1 (CDMP-1).[70,71]

Much of the gene therapy research in orthopedics is based on the use of retroviral and, more recently, adenoviral vectors. Although widely used and made relatively safe through construction of "disarmed" nonpathogenic vectors, retroviral vectors are limited by their inability to transduce nondividing cells and by size limitations of the therapeutic genes that can be transferred. In addition, retroviral vectors require ex vivo cell culture manipulations and carry safety issues of possible mutagenesis leading to host tumorgenicity. The first human gene therapy trial for the treatment of rheumatoid arthritis, using a retroviral vector encoding the IL-1 Ra, was recently performed successfully.[19] The retroviral-mediated gene transfer of β-galactosidase and IL-1 Ra has been carried out in vitro in bovine intervertebral endplate chondrocytes.[79] For safety reasons, retroviral gene therapy necessitates an ex vivo approach that involves harvesting host cells, infecting these host cells in vitro, selecting and enriching infected cells, and finally returning these cells to the host. The need for extensive cell culture manipulations, combined with these limitations, can limit the efficiency, versatility, and cost effectiveness of this method of gene transfer.

The adenovirus vector often possesses high titers and infectivity and is able to infect nondividing cells such as cells of the IVD. However, there is again a small-size limitation on the therapeutic gene as well as problems with persistent viral protein expression leading to antigenicity and host immune response against infected cells.[83] In a recent study, Nishida et al[49] demonstrated the feasibility of direct in vivo adenoviral-mediated gene transfer to NP cells using the β-galactosidase gene. Transgene expression was demonstrated for up to 12 weeks. They also showed that transfection of the TGF-β gene resulted in the stimulation of matrix synthesis.[48] More recently, Moon et al also showed that human IVD cells could be genetically modified by gene therapy using the adenovirus vector.[45] However, a long-term safety study to determine the presence of delayed immune responses has not yet been carried out.

In a feasibility study, the effectiveness of a novel gene gun–mediated gene transfer method for rabbit IVD cells in vitro was demonstrated.[11] This nonviral transfection method is suitable for use with a non-life-threatening disease, such as disc degeneration. Another in vitro study showed that transgene expression was sustained for 3 weeks without significant alterations in the metabolic activity of the cells.[11] These findings suggest that when the goal is to use growth factors to promote regeneration of disc tissues, gene gun–mediated gene transfer has great promise.

Advanced-Stage Treatment

Even when the gene therapy approach is used, the metabolic status of cells in the disc as effector cells must be considered. The cells in the degenerated disc may have impaired metabolic function and fail to respond to mechanical stresses. The injection of cells into the IVD space after microdiscectomy or even percutaneous procedures such as percutaneous discectomy and nucleus prosthetic implantation might be problematic because the cells may move out through the anular defect generated by the procedure itself. Furthermore, in severe stages of disc degeneration with tissue defects, protein or cells alone may not replenish the matrix sufficiently.

In order to replenish the matrix in the IVD after those situations, in vitro tissue engineering techniques may be used to produce functional tissue for transplantation into the defect. There is little information in the literature on tissue-engineered IVDs. Recently a novel two-step culture method, the alginate-recovered-chondrocyte (ARC) method, was developed for the production of cartilaginous tissue in vitro that does not require exogenous matrices.[37] This technique is adapted to form a cohesive disc using NP and AF cells tissue for transplantation to defects in the IVD. It is hypothesized that the gene therapy approach used in combination with the tissue engineering approach could achieve the best therapeutic result in the treatment of disc degeneration.

Growth Factors and BMPs

Advancements in molecular biology have led to the cloning and characterization of the BMPs,[80,81] including OP-1,[56,60] and BMP-like molecules such as the CDMPs.[10] With the development of and refinements in recombinant DNA technology, recombinant BMPs have become available for use in musculoskeletal research and have shown promise as therapeutic agents in skeletal tissue regeneration. Despite the promises of BMPs, the use of these recombinant growth factors in vivo has been somewhat limited partly because of difficulties with optimizing the carrier delivery system and partly because of the short half-lives of recombinant BMPs.

Osteogenic protein-1 is a member of the TGF-β superfamily that exerts potent effects on chondrocyte and osteocyte differentiation and metabolism.[6] Recombinant human OP-1 (rhOP-1) promotes growth and differentiation of osteoblasts in vitro.[60] It also causes differentiation of mesenchymal stem cells along chondrogenic and osteogenic pathways.[7] In addition, rhOP-1 promotes growth of chick sternal chondrocytes[14] and induces the synthesis of type X collagen, suggesting that OP-1 is able to affect chondrocyte maturation as well. Bovine articular chondrocytes, in contrast, did not express type X collagen in response to OP-1 but did exhibit increased synthesis of PGs and type II collagen.[13] A recent clinical study showed that the insertion of an OP-1 implant induced a sequence of cellular events that led to the formation of new bone.[17]

The effects of rhOP-1 on mature human articular chondrocytes cultured in alginate beads have been documented.[20] In this system, the synthesis of PG and type II collagen (but not of type X collagen) was significantly stimulated, with only minimal effects on cell proliferation. In another study, OP-1 stimulated the assembly of the cell-associated matrix by normal human articular chondrocytes as well as the upregulation of HA synthase, CD44, and aggrecan.[50,51]

Effect of Growth Factors or BMPs on IVD Cells: In Vitro and In Vivo Models

The rate of PG synthesis by IVD cells in vitro increases several-fold with the addition of TGF-β and epidermal growth factor.[72] Insulin-like growth factor-1 (IGF-1) stimulates proliferation and matrix synthesis by bovine IVDs in vitro.[55]

The synthesis and mRNA expression of PG and type II collagen by NP and AF cells in vitro is upregulated by rhOP-1.[38] A comparison of the effects of growth factors (i.e., OP-1, BMP-4, IGF-1) on rabbit IVD cells cultured in the presence of fetal bovine serum (FBS) showed that rhOP-1 has more potent effects on PG and collagen type II synthesis than similar concentrations of the other growth factors (unpublished data). Recombinant OP-1 also promotes IVD matrix repair in vitro through PG replenishment following both chondroitinase-ABC (C-ABC)–induced chemonucleolysis[67] and IL-1 treatment.[64] These promising preliminary data point to the potential therapeutic use of OP-1 in the treatment of degenerative disc disease. Further, these results have been confirmed in an in vitro whole disc culture system[66] and in an in vivo experiment using an injection of OP-1 into a rabbit IVD.[65] The intradiscal administration of OP-1 in vivo resulted in an increase in disc height and in the PG content of NP that was not seen in the saline injection group.[65]

The effect of growth factors on normal human IVD cells has not been well studied. Gruber et al reported that TGF-β stimulated cell proliferation early in the culture period,[22] and recently found that IGF-1 and platelet-derived growth factor have anti-apoptotic effects in vitro on human IVD cells.[23] Also, the same group studied the effect of Matrigel (reconstituted basement membrane extract) and found that it is a potent inducer of cell growth and differentiation in vitro.[18]

Effect of OP-1 on Matrix Metabolism of IVD Cells In Vitro

The synthesis and organization of a PG-rich ECM was promoted by rhOP-1 in NP and AF cells in vitro.[38] In this study, rhOP-1 stimulated PG and collagen

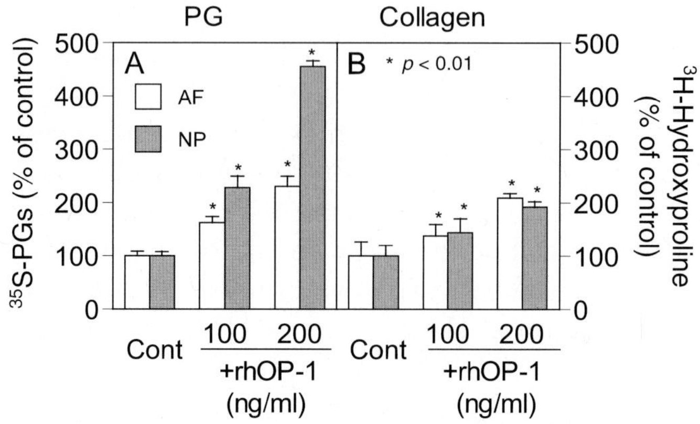

Fig. 17-1 The effect of osteogenic protein-1 on proteoglycan and collagen synthesis. (From Masuda K, Takegami K, An H, et al. Recombinant osteogenic protein-1 upregulates extracellular matrix metabolism by rabbit annulus fibrosus and nucleus pulposus cells. Orthop Res Soc Trans 24:1029, 1999.)

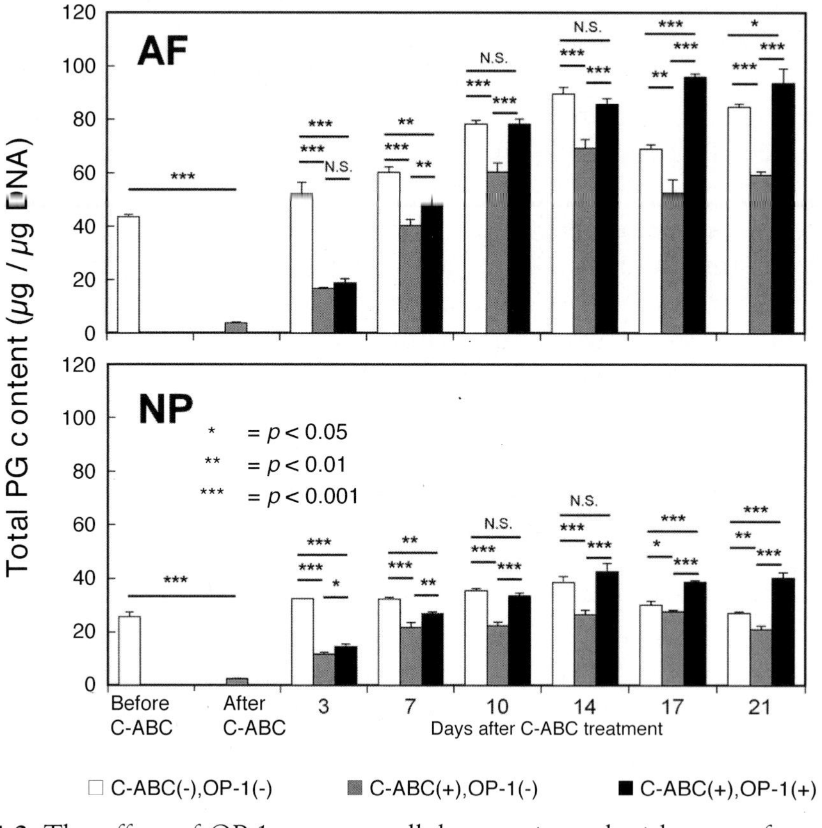

Fig. 17-2 The effect of OP-1 on extracellular matrix replenishment after the depletion of the matrix with chrondroitinase-ABC treatment. (From Takegami K, An HS, Kumano F, et al. Osteogenic protein-1 is most effective in stimulating nucleus pulposus and annulus fibrosus cells to repair their matrix after chondroitinase ABC-induced in vitro chemonucleolysis. Spine J 5:231-238, 2005.)

synthesis of both rabbit IVD cells (NP and AF) in a dose-dependent manner (Fig. 17-1). Recombinant human OP-1 had a significant mitogenic effect only at high doses, but even then the rate of PG and collagen synthesis remained significantly elevated when expressed per μg DNA. Continuous treatment with rhOP-1 at 100 ng/ml resulted in a significant increase in PG and collagen accumulation within the alginate beads especially during the second week of culture. As seen in Fig. 17-1, *A*, with respect to PG synthesis, rhOP-1-treatment resulted in a significant dose-dependent increase in proteoglycan synthesis by both AF and NP cells in alginate bead cultures maintained in the presence of 10% FBS ($p < 0.01$). Nucleus pulposus cells were more responsive than AF cells to rhOP-1 (rate of synthesis as percentage of control: AF = 230%; NP = 460%). As seen in Fig. 17-1, *B*, with respect to collagen synthesis, rhOP-1 stimulated collagen synthesis by both NP cells and AF cells in a dose-dependent manner ($p < 0.01$), but the magnitude of the response was less marked than in the case of PG synthesis.

In addition, rhOP-1 was effective in promoting, in vitro, the repair of the C-ABC-treated ECM around NP and AF cells.[68] Alginate beads containing rabbit nucleus and anulus cells were first treated with C-ABC, an enzyme that degrades the chondroitin sulfate and dermatan sulfate chains of PGs, and then maintained in media containing OP-1 (100 ng/ml) (Fig. 17-2).

The alginate beads encapsulating either AF or NP cells were cultured for 14 days to reestablish the matrix around the cells. The control treatment consisted of beads cultured for an additional 12 days in a complete medium (without C-ABC and OP-1). The beads in the other two treatment groups were first cultured for 2 hours in the presence of C-ABC (0.1 U/ml), to deplete PGs from the matrix, followed by 3 × 30-minute washes before culturing the beads for the next 21 days in complete medium either in the presence or absence of osteogenic protein-1 (OP-1) at 200 ng/ml (C-ABC with OP-1, C-ABC without OP-1, respectively). At various time points (0, 3, 7, 10, 14, and 21 days), the PG content in the beads was measured using the dimethylmethylene blue (DMMB) dye-binding method after papain digestion. The recovery and further increase of the PG content of C-ABC-treated alginate beads subsequently cultured in the presence of OP-1 were noted.

Using the same in vitro culture system (rabbit NP and AF cells in alginate beads), OP-1 effectively stimulated matrix reestablishment following matrix degradation with IL-1[69] (Fig. 17-3). These results—that rhOP-1 promoted repair after C-ABC- or IL-1-induced matrix degradation—suggest that, as shown in articular cartilage, OP-1 is still effective in counteracting the deleterious effects of C-ABC or IL-1 on aggrecan synthesis when IL-1 is still present as occurs in pathologic states.[25] It is possible that rhOP-1 could be used as a therapeutic agent to promote repair of the matrix of degenerated human IVDs or to promote matrix repair in conjunction with chemonucleolysis.

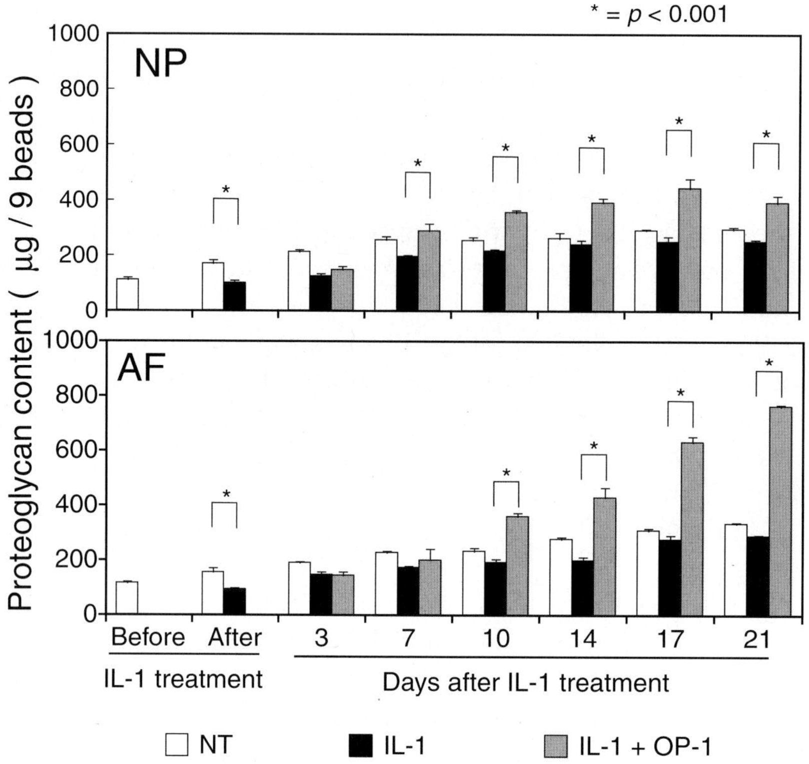

Fig. 17-3 The effect of OP-1 on extracellular matrix replenishment after the depletion of the extracellular matrix with IL-1 treatment. (From Takegami K, Thonar EJ, An HS, et al. Osteogenic protein-1 enhances matrix replenishment by intervertebral disc cells previously exposed to interleukin-1. Spine 27:1318-1325, 2002.)

After 3 days of treatment with IL-1 (IL-1α, 0.5 ng/ml), the IL-1-treated beads had a significantly lower PG content than the nontreated (NT) beads (NP: 48% of NT group; AF: 58% of NT group). During the next 21 days, the PG content of NP beads in the NT group increased during the first 7 days before reaching a plateau, whereas the PG content of AF beads continued to increase throughout the culture period. In the IL-1-treated group, the PG content of NP and AF beads showed similar changes with time but never reached the levels found in beads not treated with IL-1. Importantly, in the IL-1 + OP-1 group (200 ng/ml), the PG content of both NP and AF cells rapidly returned to the levels seen in beads not treated with IL-1 and then continued to show a pronounced progressive rise.

Effect of OP-1 on IVD Cells In Vitro in the Whole Disc Culture Model

The studies were conducted (1) to establish a new method to culture a whole disc with endplates and (2) to investigate the usefulness of this model in studying the effects of an intradiscal rhOP-1 injection on PG synthesis.[66] The tissue culture model was developed using IVDs containing endplates from rabbits. The discs were divided into three treatment groups. Discs from the NT group

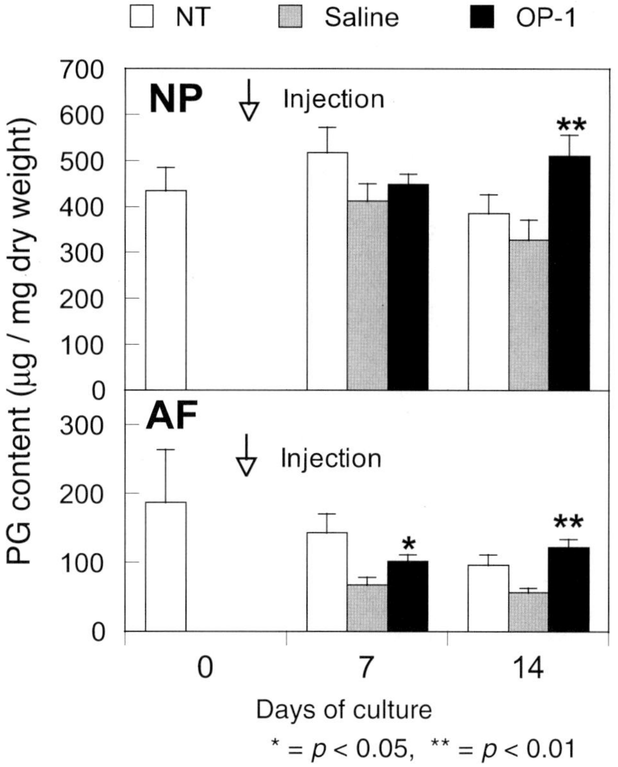

Fig. 17-4 The effect of OP-1 on the PG content of the NP and AF in the Tissue Culture System with endplate. (From Takegami K, Masuda K, An H, et al. A novel culture system for the intervertebral disc: An organ with endplates. Orthop Res Soc Trans 26:73, 2001.)

were cultured for an additional 14 days in a complete medium. Discs in the other two groups were first injected with saline solution (saline group) or with OP-1 (OP-1 group) before being cultured for the next 14 days. The culture of a whole IVD with endplates for up to 14 days followed by histologic evaluation showed both good retention of matrix in the tissue and maintenance of cell viability. The PG content of the NT group decreased significantly between days 7 and 14 in the NP but not in the AF when compared with that group's noncultured control (Fig. 17-4). Interestingly, the PG content per unit of dry weight on day 7 and day 14 was significantly lower in the saline group than in the NT group. In the OP-1 group, the PG content of the NP was significantly higher on day 14 than in the saline group (see Fig. 17-4). Also, in the OP-1 group, the PG content in the AF was higher than that in the saline group on both day 7 and day 14. Importantly, these results for the OP-1 group, when compared with those for the NT and saline groups, strongly suggest that OP-1 contributed positively to the maintenance of steady-state metabolism.

Intervertebral discs from New Zealand White rabbits were dissected with endplates. After injection with 10 µl of physiologic saline solution (saline group) or OP-1 at 0.2 µg/µl (OP-1 group) into the NP, the IVDs with endplates were cultured for the next 14 days in complete medium (DMEM/F-12 medium containing 10% FBS). On days 0, 7, or 14 of culture, the content of PG in the NP and AF was measured, using the DMMB assay. In the OP-1 injection group, the PG content of the NP was significantly higher on day 14 ($p < 0.01$) than that in the saline group. The PG content in the AF was also higher than that in the saline group on day 7 ($p < 0.05$) and day 14 ($p < 0.01$). After 14 days of culture, the PG content in the NP and AF of the OP-1 group was not statistically different from the noncultured control (day 0), whereas that of the saline group was significantly lower than the noncultured control (day 0).

In this method of culturing the whole disc with attached endplates, the swelling of the NP seen in other whole disc culture methods[15] was largely prevented. Further, the single intradiscal administration of OP-1 also largely prevented the loss of PG from the NP found in other whole disc culture methods[15] and in the control groups (NT and saline) of the culture methodology being presented here. In the OP-1 group, the retention of a high PG content was promoted in both the NP and AF and maintained for 14 days. Therefore, by using the whole IVD with attached endplates, the effects of various chemicals and growth factors could be studied before conducting in vivo experiments. The same culture system should also prove useful when investigating the effects of biomechanical loading on IVD metabolism.

Effect of OP-1 on Matrix Metabolism of IVD Cells In Vivo

To expand on the in vitro findings, the effects of OP-1 injected into a rabbit lumbar intervertebral disc on its metabolism and its resident cells were examined.[65] Osteogenic protein-1 (20 μg) was injected into the rabbit IVD and the changes in disc height and biochemical composition in the NP were determined at up to 8 weeks postinjection. As shown in Fig. 17-5, 2 weeks after the injection, the mean percentage of disc height index (DHI) of injected discs was 15% higher in the OP-1 group than in the saline group. This OP-1-induced effect was also significant at the 4- and 8-week time points. The PG content in the OP-1 group was significantly higher than in the saline group at the 2-week time point, but this difference was less marked and not statistically significant at the later time points. This might suggest that continuous or repeated local delivery of OP-1 may be needed to maximize its beneficial effects.

Under general anesthesia, rabbit lumbar intervertebral discs (L2-5) were exposed through a posterolateral retroperitoneal approach; osteogenic protein-1 (OP-1) at 2 μg in 10 μl of saline, or saline (10 μl) only was injected into the center of the NP of three consecutive IVDs (L2/3,3/4,4/5). The disc height index (DHI) was measured using the method of Lu et al[34] with a slight modification at 2, 4, and 8 weeks after the injection of saline or OP-1. By 2 weeks after the injection, the mean percentage DHI of injected discs in the OP-1 group was significantly higher than in the saline group ($p < 0.01$). This significant difference in mean percentage DHI was maintained at 4 and 8 weeks ($p < 0.01$).

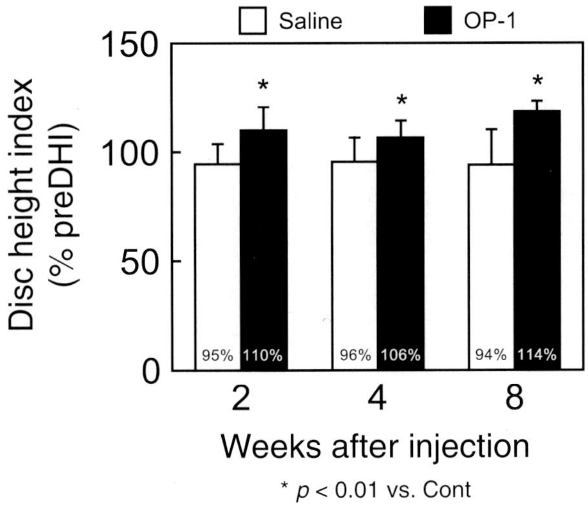

Fig. 17-5 The effect of intradiscally-injected OP-1 on the disc height.

In vivo animal models of IVD degeneration, using an anular needle puncture method[5] and an intradiscal C-ABC injection method, were recently developed (unpublished data). Preliminary results have shown that the severity of IVD degeneration is significantly less in the animals receiving OP-1 injections when compared with the control animals in both the puncture- or C-ABC-treated models (unpublished data). Therefore the coinjection of C-ABC and OP-1 might be therapeutically appealing because disc herniation may be treated with chemonucleolysis by the injection of C-ABC, and the IVD degeneration resulting from chemonucleolysis may be retarded or prevented by the coinjection of OP-1.

To summarize, these in vivo and in vitro findings illustrate the potential of OP-1 to promote nucleus pulposus regeneration in humans. The in vivo studies were performed using normal healthy rabbits, which led to the important question of the efficacy of OP-1 on metabolically impaired IVD cells such as those found in degenerative discs. Therefore to address this question, the effect of growth factors, such as OP-1, on the matrix of both the NP and AF in animal models of disc degeneration was evaluated.

Nonviral Transfection of the OP-1 Gene Using the Gene Gun System

Gene gun–mediated transfection of the OP-1 gene can induce specific metabolic changes in bovine IVD cells (NP and AF cells).[41] To determine whether gene transfection can be used to alter the metabolism of IVD cells, the human OP-1 gene was transfected using a pW24 vector. On day 3 after transfection,

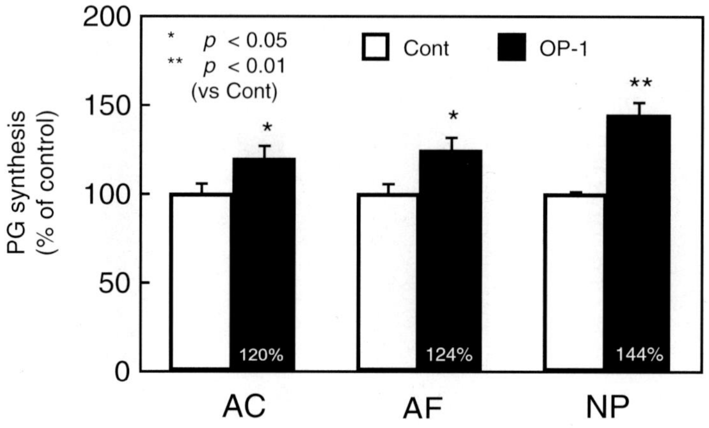

Fig. 17-6 Effect of OP-1 gene transfer on PG synthesis by bovine articular chondrocytes, AF, and NP cells.

there were no significant differences in the DNA and PG contents of the cell layer in any group. In contrast, cells transfected with the OP-1 gene synthesized PGs at a faster rate in both the AF (124% of control) and NP (144% of control) groups (Fig. 17-6). It was noteworthy that NP cells were more responsive than AF cells to the transfection of the OP-1 gene. The results in articular chondrocytes, given as a comparison, suggest that the IVD cells are comparable or better candidates for particle-mediated gene transfer.

To study whether gene transfection can alter the metabolism of bovine intervertebral disc cells (anulus fibrosus [AF], nucleus pulposus [NP], and bovine articular cartilage [AC] cells), these cells were transfected in vitro with the human osteogenic protein-1 (1 gene [pW24 vector]) using a nonviral gene gun–mediated technique. On day 3 after transfection, the rate of proteoglycan (PG) synthesis was significantly higher in all cell types (AC [120%] [$p < 0.05$], AF [124%] ($p < 0.05$), and NP [144%] ($p < 0.01$)] in the OP-1 transfected cells compared with the control nontransfected cells. Cells from the NP were more responsive than either AF cells or AC cells to the transfection of the OP-1 gene.

Cell Injection

The reinsertion of autogenous NP cells, an innovative method to delay further disc degeneration, has been successful in an experimental animal model by Nishimura and Mochida.[52] However, the preparation of NP cells for reinsertion is problematic because autogenous transplantation requires more cells than can be harvested from a single IVD. Okuma et al showed that the coculture of NP and AF cells induced a significant stimulation on cell metabolism in both cell types.[54] In a model of disc degeneration in rabbits, the reinsertion of activated autogenous NP cells delayed the formation of clusters of chondrocyte-like cells and the destruction of disc architecture.[54]

The autogenous reinsertion of the NP itself, or NP cells, into the degenerative disc is slightly problematic because of an acceleration of disc degeneration at the donor site. Nomura et al[53] also tested the effect of intact NP insertion as a tissue and NP cell transplantation on a disc degeneration model. Discs receiving an intact NP showed the least degeneration, followed by discs receiving NP cells, both of which were better than no treatment. They found that allogenic grafts did not induce any appreciable host-versus-graft response. When NP cell injection and NP tissue transplantation were compared, the injection of an intact NP was more effective than the injection of NP cells alone.

Because the transfection of the OP-1 gene stimulates IVD matrix synthesis in vitro, the introduction of gene-transfected cells by ex vivo cell expansion with gene transfection might be a practical choice for treating disc degeneration. Preliminary results showed that the injection of OP-1 transfected cells into the NP induced a significant preservation of disc height and retention of PG content when compared with the control vector-transfected group (unpublished data). Those results support the contention that the delivery of growth factor gene–transfected IVD cells to an IVD improves the maintenance of the disc matrix.

Tissue Engineering Approach to Disc Repair

The technology to produce cartilaginous tissues in vitro, without the aid of a synthetic matrix for transplantation in vivo has been developed.[37] This two-step culture method, called the *alginate-recovered-chondrocyte (ARC) method*, has shown promise in the treatment of articular cartilage defects.[42] The first step consists of culturing phenotypically stable chondrocytes under conditions optimal for the formation of a cell-associated matrix (CM). The second step allows these cells with their CM to form rapidly and become integrated into a solid mass of cartilage on a porous insert.

By combining two technologies, the ARC method and the use of OP-1 in IVD cell culture,[39] the feasibility of forming in vitro a cohesive IVD tissue for transplantation in vivo has been demonstrated.[40] Adult bovine IVD cells (AF and NP cells) were cultured in alginate gel for 10 days. The cells and their associated matrix were recovered and seeded onto a tissue culture insert in the presence of 20% FBS and 200 ng OP-1/ml. After 2 weeks, the tissues were weighed (dry and wet) and examined histologically, biochemically, and biomechanically. After 2 weeks on a tissue culture insert engineered from both NP and AF, cells had a disk-like structure and were easy to separate from the porous insert mem-

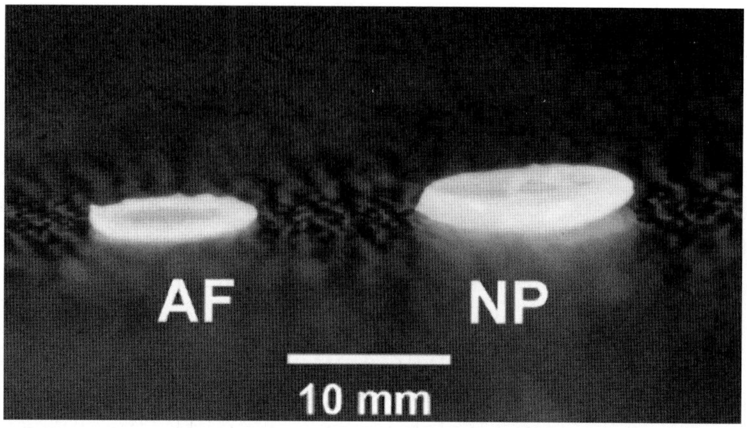

Fig. 17-7 Alginate recovered chondrocyte method and tissue engineered IVD tissue (2 weeks). (From Matsumoto T, Musuda K, An H, et al. Formation of transplantable disc-shaped tissues by nucleus pulposus and annulus fibrosus cells: Biochemical and biomechanical properties. Orthop Res Soc Trans 16:897, 2001.)

brane (Fig. 17-7). Preliminary data has shown that the mechanical strength of the tissues increased significantly with a prolonged culture period (unpublished data).

The ARC method offers several advantages over other approaches to engineering skeletal tissues. The mechanical properties, and therefore the performance, of skeletal tissues are determined by the molecular composition and organization of the ECM, which is only possible if the cells express the appropriate phenotype. The phenotype is affected by the physical conformation and distribution of cells within the tissue. The ARC method of culture, by establishing the proper cellular conformation and distribution, promotes proper phenotypic expression and, therefore matrix production. Cells cultured using the ARC method produce, in vitro, an ECM with sufficient mechanical properties to allow handling and suturing. Unlike several other engineered tissues under development, no exogenous matrix material or scaffold material is necessary. The cells are maintained in a biologically optimal environment, not subjected to influences of extrinsic matrix materials and their degradation products that might negatively impact the expression of the appropriate phenotype. Furthermore, in a clinical setting the patient will not be subjected to what are as yet unclear effects of breakdown products of artificial scaffold materials, such as chronic inflammation.

Preliminary data indicate that the ECM of tissue produced using the ARC method is relatively immature, that is, fetal-like, at time points from 2 to 4 weeks of culture, after which the matrix undergoes a relatively rapid maturation process. This characteristic of the tissue development process is advantageous because tissues surgically implanted at an immature stage have a greater capacity for integration with surrounding host tissues and for remodeling in situ than tissues implanted at a fully mature stage. Cells cultured by the ARC method maintain the normal phenotype during the culture process, and in vitro tissue production proceeds rapidly allowing harvesting at an early, immature stage of tissue organization.

In summary, a tissue engineering approach to lumbar disc disease in young patients merits investigation because it offers the potential for long-term restoration of disc function that can reduce or eliminate symptoms and prevent degeneration of discs at other levels.

The surgical treatment of a herniated NP is highly effective for relief of symptoms related to nerve root compression (sciatica), but currently does not address the permanent change in the status of the IVD. Repair of the AF and regeneration of the NP may readily be applied as an adjunct to the current surgical management, thereby more completely addressing the pathology and preventing the long-term degenerative sequelae of lumbar disc herniation. The investigation of the treatment of anular lesions is a logical initial step, because no method of restoration of the NP is likely to be successful in the setting of a compromised AF. Once anular repair is possible, a logical approach to the treatment of the spectrum of disc disease is possible.

For the production of a tissue-engineered IVD, the cell sources will likely be allogenic cells because of their availability. Future studies on the immunologic reaction to allogenic cells by spine tissues will be important for the clinical application of this technology. The tissue-engineered disc with a maximum viability will not be available as an off-the-shelf product because the properties of the tissue change with time. Therefore the tissue implant must be prepared on a made-to-order basis when the surgeon schedules the patient for surgery. The enhancement of tissue formation and preservation of steady state of tissue metabolism with growth factors might be an important consideration. The combination of two therapeutic approaches, gene therapy and tissue engineering, may provide benefits to the patient. Ultimately, disc restoration will become a routine component of surgery for the herniated NP.

Conclusion

In this chapter we have outlined our strategic approaches to the biologic repair or regeneration of the IVD. In the future, the use of growth factors, BMPs, cells, genes, tissues, or a combination of these agents is expected to be a common therapeutic practice in treating IVD degeneration. More research is needed to further define the effects of these potential therapeutic agents in different models and eventually in humans. Comprehensive research is needed in the areas of epidemiology, ergonomics, biomechanics, imaging, and biology to improve diagnosis and treatment as well as prevention of lumbar disc disease.

The biologic repair or regeneration of the IVD is feasible by injecting growth factors or BMPs or by transplanting cells that are transfected with therapeutic genes by viral or nonviral gene therapy. Molecular biology will also help identify candidate genes responsible for disc degeneration and repair. Tissue engineering of the intervertebral disc may help treat lumbar disc disease biologically rather than by surgery.

REFERENCES

1. Aguiar DJ, Johnson SL, Oegema TR. Notochordal cells interact with nucleus pulposus cells: Regulation of proteoglycan synthesis. Exp Cell Res 246:129-137, 1999.
2. An HS, Andersson G, Lieberman I, et al. Minimally invasive surgery for lumbar degenerative disorders: Part II. Degenerative disc disease and lumbar stenosis. Am J Orthop 29:937-942, 2000.
3. An HS, Simpson JM, Stein R. Outpatient laminotomy and discectomy. J Spinal Disord 12:192-196, 1999.
4. Antoniou J, Steffen T, Nelson F, et al. The human lumbar intervertebral disc: Evidence for changes in the biosynthesis and denaturation of the extracellular matrix with growth, maturation, ageing, and degeneration. J Clin Invest 98:996-1003, 1996.
5. Aota Y, Masuda K, Nguyen C, et al. Radiological and MRI analyses of a novel rabbit model: A mild, progressive disc degeneration. Orthop Res Soc Trans 27:118, 2002.
6. Asahina I, Sampath TK, Hauschka PV. Human osteogenic protein-1 induces chondroblastic, osteoblastic, and/or adipocytic differentiation of clonal murine target cells. Exp Cell Res 222:38-47, 1996.
7. Asahina I, Sampath TK, Nishimura I, et al. Hauschka PV. Human osteogenic protein-1 induces both chondroblastic and osteoblastic differentiation of osteoprogenitor cells derived from newborn rat calvaria. J Cell Biol 123:921-933, 1993.
8. Buckwalter JA, Kuettner KE, Thonar EJ. Age-related changes in articular cartilage proteoglycans: Electron microscopic studies. J Orthop Res 3:251-257, 1985.
9. Buckwalter JA, Pedrini MA, Pedrini V, et al. Proteoglycans of human infant intervertebral disc. Electron microscopic and biochemical studies. J Bone Joint Surg Am 67:284-294, 1985.
10. Chang SC, Hoang B, Thomas JT, et al. Cartilage-derived morphogenetic proteins. New members of the transforming growth factor-beta superfamily predominantly expressed in long bones during human embryonic development. J Biol Chem 269:28227-28234, 1994.
11. Chang S, Masuda K, Takegami K, et al. Gene gun-mediated gene transfer to intervertebral disc cells. Orthop Res Soc Trans 25:231, 2000.
12. Chelberg MK, Banks GM, Geiger DF, et al. Identification of heterogeneous cell populations in normal human intervertebral disc. J Anat 186:43-53, 1995.
13. Chen P, Vukicevic S, Sampath TK, et al. Bovine articular chondrocytes do not undergo hypertrophy when cultured in the presence of serum and osteogenic protein-1. Biochem Biophys Res Commun 197:1253-1259, 1993.
14. Chen P, Vukicevic S, Sampath TK, et al. Osteogenic protein-1 promotes growth and maturation of chick sternal chondrocytes in serum-free cultures. J Cell Sci 108:105-114, 1995.
15. Chiba K, Andersson GB, Masuda K, et al. A new culture system to study the metabolism of the intervertebral disc in vitro. Spine 23:1821-1827, 1998.
16. Cole TC, Ghosh P, Taylor TK. Variations of the proteoglycans of the canine intervertebral disc with ageing. Biochim Biophys Acta 880:209-219, 1986.
17. Cook SD. Preclinical and clinical evaluation of osteogenic protein-1 (BMP-7) in bony sites. Orthopedics 22:669-671, 1999.

18. Desai BJ, Gruber HE, Hanley EN Jr. The influence of Matrigel or growth factor reduced Matrigel on human intervertebral disc cell growth and proliferation. Histol Histopathol 14:359-368, 1999.
19. Evans CH, Ghivizzani SC, Robbins PD. Blocking cytokines with genes. J Leukoc Biol 64:55-61, 1998.
20. Flechtenmacher J, Huch K, Thonar EJ, et al. Recombinant human osteogenic protein 1 is a potent stimulator of the synthesis of cartilage proteoglycans and collagens by human articular chondrocytes. Arthritis Rheum 39:1896-1904, 1996.
21. Fujita K, Nakagawa T, Hirabayashi K, et al. Neutral proteinases in human intervertebral disc. Role in degeneration and probable origin. Spine 18:1766-1773, 1993.
22. Gruber HE, Fisher EC Jr, Desai B, et al. Human intervertebral disc cells from the annulus: three-dimensional culture in agarose or alginate and responsiveness to TGF-beta 1. Exp Cell Res 235:13-21, 1997.
23. Gruber HE, Norton HJ, Hanley EN Jr. Anti-apoptotic effects of IGF-1 and PDGF on human intervertebral disc cells in vitro. Spine 25:2153-2157, 2000.
24. Horner HA, Roberts S, Bielby RC, et al. Cells from different regions of the intervertebral disc: effect of culture system on matrix expression and cell phenotype. Spine 27:1018-1028, 2002.
25. Huch K, Wilbrink B, Flechtenmacher J, et al. Effects of recombinant human osteogenic protein 1 on the production of proteoglycan, prostaglandin E_2, and interleukin-1 receptor antagonist by human articular chondrocytes cultured in the presence of interleukin-1 beta. Arthritis Rheum 40:2157-2161, 1997.
26. Jahnke MR, McDevitt CA. Proteoglycans of the human intervertebral disc. Electrophoretic heterogeneity of the aggregating proteoglycans of the nucleus pulposus. Biochem J 251:347-356, 1988.
27. Kang JD, Georgescu HI, McIntyre-Larkin L, et al. Herniated cervical intervertebral discs spontaneously produce matrix metalloproteinases, nitric oxide, interleukin-6, and prostaglandin E2. Spine 20:2373-2378, 1995.
28. Kang JD, Georgescu HI, McIntyre-Larkin L, et al. Herniated lumbar intervertebral discs spontaneously produce matrix metalloproteinases, nitric oxide, interleukin-6, and prostaglandin E2. Spine 21:271-277, 1996.
29. Kang JD, Stefanovic-Racic M, McIntyre LA, et al. Toward a biochemical understanding of human intervertebral disc degeneration and herniation. Contributions of nitric oxide, interleukins, prostaglandin E2, and matrix metalloproteinases. Spine 22:1065-1073, 1997.
30. Klara PM, Ray CD. Artificial nucleus replacement: clinical experience. Spine 27:1374-1377, 2002.
31. Lemaire JP, Skalli W, Lavaste F, et al. Intervertebral disc prosthesis. Results and prospects for the year 2000. Clin Orthop 337:64-76, 1997.
32. Lipson SJ, Muir H. Experimental intervertebral disc degeneration: Morphologic and proteoglycan changes over time. Arthritis Rheum 24:12-21, 1981.
33. Liu J, Roughley PJ, Mort JS. Identification of human intervertebral disc stromelysin and its involvement in matrix degradation. J Orthop Res 9:568-575, 1991.
34. Lu DS, Shono Y, Oda I, et al. Effects of chondroitinase ABC and chymopapain on spinal motion segment biomechanics. An in vivo biomechanical, radiologic, and histologic canine study. Spine 22:1828-1834, 1997.
35. Maeda S, Kokubun S. Changes with age in proteoglycan synthesis in cells cultured in vitro from the inner and outer rabbit annulus fibrosus. Responses to interleukin-1 and interleukin-1 receptor antagonist protein. Spine 25:166-169, 2000.
36. Maldonado BA, Oegema TR, Jr. Initial characterization of the metabolism of intervertebral disc cells encapsulated in microspheres. J Orthop Res 10:677-690, 1992.

37. Masuda K, Sah R, Hejna M, et al. A novel two-step method for the formation of tissue-engineered cartilage by mature bovine chondrocytes: The Alginate-Recovered-Chondrocyte (ARC) method. J Orthop Res 21:139-148, 2003.
38. Masuda K, Takegami K, An HS, et al. The effect of recombinant osteogenic protein-1 on proteoglycan and collagen synthesis by rabbit intervertebral disc cells. Presented at the Annual Meeting of the North American Spine Society, Chicago, Oct 1999.
39. Masuda K, Takegami K, An HS, et al. Recombinant osteogenic protein-1 upregulates extracellular matrix metabolism by rabbit annulus fibrosus and nucleus pulposus cells. Orthop Res Soc Trans 24:1029, 1999.
40. Matsumoto T, Masuda K, An H, et al. Formation of transplantable disc-shaped tissues by nucleus pulposus and annulus fibrosus cells: Biochemical and biomechanical properties. Orthop Res Soc Trans 16:897, 2001.
41. Matsumoto T, Masuda K, Chen S, et al. Transfer of osteogenic protein-1 gene by gene gun system promotes matrix synthesis in bovine intervertebral disc and articular cartilage cells. Orthop Res Soc Trans 26, 2001.
42. Matsuzaka S, Miyachi Y, Mizutani A, et al. Formation of cartilaginous tissue by the alginate-recovered-chondrocyte method and in vivo transplantation to full-thickness defects in swine articular cartilage—feasibility study. Orthop Res Soc Trans 27:453, 2002.
43. Mayne R, Brewton RG. Extracellular matrix of cartilage: Collagen. In Woessner JF, Howell DS, eds. Joint Cartilage Degradation. Marcel Dekker: New York, 1993, pp 81-108.
44. Melrose J, Ghosh P, Taylor TK, et al. A longitudinal study of the matrix changes induced in the intervertebral disc by surgical damage to the annulus fibrosus. J Orthop Res 10:665-676, 1992.
45. Moon SH, Gilbertson LG, Nishida K, et al. Human intervertebral disc cells are genetically modifiable by adenovirus-mediated gene transfer: implications for the clinical management of intervertebral disc disorders. Spine 25:2573-2579, 2000.
46. Nerlich AG, Schleicher ED, Boos N. 1997 Volvo Award winner in basic science studies. Immunohistologic markers for age-related changes of human lumbar intervertebral discs. Spine 22:2781-2795, 1997.
47. Nguyen-Minh C, Riley L 3rd, Ho KC, et al. Effect of degeneration of the intervertebral disk on the process of diffusion. Am J Neuroradiol 18:435-442, 1997.
48. Nishida K, Kang JD, Gilbertson LG, et al. Modulation of the biologic activity of the rabbit intervertebral disc by gene therapy: An in vivo study of adenovirus-mediated transfer of the human transforming growth factor beta 1 encoding gene. Spine 24:2419-2425, 1999.
49. Nishida K, Kang JD, Suh JK, et al. Adenovirus-mediated gene transfer to nucleus pulposus cells. Implications for the treatment of intervertebral disc degeneration. Spine 23:2437-2442, 1998.
50. Nishida Y, Knudson CB, Eger W, et al. Osteogenic protein-1 stimulates cells-associated matrix assembly by normal human articular chondrocytes: Up-regulation of hyaluronan synthase, CD44, and aggrecan. Arthritis Rheum 43:206-214, 2000.
51. Nishida Y, Knudson CB, Kuettner KE, et al. Osteogenic protein-1 promotes the synthesis and retention of extracellular matrix within bovine articular cartilage and chondrocyte cultures. Osteoarthritis Cartilage 8:127-136, 2000.
52. Nishimura K, Mochida J. Percutaneous reinsertion of the nucleus pulposus. An experimental study. Spine 23:1531-1538, 1998.
53. Nomura T, Mochida J, Okuma M, et al. Nucleus pulposus allograft retards intervertebral disc degeneration. Clin Orthop 389:94-101, 2001.
54. Okuma M, Mochida J, Nishimura K, et al. Reinsertion of stimulated nucleus pulposus cells retards intervertebral disc degeneration: An in vitro and in vivo experimental study. J Orthop Res 18:988-997, 2000.

55. Osada R, Ohshima H, Ishihara H, et al. Autocrine/paracrine mechanism of insulin-like growth factor-1 secretion, and the effect of insulin-like growth factor-1 on proteoglycan synthesis in bovine intervertebral discs. J Orthop Res 14:690-699, 1996.
56. Ozkaynak E, Rueger DC, Drier EA, et al. OP-1 cDNA encodes an osteogenic protein in the TGF-beta family. EMBO J 9:2085-2093, 1990.
57. Pearce RH, Grimmer BJ, Adams ME. Degeneration and the chemical composition of the human lumbar intervertebral disc. J Orthop Res 5:198-205, 1987.
58. Rufai A, Benjamin M, Ralphs JR. The development of fibrocartilage in the rat intervertebral disc. Anat Embryol (Berlin) 192:53-62, 1995.
59. Saal JA, Saal JS. Intradiscal electrothermal treatment for chronic discogenic low back pain: Prospective outcome study with a minimum 2-year follow-up. Spine 27:966-973, 2002.
60. Sampath TK, Malikal JC, Hauschka PV, et al. Recombinant human osteogenic protein-1 (hOP-1) induces new bone formation in vivo with a specific activity comparable with natural bovine osteogenic protein and stimulates osteoblast proliferation and differentiation in vitro. J Biol Chem 267:20352-20362, 1992.
61. Schmidt TA, An HS, Lim TH, et al. The stiffness of lumbar spinal motion segments with a high-intensity zone in the annulus fibrosus. Spine 23:2167-2173, 1998.
62. Shinmei M, Kikuchi T, Yamagishi M, et al. The role of interleukin-1 on proteoglycan metabolism of rabbit annulus fibrosus cells cultured in vitro. Spine 13:1284-1290, 1988.
63. Takahashi H, Suguro T, Okazima Y, et al. Inflammatory cytokines in the herniated disc of the lumbar spine. Spine 21:218-224, 1996.
64. Takegami K, Masuda K, An H, et al. The effect of osteogenic protein-1 on intervertebral disc cells pre-exposed to interleukin-1. Orthop Res Soc Trans 25:1040, 2000.
65. An H, Takegami K, Kamala H, et al. Infradiscal administration of osteogenic protein-1: Increased intervertebral disc height and proteoglycan content in the nucleus pulposus in normal adolescent rabbit. Spine 30:25-32, 2005.
66. Takegami K, Masuda K, An H, et al. A novel culture system for the intervertebral disc: An organ with endplates. Trans Orthop Res Soc 26:73, 2001.
67. Takegami K, Masuda K, Kumano F, et al. Osteogenic protein-1 is most effective in stimulating nucleus pulposus and annulus fibrosus cells to repair their matrix after chondroitinase ABC-induced chemonucleolysis. Orthop Res Soc Trans 24:201, 1999.
68. Takegami K, Masuda K, Kumano F, et al. The effect of osteogenic protein-1 on proteoglycan replenishment following chondroitinase ABC-induced chemonucleolysis of the matrix of cultured intervertebral cells. Presented at the Annual Meeting of the North American Spine Society, Chicago, Oct 1999.
69. Takegami K, Thonar EJ, An HS, et al. Osteogenic protein-1 enhances matrix replenishment by intervertebral disc cells previously exposed to interleukin-1. Spine 27:1318-1325, 2002.
70. Thomas JT, Kilpatrick MW, Lin K, et al. Disruption of human limb morphogenesis by a dominant negative mutation in CDMP1. Nat Genet 17:58-64, 1997.
71. Thomas JT, Lin K, Nandedkar M, et al. A human chondrodysplasia due to a mutation in a TGF-beta superfamily member. Nat Genet 12:315-317, 1996.
72. Thompson JP, Oegema TJ, Bradford DS. Stimulation of mature canine intervertebral disc by growth factors. Spine 16:253-260, 1991.
73. Thonar EJ, Manicourt DH. Body fluid markers of cartilage changes in osteoarthritis (review). Rheumatol Dis Clin North Am 19:635-657, 1993.
74. Trout J, Buckwalter J, Moore K, et al. Ultrastructure of human intervertebral disc. I. Changes in notochordal cells with age. Tissue Cells 14:359-369, 1982.
75. Urban JP, Holm S, Maroudas A, et al. Nutrition of the intervertebral disk. An in vivo study of solute transport. Clin Orthop 129:101-114, 1977.

76. Urban JP, McMullin JF. Swelling pressure of the intervertebral disc: Influence of proteoglycan and collagen contents. Biorheology 22:145-157, 1985.
77. Urban JP, McMullin JF. Swelling pressure of the lumbar intervertebral discs: Influence of age, spinal level, composition, and degeneration. Spine 13:179-187, 1988.
78. Wang JY, Baer AE, Kraus VB, et al. Intervertebral disc cells exhibit differences in gene expression in alginate and monolayer culture. Spine 26:1747-1751, 2001.
79. Wehling P, Schulitz KP, Robbins PD, et al. Transfer of genes to chondrocytic cells of the lumbar spine. Proposal for a treatment strategy of spinal disorders by local gene therapy. Spine 22:1092-1097, 1997.
80. Wozney JM. Bone morphogenetic proteins. Prog Growth Factor Res 1:267-280, 1989.
81. Wozney JM, Rosen V, Celeste AJ, et al. Novel regulators of bone formation: Molecular clones and activities. Science 242:1528-1534, 1988.
82. Wu JJ, Eyre DR, Slayter HS. Type VI collagen of the intervertebral disc. Biochemical and electron-microscopic characterization of the native protein. Biochem J 248:373-381, 1987.
83. Yang NS, Burkholder J, Roberts B, et al. In vivo and in vitro gene transfer to mammalian somatic cells by particle bombardment. Proc Natl Acad Sci USA 87:9568-9572, 1990.
84. Zeegers WS, Bohnen LM, Laaper M, et al. Artificial disc replacement with the modular type SB Charite III: 2-year results in 50 prospectively studied patients. Eur Spine J 8:210-217, 1999.

CHAPTER

18

THE "SMART" INTERVERTEBRAL DISC

Lisa A. Ferrara

Merging smart technologies with living systems should not be viewed as replacing man with machine, but as creating an environment where man and machine live, evolve, and flourish together.

Intervertebral Disc Anatomy

The intervertebral disc is the highly viscoelastic tissue situated between the vertebral bodies and is subject to multiple complex forces and bending moments. The disc and the facet joints function to fully support the compressive loads on the spine, where the disc is responsible for 20% to 33% of the entire height of the spinal column. The work by Nachemson and colleagues quantified the internal disc pressures for numerous spinal loading paradigms.[24] Their in vivo measurements demonstrated significantly greater loads and pressures in the lumbar disc with the patient in a sitting position, and lower loads and pressures in the supine position. In addition, the daily dynamic cyclical loading of the spine under normal activities will yield twice the loads on the intervertebral disc that are created with static positions. Normal motions will induce bending moments on the spine and create tensile forces in the disc under flexion, extension, and lateral bending. Rotation of the spine in the torso region will cause torsional loads that will translate into shear loads upon the lumbar disc. Overall, these combined forces exert a series of stresses on the disc that are a combination of tensile, compressive, and shear stresses. If beyond the tolerance threshold of injury, these stresses can result in acute or chronic injury to the disc structures (Fig. 18-1). Furthermore, the rate and duration of forces applied to an intervertebral disc can alter the stress response of the disc. Acute injury to the disc can occur from short-duration, high-magnitude loads at forces greater than the ultimate strength of the disc, resulting in irreparable structural damage. Alternatively, long-duration, low-magnitude loads can inflict injury to the disc through fatigue failures, such as tearing and disc degeneration.[27]

The anatomy of the intervertebral disc correlates with the biomechanical function of the disc. It is the viscoelastic behavior of the intervertebral disc that is

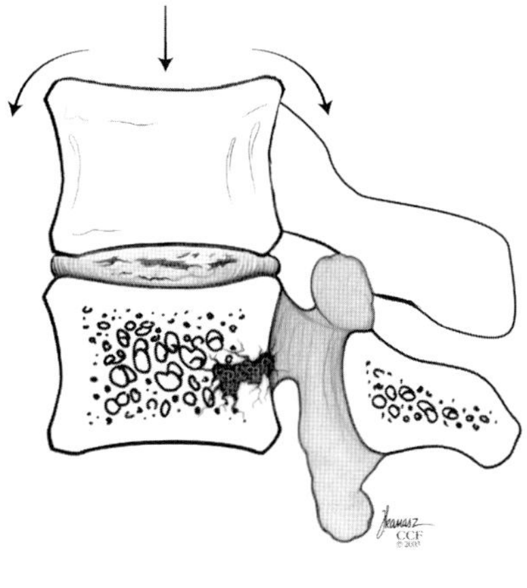

Fig. 18-1 Forces on the spine beyond the injury threshold can cause acute or chronic injury, such as degenerative disc disease.

reflected in the composite structural nature of the disc. The three major components of the disc that contribute to this overall mechanical performance are the nucleus pulposus, the anulus fibrosus, and the cartilaginous endplate.

Nucleus Pulposus

The nucleus pulposus, a remnant of the notochord, is the centrally located gelatinous network of fine fibrous strands that lie within a mucoprotein gel.[27] The function of the nucleus is to prevent buckling of the anulus and maintain disc height through osmotic pressure differentials. The water content of the nucleus pulposus ranges from about 90% at birth to 70% by age 70.[8,27] It is the proteoglycans housed within a collagen fibrous matrix in the nucleus pulposus that is responsible for the attraction of water molecules into this space. The tensile properties of the collagen fibers contribute to the maintaining of the water molecules within the matrix. However, the water content of the disc is dynamic and will change in response to weight bearing, resulting in a hydrostatic pressure effect. In the supine position, water enters the disc and increases the natural height of the disc. Under axial load-bearing conditions, the disc is compressed and water escapes through a semipermeable membrane from the collagenous matrix via hydrostatic forces.[27] During equilibrium, the sum of the extradiscal hydrostatic pressure and the intradiscal oncotic pressure is equivalent and in balance with the sum of the intradiscal hydrostatic pressure and the extradiscal oncotic pressure.[8] If this equilibrium is disrupted, fluid is forced to move across the semipermeable membrane.

Anulus Fibrosus

The anulus fibrosus is composed of 10 to 20 lamellae of collagen fibers concentrically arranged into bands around the borders of the disc. It encompasses the nucleus pulposus and is gradually differentiated from the periphery of the nucleus to the cortical margins of the vertebral bodies. The collagen fibers align along a 65 degree angular orientation to the long axis of the spine. In the successive lamellae, the fibers are opposite in direction.[27] The inner anular fibers encapsulate the nucleus pulposus and insert into the vertebral endplates. The outermost anular fibers insert into the ring apophysis, thus forming the more ligamentous portion of the intervertebral disc.[11] The collagen fibers within the lamellae can resist tension, and the multiple layers of closely packed lamellae rings are able to resist compression (Fig. 18-2). Provided the anular fibers do not buckle, the anulus is capable of bearing the axial loads to which the vertebral bodies are subjected.

Vertebral Endplate

The vertebral endplates are the cartilaginous plates that sandwich the intervertebral disc. During development, the endplates form the growth plates of the vertebral bodies, eventually resulting in secondary ossification along the cortical margin of the vertebra at maturity.[27] This circumferential ring of denser endplate bone is termed the *ring apophysis,* with the weakest portion of the vertebral endplates centered over the nucleus pulposus. At maturity, the endplate is centralized and covers approximately 70% of the vertebral surface, with the remaining 30% of the endplate surface consisting of cortical bone and covering the peripheral ring of the vertebra. Therefore the peripheral margin or "cortical margin" is the denser bone along the periphery of the vertebral body, and is significantly stronger than the centrum of the vertebral body. The central portion of the vertebral endplate is composed of compressed cancellous bone with polygonal lacunae.[11] This morphology at the central portion of the endplate contributes to a significantly weaker region of bone than the cortical margin.[15] It also creates an environment that is highly susceptible to implant subsidence if implants with higher moduli of elasticity are used improperly. Therefore a large footprint that will incorporate the cortical margin of the vertebral body is encouraged in interbody implant design.[9,10,16]

The viscoelastic properties of the vertebral endplates can further complicate the biomechanics of interbody fusion or motion preservation. The endplates

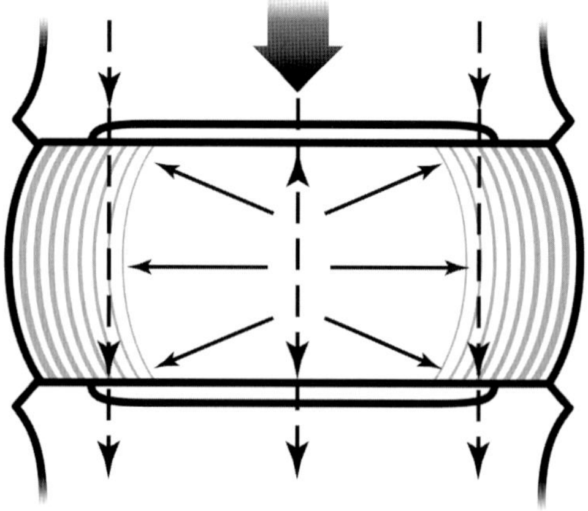

Fig. 18-2 The collagen fibers within the lamellae can resist tension, and the multiple layers of closely packed lamellae rings are able to resist compression.

demonstrate deformations during spinal loading.[12,21,25] Researchers have demonstrated the effects of endplate removal on the structural properties of the vertebral bodies as well as the deformations that occur with the implantation of an interbody device. The endplates respond differently to different interbody implants with dissimilar moduli of elasticity. Furthermore, loss of the entire endplate, as shown by Oxland et al,[25] will significantly decrease the mean failure load of the vertebral bodies. Finally, if an implant is centralized and does not adequately incorporate a portion of the cortical margin, there are heightened risks of vertebral endplate fracture surrounding the implant, or implant subsidence caused by repetitive cycling through the central portion of the endplate.[20]

Biomechanical Motions of the Intervertebral Disc

The spine moves about three planes, with six degrees of freedom based on the Cartesian coordinate system.[27] Therefore, there are six basic types of motion that a spinal segment may experience. These motions are described as flexion and extension along the sagittal plane, rotation about the coronal plane causing lateral bending to the right or left, and rotation about the horizontal plane. Combinations of these motions with compressive, tensile, translational, and/or rotational forces result in a variety of stresses placed on the anular fibers of the disc. Bending creates compression of the anular fibers on the concave side, and tension of the fibers on the convex side. Bending moments also have a direct effect on the nucleus pulposus. A bending moment in flexion will displace the nucleus dorsally; a bending moment in extension will displace the nucleus ventrally (Fig. 18-3). Lastly, translation will produce shear forces to the anular fibers.

In any loading mode, exceeding the yield strength of the material could result in the ultimate failure of the material. However, ultimate failure of the intervertebral disc can result by two means: (1) an acute incident at forces greater than the ultimate strength, or (2) through repetitive long-term combinational cycling resulting in a fatigue failure of the disc. Finally, the intervertebral disc is a difficult material to mimic because of its complex composite nature, viscoelastic nonlinear behavior, and dynamic molecular composition that changes with aging and loading conditions.

Motion Preservation: The Total Artificial Disc and the Nuclear Replacement Prosthesis

The goal of a motion preservation system is to develop a spinal implant that will maintain the necessary motion to a spinal segment without compromising the biomechanics of the surrounding spinal elements and adjacent spinal segments. The design of a motion preservation system, either that of a total artificial disc or a nuclear replacement device, can be quite complicated because of the complex biomechanical nature of the natural and dynamically changing intervertebral disc. The total artificial disc prosthesis is a total prosthetic re-

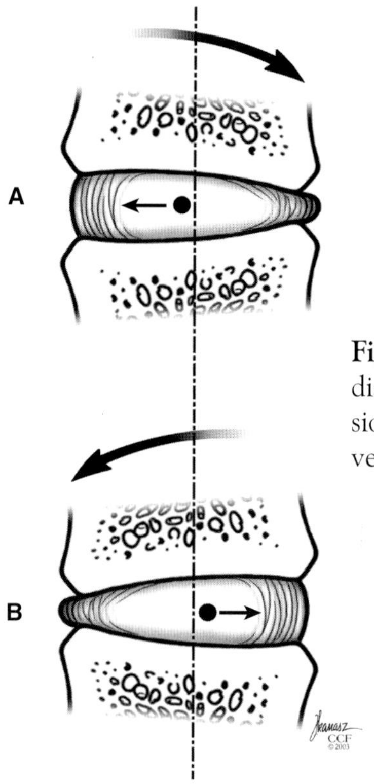

Fig. 18-3 A, Flexion bending moment displaces the nucleus dorsally. **B,** An extension bending moment displaces the nucleus ventrally.

placement of the anulus fibrosus and nucleus pulposus with an endplate that interfaces with the host vertebral endplates. Therefore it is essential that the mechanics and kinematics of these structures be closely imitated in the design of the prosthesis. Capturing and securing the total artificial disc prosthesis to the vertebral endplate can be challenged by the asymmetrical and cyclic loads placed upon the spine. As described in the previous sections, a combination of bending moments, compression, and rotation could place excessive stresses on the disc either acutely or through repetitive cycling, contributing to disc herniation.[5,13] With respect to the total artificial disc prosthesis, these combinational forces can place excessive stresses at the host bone and prosthetic endplate interface and result in early loss of fixation.

The function of the nuclear replacement device is to replace the damaged nucleus pulposus with a device that restores disc height while maintaining the gel-like kinematics of the healthy intact nucleus pulposus. Unlike the total artificial disc prosthesis, it is surgically less invasive to the spine. Minimally invasive surgical techniques are currently under development to provide implantation of these nuclear replacement devices into the nucleotomized space resulting in minimal tissue damage. However, implant extrusion, migration, and endplate subsidence with nuclear replacement devices are still current issues that continue to exist and require further investigation.

The dorsal elements of the spine, in particular the facets, play a major role in spinal stabilization and motion preservation. The resistance to torsional forces, compressive forces, and combinational bending moments prevent injury caused by hyperloading (acutely or chronically) of the spinal elements. The intervertebral disc supplies a 35% resistance to torsional load and the remaining 65% resistance is provided by the facets, the load-sharing behavior of the disc, and the dorsal elements.[17] Numerous biomechanical studies have examined facet behavior and the interaction of the intervertebral disc with the facets. Dooris et al[14] demonstrated that the facet loads were less sensitive to the amount of anular material removed and more sensitive to the dorsoventral location. In addition, disc degeneration is codependent with facet degeneration.[17,18] Clinical evidence suggests that the intact intervertebral disc protects the facets from hyperloading and degeneration. Often, adjacent disc degeneration contributes to the initiation of the facet degenerative cascade and facet arthroses.[18] Therefore one of the concerns in the development of a motion preservation device is that of the natural degenerative cascade of the aging spine. It is in this manner that a smart disc implant (SDI) could potentially compensate for the changes that occur with adjacent level discs because of aging and other related etiologies responsible for changing the force distributions along the spinal column.

Smart Technology

The concept of smart technology or "smart systems" is to design systems capable of imitating human intelligence. A better definition for the application of this technology to orthopedic implants is a system that can provide physical, chemical, and/or mechanical diagnostics and respond appropriately and dynamically to the changing stimuli. Smart technology includes innovations such as smart biomaterials, microelectromechanical systems (MEMS), nanoelectromechanical systems (NEMS), and robotics. Numerous research studies are under way to merge these new technologies with medical applications to significantly advance medicine into a new era. The ability to manipulate cells, genes, molecules, and atoms will revolutionize medicine and the treatment of currently incurable diseases. Materials that are safe and efficacious, yet behave in a "smart" manner, may be biodegradable or bioresorbable such that the existing biomaterial is replaced by bone or fibrous tissue. Smart material should be capable of nonlinear responses to mechanically imitate a living tissue or fluidic substance, and is currently gaining ground in the field of orthopedic and spinal implants. The incorporation of MEMS or NEMS sensors and actuators could allow enhanced precision in cutting, tissue manipulation, tissue identification, and the precise navigation of surgical tools through various densities of tissue producing minimal tissue damage. Additionally, microscopically sized sensors, transducers, and actuators implanted into a spinal implant or living tissue could ultimately provide the surgeon with real-time, continuous biofeedback regarding the tissue responses to the stimuli, or in particular, the mechanical behavior of spinal implants.

Finally, incorporating robotic technology and haptic feedback (i.e., pertaining to tactile sensation) into surgical tools and spinal implants will contribute to the development of the next generation of surgical tools and implants. Smart tools and implants that are capable of providing feedback related to tool or implant performance can enhance the capabilities of minimally invasive surgical procedures or warn the surgeon of early risks to implant failures.

Smart Biomaterials and Tissue Engineering: Their Potential Use in the Smart Disc

The development of new materials that are biocompatible within a living system and can drive and maintain a required and appropriate cellular and tissue response is desirable for medical applications. Materials capable of replacing degenerative tissues and diseased organs are being vigorously researched, but still face numerous years of testing before they can be implanted into humans. Potential advances in this field are mainly theoretical or in the early stages of development and lack the clinical information needed to further the design and implementation of such materials. However, the design of organic protein or chemically based materials could rapidly advance the use of such materials in vivo. Being able to simulate the natural and chemical environment to imitate human tissue with materials that are inert and live symbiotically with existing cells, tissues, and organs would provide a safe environment with minimal adverse foreign-body responses.

Numerous research facilities are developing smart biomaterials based on nanoscale information taken from fundamental techniques and theories in order to assemble organic compounds.[1] Specific coatings for biomedical applications, aimed at biocompatibility and biologic functionality, are being developed and evaluated to form controllable structures consisting of protein-based materials. The potential use of these smart materials will be to control cell adhesion, especially pertaining to orthopedic or vascular implants, and to control cellular responses in the local setting during tissue repair. Stable fiber matrices can be formed from these adhesion-promoting proteins to create highly organized "mat" structures that exhibit their own controllable nanoscale topography. These fibrous modules can be enhanced with growth factors or chemically synthesized drugs. The potential of such smart biomaterials is obvious: the development of a protein-based fibrous material that could be formed into lamellae to replace a degenerative anulus fibrosus.

Bioactive Composites, Bioceramics, and Synthetic Tissue Scaffolds

The development of bioactive composites, bioceramics, bioactive bone cements, and temporary scaffolds for tissue-engineered implants is under way for bone and joint replacement systems.[1,2] Ceramics, glasses, and glass-ceramics are generally used to repair or replace skeletal hard connective tissue such as bone.[6] The effectiveness of these materials is based upon a successful attachment to the connective tissue, further enriched by the eventual creep substitution of bone. Bioactive composites can form scaffolding structures that can be seeded with mesenchymal cells, growth factors, or other factors that would enhance tissue regeneration and replacement into the structure. Bone substitution and tendon regeneration are areas of active tissue engineering and currently rely upon bioactive agents to induce or augment the regenerative process. The research is driven by optimizing the chemistry of the materials as well as developing an ideal porosity for optimal osteoinduction. Although understanding the macroporosity issues of a synthetic bone scaffold is essential to provide adequate surface area for cellular attachment, understanding the microporosity of the scaffold is equally important. Optimal microporosity will allow transport of the nutrients and mechanical signals necessary to promote remodeling of the tissue matrix.[7]

The key concept behind bioactivation of a biocompatible ceramic material would be to alter the physical and chemical characteristics of the ceramic structure to initiate rapid healing in diseased tissue. Use of these synthetic bone scaffolds would provide immediate mechanical support while converting to host skeletal tissue. HAPEX™ is a second-generation biomaterial that has been shown in vivo to produce direct bone contact.[3] Growth factors, bone morphogenetic proteins, and drug-delivery mechanisms can be added to the synthetic bone scaffolds to augment bony fusion or ingrowth for difficult, high-risk patients. These novel synthetic tissue-replacement and tissue-regenerative products could essentially be applied to spinal implants to improve long-term adherence to the bone for improved fixation. For example, the application of these bone-substitute scaffolds within the keel or plate of a spinal implant would significantly improve the osteo-adhesive properties to the implant for long-term stability and purchase within the bone. The implant would essentially "meld" into its surrounding host bone environment.

Biodegradable and Bioerodable Materials

Degradable polymeric implants are of value for short-term medical applications such as sutures, drug-delivery devices, adhesion, temporary vascular grafts and stents, and orthopedic fixation systems.[6] One of the advantages of using biodegradable materials is that complications related to the long-term safety of permanently implanted devices may be avoided by using a device that degrades gradually. Furthermore, these materials can be used as ideal temporary scaffolds, temporary barriers, and drug-delivery devices. Biodegradable materials include polyhydroxybutyrate (PHB) and polyhydroxyvalerate (PHV), which are both capable of storing a reserve of carbon and energy; polycaprolactone, a synthetic polymer that can be degraded by microorganisms and can be used for long-term drug-delivery systems; polyanhydrides are hydrolytically unstable with a rapid degradation rate; poly(orthoesters) are ideal because of the surface erosion properties of this polymer for the release of drugs at a constant rate; polycyanoacrylates as bioadhesives; polyphosphazenes for their use in controlled drug-delivery systems; and poly(amino acids), which are promising candidates for the attachment of drugs and cross-linking agents. Polylactic acid (PLA) and polyglycolic acid (PGA) function as bioerodable polymers and are currently the most widely investigated and commonly used synthetic bioerodable polymers.[6] For orthopedic devices, PLA is favored because of its high mechanical strength and durability. However, its rate of degradation can alter the pH of the surrounding tissues, eventually increasing the acidity surrounding the device and resulting in the formation of a seroma within the tissues. This complication should not hinder future research and development into the use of biodegradables for spinal fixation systems. Further research can look into minimizing or eliminating these negative tissue responses.

Incorporating bioactive components, bioglasses, biodegradable or bioerodable substances, and/or bioceramics into spinal implant design could minimize the stresses placed on the host bone, while allowing for the natural progression of bone remodeling around the implant to occur and to enhance the purchase within the bone. Surface coating the implant interface can enhance the biologic bonding of the bone to the implant surface for superior fixation and stability to the bone. Calcium phosphate coatings can be electrochemically bonded to metallic surfaces to encourage biologic tissue ingrowth.[22]

To date, the endplates of a total artificial disc prosthesis have been constructed from metallic materials, and coated for increased bone attachment. Titanium, cobalt chromium, and 316L stainless steel are some of the standard metals used in spinal implants. The major disadvantage for their use in interbody spinal devices, such as the total artificial disc prosthesis, is the high modulus of elasticity they possess in comparison to the host bone. The higher stiffnesses of the metallic devices impose higher stresses on the bone and surrounding tissues when exposed to both static and dynamic spinal-loading paradigms. Matching environmental integrities, that is, closely matching the modulus of elasticity of the host bone and the implant without compromising the overall strength, provides a mechanically sound situation. The elastic behavior of both the host bone and implant would respond similarly, thus minimizing stress-risers imposed onto the bone or the implant that can result in early loss of fixation.

Smart Polymers and Foams

In the past, polymeric materials have had a limited use in dental and orthopedic applications because of their strength limitations. However, because of their resistance to wear debris they perform well when used as a bearing surface of an artificial joint device. Numerous technologic advancements have been made in the field of polymer science. Polymers display a better balance between chemical, physical, mechanical, and weight properties when compared to metals and ceramics.[3] Polymers have been used extensively in the development of prosthetic devices such as heart valves, contact lenses, replacement arteries and veins, artificial kidneys, artificial lungs, artificial heart, and breast implants. They serve as ideal candidates for sutures, adhesives, cements, drug-delivery systems and even intervertebral disc replacement systems (also known as motion preservation systems). Their elastic properties are more similar to the natural disc and some polymers and foams behave in a nonlinear fashion. Significant differences in the loading rate to a smart polymer will elicit different stiffness responses, much like that of the natural disc. The development of novel polymers that can respond to stimuli, change their chemical and mechanical properties, and deform through macroscopic displacements is already a bioengineering possibility.

Electroactive polymers (EAP) and EAP actuators, whose properties change drastically upon stimuli, are currently being investigated for their potential use in the biomedical arena.[4] Polymers such as hydrogel, polyacrylamide gel (PAAm), polyacrylonitrile gel (PAN), polyvinyl alcohol gel (PVA), and perfluorinated sulfonic gel (Nafion) can respond to changes in pH, electric field, photon, temperature, and stress. These polymers can be shaped into pillars, actuators, levers, and spheres, producing an actuation mode that responds by large axial displacements. Ideally, these pillars could be formed into lamellar sheets to simulate the anulus fibrosus. They can be programmed or conditioned to respond to changes in loading of the spine and respond by lengthening or contracting. Fast strain rates imposed upon the smart disc would elicit a stiffening response from the polymer whereas slow strain rates would elicit a greater elastic response, thus imitating the natural intervertebral disc.

Microelectromechanical Systems, Nanoelectromechanical Systems, and Robotics

Electromechanical devices originated in 1785 when Charles-Augustin de Couloumb created an apparatus that measured electrical charge. His invention was an electrical torsion balance consisting of two spherical metal balls, one fixed, and the other attached to a moving rod. The two balls performed as a capacitive plate that converted the charge to an attractive force. This invention represented the two main components of mechanoelectrical systems: (1) a mechanical element and (2) transducers, both common to most electro mechanical systems. Microsizing these mechanoelectrical systems through recent micromachining fabrication technologies and combining these systems with integrated circuit technology has led to the development of microelectromechanical and nanoelectromechanical systems (nanotechnology or NEMS).

Sensors and transducers have contributed to the advancement, productivity, and efficiency of many industries. There are tactile sensors, chemical sensors,

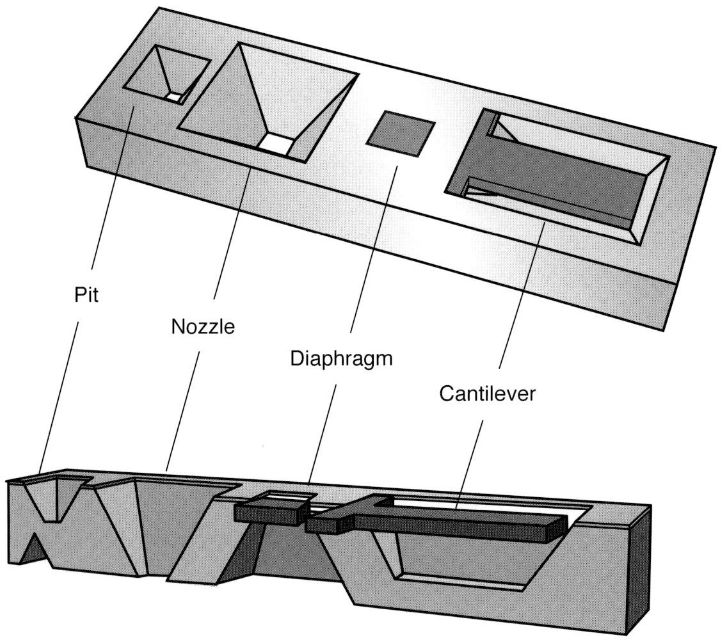

Fig. 18-4 Schematic depiction of a series of microstructures fabricated by bulk micromachining techniques onto a silicon substrate. Structure includes a pit, nozzle, diaphragm, and a cantilever. Bulk micromachining is a fabrication technique used to create MEMS structures.

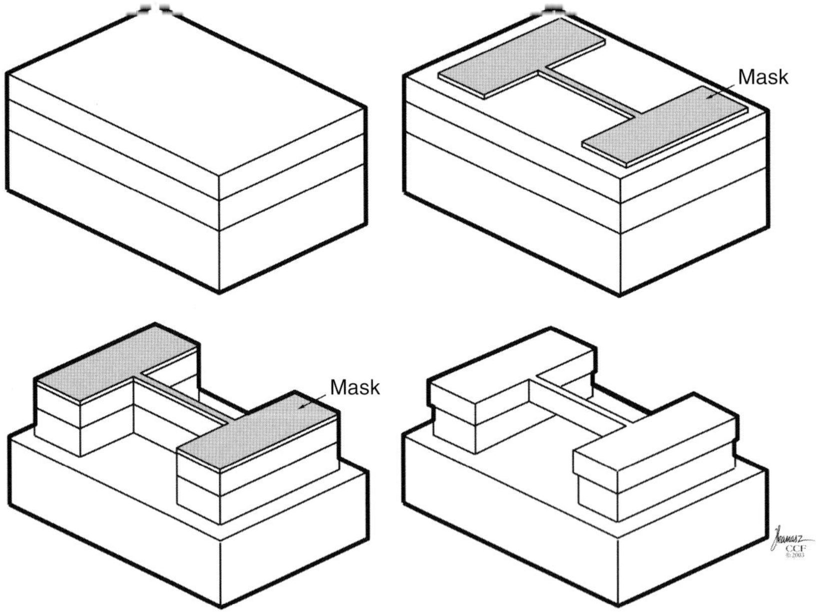

Fig. 18-5 The silicon substrate serves as the mechanical support on which alternating layers of structural and sacrificial materials are deposited and patterned. The desired design is "carved" from repetitive layering of structural and sacrificial layers.

pressure sensors, optical sensors, mechanical sensors, electrical sensors, and numerous other types that perform the full range of tasks, from the mundane to the complex. These sensors may generate a voltage response to a certain pressure level, tactile sensations, and various chemical or optical stimuli. Advances in microprocessor technology have enabled the sensor and processing technology to be housed onto a single chip, such as that found in integrated chip technology within a computer. The onset of microelectromechanical systems (MEMS) has enabled integrated chip technology to merge with microfabrication techniques to produce precise microsized devices that may house a sensor, actuator, data processing unit, and a power source all on a chip that is less than 4 mm^2 in area. MEMS technology is capable of constructing machines that are microscopic in size. Devices such as pumps, cantilever arms, gripping systems, diaphragms that deform, valves, and pores can be constructed using surface micromachining or bulk micromachining methods onto a silicon substrate (Fig. 18-4).

Surface micromachining is a versatile technology because it enables the creation of integrated multilevel structures using multiple layers of structural and sacrificial material (Fig. 18-5; see also Fig. 18-4).[26] The silicon substrate (conventionally a wafer 4 inches in diameter composed of silicon glass) serves as the mechanical support on which alternating layers of structural and sacrificial materials are deposited and patterned. Conventional photolithographic and etching techniques are used to create micromechanical structures by eventually "carving out" the desired device design from repetitive layering of structural and sacrificial layers.

Bulk micromachining is a second fabrication technique used to create MEMS structures in which the bulk of the silicon substrate is etched away, leaving behind the desired micromechanical elements. The electrical components to power the device and conduct the data processing can also be housed on the same microsized chip. The successful development of smart, implantable devices using MEMS technology will be further enhanced with on-chip wireless telemetry. Wireless telemetry to transmit and receive information from the device is ideal, and will eliminate the risk of corrosion and breakage to wires while improving the life span of these devices.

The use of MEMS and NEMS sensors and actuators integrated with electronics and wireless telemetry will revolutionize medicine. Numerous neurosurgical and orthopedic applications would benefit with the addition of MEMS and NEMS technologies. The difference between the two technologies is simply based on the size of the fabricated structures, and some differences in machining and fabrication. MEMS is capable of manipulating cells; NEMS is capable of manipulating molecules and atoms.

The micro-sized sensors with on-board telemetric data transmission could be implanted into the smart disc at various locations to monitor the stresses and strains placed upon the implant and the bone-implant interface.[26] Pressure sensors (Fig. 18-6) on the implant at the host bone interface could potentially monitor the biologic bonding of bone to the implant. These sensors could provide feedback to the surgeon pertaining to implant performance through continuous monitoring of the mechanical actions of the devices. Therefore it is feasible that other sensors housed within the same device would also enable the artificial prosthesis to respond to these changing loads, moments, strains, and pressures by counteracting these forces, realigning the device through disc height and angle alterations, and changing the stiffnesses in response to the altered loads, if the prosthesis material allows for such actions.

Nanotechnology is the ability to fabricate devices that challenge even the microtechnology world. It is the ultimate in flexibility, allowing molecular and atomic manipulation to occur to develop precision technology.[23] Scanning tunneling microscopy uses an extremely sharp probe to scan a surface, allowing the visualization and manipulation of the atoms on it.[23] Consequently, the manipulation of atoms using nanostructures will allow us to arrange and stack them to build and change systems. We are still decades away from building nanostructures that can manipulate atoms responsible for altering entire disease pathways. At the present time, nanochannels and nanopores have been constructed that are capable of filtering and selecting molecules through pore and channel size designs. The applications for this technology are endless. For example, regeneration of the intervertebral disc through tissue engineering and nanotechnology is theoretically feasible. Precise nanopores can be integrated into a tissue scaffold design that would selectively allow for the inclusion of particular molecules capable of regenerating the anular and nuclear material within a disc, while excluding the undesirable molecules. These devices are significantly smaller than a human cell. To give an example of nanosize, a mitochondrion is approximately 1-2 × 0.1-0.5 microns, a cell is typically 20 microns, and a fabricated NEMS robotic arm could be approximately 100

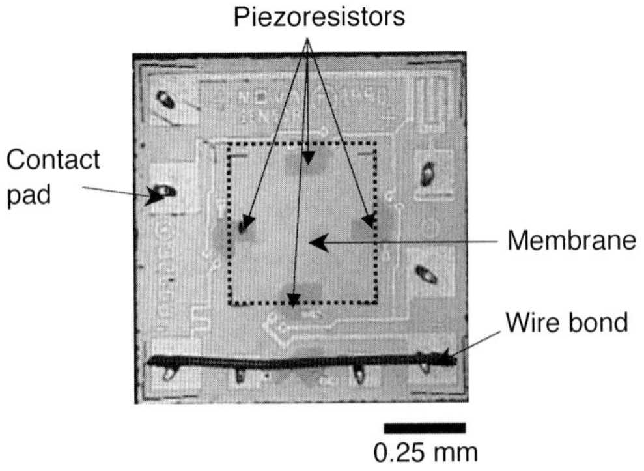

Fig. 18-6 The GE NovaSensor (*http://www.novasensor.com/catalog_5psi_fr.html*) is a commercially available MEMS pressure sensor that uses a diaphragm surrounded by four doped piezoresistors. It is a 1 × 1 × 0.6 mm^3 device constructed by bulked micromachining techniques onto a silicon substrate.

nanometers. Multiple robotic arms could fit into one mitochondrion. Furthermore, NEMS devices could provide molecular transport to specialized tissue sites, such as that of the proteoglycans in the nucleus pulposus.

Using nanorobots, or NEMS devices that can be powered to perform tasks, in the spine is still a futuristic concept, but one that can become a reality. Nanorobots could some day be used to deliver drugs and molecules to specialized sites within the spine (bone or soft tissue). Drugs could be delivered to reproduce pain in a mechanically compromised disc, thus making conventional discogram methods obsolete, or used to alleviate localized pain.[19] Bone-growth-enhancing substances, such as bone morphogenetic proteins, could be delivered to fracture sites or sites of stress-risers to strengthen a biomechanically compromised region of bone and improve fixation of the spinal implant to the host bone. Noninvasive surgical procedures of the spine could be performed by microrobots and nanorobots; these robots could repair the anulus through drug delivery or mechanical means after a surgical procedure such as nuclear replacement.

Conclusion

The ideal artificial disc prosthesis is one that can imitate the natural intact disc. It must also conform to the natural aging process, possessing the ability to dynamically change to match the naturally degenerative cascade of the living human disc. However, this is a difficult task to achieve with the current existing motion preservation technologies.

The smart disc should realign itself to the dynamically changing biomechanics of the spine. It should possess a structure similar to the natural intervertebral disc and vertebral endplate complex. Ideally, the total artificial disc will have endplates that can bond and eventually remodel into the surrounding bony environment they are fixed to. The artificial disc will possess numerous microsensors and/or nanosensors that can provide feedback about the implant and tissue performances, and can correct the performance of the implant and surrounding tissue according to its altered biomechanical environment. The sensors would possess actuators that would alter the mechanical responses of the nonlinear material and mimic the functions of the anulus fibrosus. These sensors could also be designed to monitor disc height, and maintain or readjust disc height if it falls below threshold. Finally, the disc could be monitored according to changes in osmotic pressures, axial loading, and intradiscal pressures.

References

1. http://www.nanoscience.cam.ac.uk/irc/.
2. http://www.irc-biomed-materials.qmw.ac.uk.
3. http://www.irc-biomed-materials.qmw.ac.uk/pages/research/BoneTissueEng/Research-BoneTissueEng.htm.

4. http://depts.Washington.edu/cims/research/electroactive.htm.
5. Adams MA, Dolan P. A technique for quantifying the bending moment acting on the lumbar spine in vivo. J Biomech 24:117-126, 1991.
6. Alexander H, Brunski JB, Cooper ST, et al. Classes of materials used in medicine. In Ratner BD, Hoffman AS, Schoen FJ, et al, eds. Biomaterials Science: An Introduction to Materials in Medicine. New York: Academic Press, 1996.
7. Bauer TW. Scaffolds, cells, and signals: Advances in synthetic bone graft materials for orthopedic surgery. Orthopedics 5, 2002.
8. Benzel EC. Biomechanics of Spine Stabilization. Rolling Meadows, IL: American Association of Neurological Surgeons, 2001.
9. Benzel EC, Ferrara LA, Kowalski R. Biomechanics of Bone Fusion. Neurosurg Focus 1044/01Article 2.
10. Benzel EC, Lastra JJ, Kalfas I, et al. The biomechanics of interbody fusion and the shortcomings of lumbar fusion with cages and interbody bone dowels. Clin Neurosurg 47:557-588, 2000.
11. Bogduk N. Clinical Anatomy of the Lumbar Spine and Sacrum, 3rd ed. Philadelphia: WB Saunders, 1997.
12. Brinckmann P, Frobin W, Hierholzer E, et al. Deformation of the vertebral end-plate under axial loading of the spine. Spine 8:851-856, 1983.
13. Buckwalter JA, Einhorn TA, Simon SR. Orthopaedic basic science. Rosemont, Ill: AAOS, 1999.
14. Dooris AP, Goel VK, Grosland NM, et al. Load-sharing between anterior and posterior elements in a lumbar motion segment implanted with an artificial disc. Spine 26:E122-E129, 2001.
15. Edwards WT, Zheng Y, Ferrara LA, et al. Structural features and thickness of the vertebral cortex in the thoracolumbar spine. Spine 26:218-225, 2001.
16. Ferrara LA, Benzel EC. The biomechanics of interbody fusion and the shortcomings of lumbar fusion with cages and interbody bone dowels. Clin Neurosurg 47:577-588, 2003.
17. Gries NC, Berlemann U, Moore RJ, et al. Early histologic changes in lower lumbar discs and facet joints and their correlation. Eur Spine J 9:23-29, 2000.
18. Haher TR, O'Brien M, Dryer JW, et al. The role of lumbar facet joints in spinal stability. Identification of alternative paths of loading. Spine 19:2667-2670, 1994.
19. Hochschuler SH. Nanorobots in Spine Orthopedics. SpineLine (North American Spine Society) Jan/Feb:28-29, 2003.
20. Jin BH, Ferrara LA, Secor J, et al. Cortical margining capabilities of fins associated with ventral cervical spine instrumentation. J Neurosurg 2003.
21. Lim TH, Kwon H, Jeon CH, et al. Effect of endplate conditions and bone mineral density on the compressive strength of the graft-endplate interface in anterior cervical spine fusion. Spine 26:951-956, 2001.
22. McAfee PC, Cunningham BW, Orbegoso CM, et al. Analysis of porous ingrowth in intervertebral disc prostheses: A nonhuman primate model. Spine 28:332-334, 2003.
23. Merkle RC. Nanotechnology and Nanomedicine. SpineLine (North American Spine Society) Jan/Feb:7-10, 2003.
24. Nachemson A. The load on lumbar disks in different positions of the body. Clin Orthop Relat Res 45:107-122, 1966.
25. Oxland TR, Grant JP, Dvorak MF, et al. Effects of endplate removal on the structural properties of the lower lumbar vertebral bodies. Spine 28:332-340, 2003.
26. Roy S, Ferrara LA, Fleischman AJ, et al. Microelectromechanical systems and neurosurgery: A new era in a new millennium. Neurosurgery 49:779-797, 2001.
27. White AA, Panjabi MM. Clinical Biomechanics of the Spine, ed 2. Philadelphia: Lippincott Williams & Wilkins, 1990.

INDEX